Prolactinomas

Prolactinomas

An Interdisciplinary Approach

Edited by

L. M. Auer, G. Leb, G. Tscherne
W. Urdl, G. F. Walter

Walter de Gruyter
Berlin · New York 1985

Prof. Dr. med. Ludwig M. Auer
Universitätsklinik für Neurochirurgie
Landeskrankenhaus
A-8036 Graz

This book contains 157 illustrations and 118 tables.

CIP-Kurztitelaufnahme der Deutschen Bibliothek

Prolactinomas : an interdisciplinary approach ; [proceedings of the Internat. Symposium on Prolactinomas, Graz (Austria), April 29–May 2, 1984] / ed. by L. M. Auer ... – Berlin ; New York : de Gruyter, 1985.
ISBN 3-11-010153-X
NE: Auer, Ludwig M. [Hrsg.]; International Symposium on Prolactinomas ⟨1984, Graz⟩

Library of Congress Cataloging in Publication Data

International Symposium on Prolactinomas (1984 : Graz, Austria)
Prolactinomas.
Includes bibliographies and indexes.
1. Prolactinoma–Congresses. I. Auer, Ludwig M., 1948–
II. Title. [DNLM: 1. Pituitary Neoplasms–congresses. 2. Prolactin–secretion–congresses.
WK 585 I615p 1984]
RC280.P5I55 1984 616.99'247 84-22998
ISBN 0 89925 039 4

ISBN 3 11 010153 X Walter de Gruyter Berlin New York
ISBN 0 89925 039 4 Walter de Gruyter, Inc., New York

 Typesetting and Printing: Arthur Collignon GmbH, Berlin. – Binding: Lüderitz & Bauer GmbH, Berlin. – Cover design: Rudolf Hübler. –
Printed in Germany.

Preface

In this volume an attempt is made to provide an up to date survey of the physiology and the pathophysiology of prolactin. Furthermore, new pharmacological developments which may have a favourable effect on diseases resulting from a pathologically high production of prolactin are discussed. Interesting new morphological aspects on the differentiation of pathological entities in the sellar region, such as DNA and S–100 protein, are also presented. We believe that this will mean a promising start towards our efforts to differentiate between hyperplasia and adenoma. A substantial amount of information from follow-up studies has been collected so as to observe the effect of both medical treatment and surgical or combined treatment.

It is demonstrated in patients with microadenomas that the risks of each type of treatment are equally low. As long as the sellar structure is normal, it seems to be commonly accepted to treat very small microadenomas medically, although some favour surgical treatment. It is absolutely essential for hyperprolactinaemia to be treated, because of the danger of osteoporosis as an additional complication of elevated serum prolactin.

For larger microadenomas both medical and surgical treatment are advisable. In this respect, it might be useful to distinguish between women who would like to become pregnant and those who do not; some of us favour surgery in the first category.

For large, and especially for invasive adenomas, it is becoming increasingly difficult to establish a clear concept: medical treatment, especially during pregnancy, is known to cause complications. However, complications do tend to accompany surgery as well. Probably the most important thing we have learned about macroadenomas is the fact that a combination of surgical and medical treatment and radiation therapy is likely to give better results, both from the endocrinological and the clinical point of view.

The present state of knowledge thus highly suggests cooperation of the disciplines involved in this field. Any type of treatment may be ideal for an individual patient, provided the decision is taken jointly by surgeons, endocrinologists and gynecologists at an early stage. Only in such rare cases of apoplectic adenomas should an immediate decision in favour of surgery be taken, assuming joint agreement.

We would like to express our thanks to D. Linnette Iliff, Ph. D. for taking care of the language editing and to Ms. Elfriede Meier for editorial assistance.

The Editors

Contents

I Morphology

II Radiology

I Morphology

Structure and ultrastructure of prolactinomas

A. M. Landolt

Introduction

Before to serum prolactin (PRL) determinations were included routinely in evaluation of all patients with pituitary adenomas, PRL-secreting pituitary adenomas (prolactinomas) were considered rare, and there were few reports describing the histology and ultrastructure of these tumours [6, 11, 12, 17, 31, 32, 38, 41, 45, 48, 56, 57]. Since that time, however, the picture has changed considerably. Hyperprolactinaemia is now the most common clinical syndrome seen in our patients with pituitary adenomas. Among 311 patients operated by the author in the past 5 years, 46% had prolactinomas [24]. The results obtained from examination of this large number of prolactinomas has made it possible to arrive at a characteristic histological description of this tumour type [14, 18, 29, 42, 47].

The histological classification of tumours is a process of defining individual adenomas by morphological methods (histology, immunocytochemistry, electron microscopy) and forming categories of tumours that bear common characteristics. When making a diagnosis, we must bear in mind that a practical and useful classification embraces only *distinguishing* features. Minor differences must not be weighed too heavily because the light and electron microscopic pictures of tumours, prolactinomas in this context, have a certain variability that can be attributed both to naturally occurring differences among tumours and to the results of external influences on the tumour. The implications of such differences must not be overestimated, and the temptation to create new and confusing subdivisions in the classification system must be resisted. To refine the differentiation of prolactinomas it is necessary to focus on changes caused by extratumoral factors. These changes can best be defined with quantitative, morphometric studies and statistical methods.

Light microscopy

Most prolactinomas consist of uniform, oval or polygonal cells with large, oval nuclei and prominent nucleoli (fig. 2a) [42, 47]; a structure that is typical of cells engaged in protein synthesis. Polymorph nuclei, multinuclear cells, and mitoses are rare. Staining with haematoxylin-eosin or PAS-orange G usually shows no secretory granules. Prolactinomas were classified as "chromophobic" in the now obsolete nomenclature that distinguished eosinophilic, basophilic, and chromophobic adenomas. Herlant's erythrosine and Brookes' carmosine, however, stain fine, bright red, secretory granules in a large number of prolactinoma specimens [14, 49]. The immunoperoxidase reaction with anti-PRL shows a positive result in 93–100% of biopsy specimens studied [10, 23, 47]. About half of these specimens show a concomitant positive reaction with anti-adrenocoticotrophic hormone (ACTH), anti-growth hormone (GH), and anti-luteinizing hormone (LH) in a few prolactinoma cells [23], although sample testing in patients from whom these specimens were obtained showed normal blood levels of these hormones.

Frequently, characteristic variations involving signs of degeneration are found on light microscopic examination: Intraadenomatous microcalcispherites are found in 19–30% of biopsy specimens. Because these components are rare in other types of pituitary adenomas, they are useful in establishing a diagnosis [22, 28, 42, 47]. The presence and extent of calcification in the specimen is not related to tumour size; calcification occurs in microadenomas as well as in large tumours; calcium deposition starts in isolated necrotic cells that are surrounded by apparently healthy adenoma cells rather than in large areas of necrosis.

Amyloid bodies are rarely found in prolactinomas [1, 15, 22, 47]. It appean in these rare cases that the fibrillary substance, showing the typical congo red reaction and birefringence is secreted by the prolactinoma cells.

Table 1 Intraadenomatous cysts observed during surgery or on CT scans of 115 prolactinomas

	Number of patients examined	Number of patients with cysts
Women		
Microadenomas	53	9 (17%)
Macroadenomas	40	9 (22%)
Men		
Macroadenomas	22	3 (13%)
Total	115	21 (18%)

Signs of old or recent microscopic, intratumoral haemorrhage are seen in about 18% of the cases; however, the percentage is much higher (up to 40–60%) in women who have had an oestrogen treatment, and during and after pregnancy [42, 43]. Intratumoral cysts, possibly originating from previous, more extensive, intratumoral haemorrhage, are seen in 18% of the cases (tab. 1); they are somewhat more frequent in women than in men, and in microadenomas than in macroadenomas, but these differences are not statistically significant.

Diffuse, sinusoidal, and papillary adenomas have been differentiated on the basis of the amount and arrangement of their connective tissue [3, 18, 39, 49, 51]. The majority of the biopsy specimens is in the group of diffuse or medullary adenomas that contain only little collagen tissue around the blood vessels [27]. Several architectural types may occur, in a single adenoma, however. A semiquantitative study performed by Robert [47] showed a higher content of intraadenomatous fibrous tissue in prolactinomas obtained from women than from men, and in invasive than in noninvasive adenomas.

Microprolactinomas are only rarely invasive. Focal invasion was seen in only 2% of intrasellar adenomas in one study [47]. However, routine examination of biopsy specimens removed from the basal sellar dura during transsphenoidal surgery demonstrated microscopic invasion in about one-third of a small group microadenomas [19]. Invasive growth is observed frequently in larger adenomas. The invasion, particularly if it is microscopic, may be undetectable on radiographs or CT scans obtained with techniques that are currently available. However, such invasive behaviour may explain the low cure rate observed in patients with macroprolactinomas, particularly in the group producing serum prolactin levels above 200 ng/ml [20]. Invasion into the cavernous sinus is seen in patients with preoperative PRL levels above 1000–2000 ng/ml. But of course, lower levels do not exclude invasion into the cavernous sinus [21, 52].

Electron miscroscopy

An examination of the ultrastructure of prolactinomas with electron microscopy confirms the light microscopy findings with cytological features typical of cells engaged in active protein synthesis (fig. 1). The cytoplasm of biopsy specimens from prolactinomas contains differentiated complexes of the rough surfaced endoplasmic reticulum, the cell organelle engaged in protein synthesis, and a prominent Golgi apparatus engaged in the formation of the secretory granules. Annulate lamellae, a form of specially differentiated rough-surfaced endoplasmic reticulum that is considered an indicator of very active protein synthesis, are found in some specimens [17, 50]. The secretory granules are usually 100–300 nm in diameter. Only few secretory granules remain stored in the cytoplasm; most are released rapidly after their formation, and ongoing granule release can be observed along the entire cell circumference in about 60% of the biopsy specimens [47]. However, a dense accumulation of larger secretory granules (diameter 600 nm or greater) can be observed in a few cases [14, 17, 18, 41, 61]. Lysosomes engaged in crinophagy are found in most specimens. Cytoplasmic microtubules may be seen, primarily in the region of the Golgi apparatus. In rare cases, a few cells contain small bundles of fine (type I) microfilaments [14]. Desmosomes and the formation of abortive follicles are rare, but they are more frequent in prolactinomas than in the GH-secreting

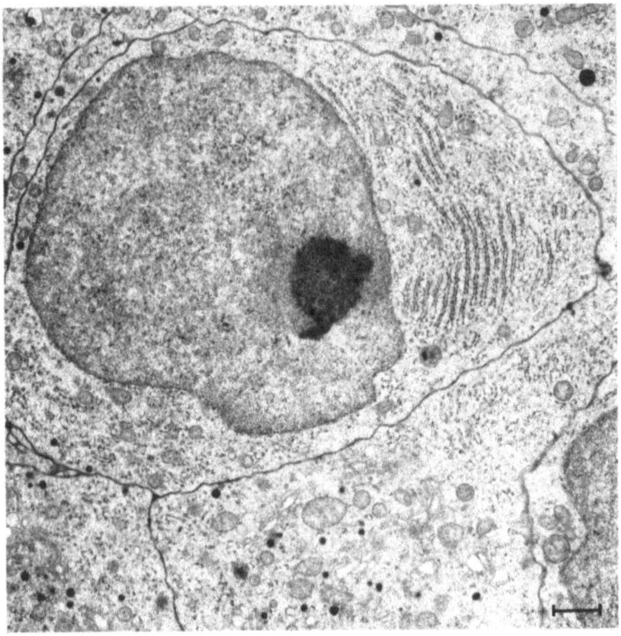

Fig. 1 Electron micrograph. Prolactinoma demonstrating oval nuclei with large nucleoli and large cytoplasma areas with a well differentiated rough-surfaced endoplasmic reticulum and few secretory granules. Osmium fixation, scale 1 μ.

adenomas [18]. Follicle formation is exaggerated in the very rare variant that is called cystic prolactinoma [16]. This type of adenoma, which must not be confused with adenomas containing an intratumoral cyst, consists of two cell types: (1) Cuboidal cells lining multiple microscopic, mucin-containing cysts, and (2) the usual prolactin cells.

The presence of oncocytes is generally interpreted as a sign of cell degeneration. Oncocytes dispersed in an actively secreting adenoma can only be detected with the electron microscope. They occur only in macroadenomas and not in microadenomas [19].

Changes in prolactinoma morphology caused by bromocriptine

Bromocriptine has been introduced as an alternative to the surgical extirpation of prolactinomas [53]. A number of reports published since 1979 have documented not only that this drug is able to normalize hyperprolactinaemia within a few days in about 66% of the patients, but also that is shrinks the tumour effectively in about 62% of the cases [2, 7, 9, 13, 30, 33, 36, 37, 58, 60]. Clinical experience has shown, however, that an ostensible cure achieved with bromocriptine seldom persists after treatment with the drug is discontinued; recurrence of hyperprolactinemia and reenlargement of the tumour usually occur within 1 or 2 weeks [54]. This observation casts some doubt on a previous assumption, based on experimental work in vitro [4, 40, 44], that bromocriptine exerts a cytostatic or even cytocidal effect on prolactinomas.

Light and electron microscopic studies of bromocriptine treated prolactinomas confirm that the drug causes pronounced shrinkage of adenoma cells (figs. 1–3). The nuclei are surrounded by a narrow rim of cytoplasm only, causing a dense accumulation of the cell nuclei that produces a lymphocyte-like picture [26, 46, 55]. A quantitative comparison of untreated and bromocriptine treated adenomas shows that the size of the nucleolus is most severely affected by the drug (tab. 2), and that the cell body, the cytoplasm, and the nucleus shrink less. The complexes of the rough-surfaced endoplasmic reticulum are reduced to single, dispersed tubules and vesicles. The Golgi cisterns become inconspicuous. Secretory granules may become rare. The cells present the morphological pattern of elements with reduced protein synthesis. The intensity of immunostaining and the number of immunostainable cells are markedly reduced [55].

These changes are caused by the bromocriptine-induced inhibition of prolactin gene transcription from DNA to messenger RNA [34, 35]. As the nucleolus is the site of the DNA to messenger RNA transcription, the pronounced reduction in the size of the nucleolus is a direct consequence of this inhibition by the drug. The reduction in the size of the rough-surfaced endoplasmic reticulum, the site of messenger RNA action during protein synthesis, is a secondary effect that leads ultimately to the reduction in prolactin synthesis and lowering or normalization of hyperprolactinaemia.

In a study by Gen et al. [8], microscopic examination of biopsy specimens from only one bromocriptine treated prolactinoma showed signs of tumour cell necrosis.

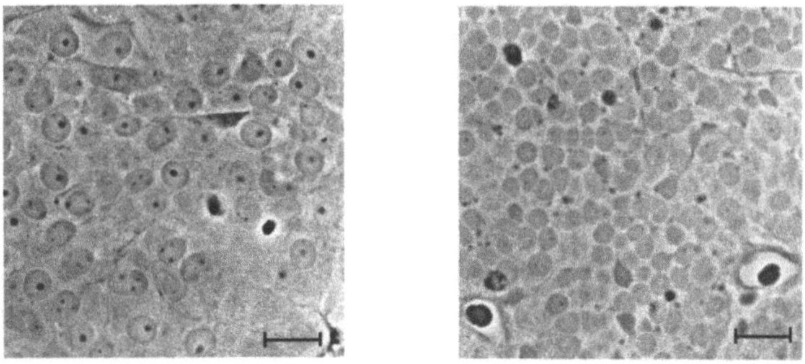

a b

Fig. 2a, b Phase contrast micrographs of osmium fixed, Epon embedded biopsy specimens of an untreated (a) and a bromocriptine-treated (6 weeks, 7.5 mg per day) prolactinoma (b). Scale 20 μ.

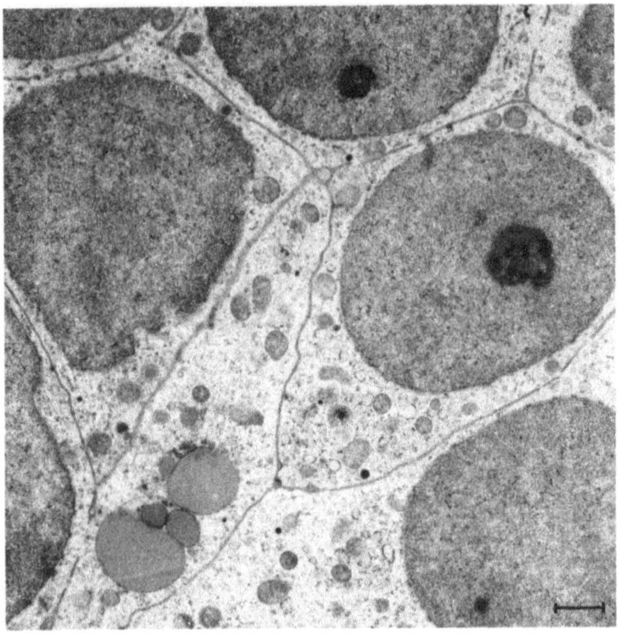

Fig. 3 Electron micrograph. Bromocriptine-treated prolactinoma with small adenoma cells demonstrating a narrow rim of cytoplasm with a reduced rough-surfaced endoplasmic reticulum. The nucleoli are reduced. Some lipid bodies are present. Note that the magnification is the same as in figure 1. Osmium fixation, scale 1 μ.

Table 2 Bromocriptine-induced changes in prolactinoma cell size*

Morphological structure	Percent decrease in size, as compared with untreated controls, caused by bromocriptine treatment of a least 4 weeks' duration
Cell size	−23
Cytoplasm area	−29
Cell nucleus	−18
Nucleolus	−49

* Data from Landolt et al. [26].

Our study has shown neither necrotic cells nor macrophages in the biopsy specimens from our cases, nor have we seen an increase in intraadenomatous calcification.

The rapid shrinkage of the prolactin cells after bromocriptine treatment is initiated causes the intercellular spaces to increase and the tissue structure of the adenoma to break up. Because the softened tissue facilitates surgical removal of the tumour, bromocriptine can be instrumental in improving surgical results in patients with prolactinomas [25, 59]. Prolonged bromocriptine treatment, however, causes deposition of fibrous tissue in the intercellular spaces. This can be measured in the perivascular area: a significantly increased perivascular fibrosis is observed in biopsy specimens obtained from prolactinomas that are treated with bromocriptine for periods of 3 months or longer [27]. The intraadenomatous fibrosis causes the adenoma to develop a rubber-like consistency, rending surgical removal more difficult at this stage because the adenoma has become more adherent to the surrounding normal tissue. In our series reported in 1982, postoperative normalization of prolactin levels was not achieved in patients who had been treated with bromocriptine for 1 year or more [25].

Prolactin levels maintained after the completion of bromocriptine therapy may be lower after withdrawal than were the pretreatment values. Although this effect has been interpreted as the result of an antiproliferative effect of the drug [5], we suspect that it may rather be a consequence of the perivascular fibrosis, which acts as a diffusion barrier between the secreting adenoma cells and the blood stream.

Discontinuation of bromocriptine treatment is followed by a rapid reenlargement of the adenoma. The cell increases to its pretreatment size within I week [26], and the ultrastructural features typical of untreated adenomas reappear [54].

Summary and conclusions

Most prolactinomas have the light and electron microscopic features typical of cells engaged in active protein synthesis. They often show secondary changes, however, such as intratumoral haemorrhage. calcification, amyloid deposition, and the appearance of dispersed oncocytes. Intraadenomatous fibrosis is present in some biopsy specimens, particularly those from invasive adenomas. Bromocriptine treatment changes the structure and ultrastructure of prolactinomas by blocking the transcription of the prolactin gene from DNA to messenger RNA. This causes a pronounced shrinkage of the nucleolus, the rough-surfaced endoplasmic reticulum, and the Golgi cisterns. The cells shrink by an average of 25% in comparison with cells in untreated samples, and the simultaneous enlargement of the intercellular spaces results in softening of the tumour tissue. Prolonged treatment, however, causes intraadenomatous, particularly perivascular, fibrosis. The fibrosis renders radical and selective removal of the adenoma difficult, if not impossible. We conclude that bromocriptine should not be used in patients suffering from prolactinoma – except briefly, to obtain preoperative tumour shrinkage – unless both the patient and physician accept that such treatment may render later surgery less effective and make continuation of the drug treatment necessary, perhaps for a lifetime.

Acknowledgements

The author thanks Prof. Ph. U. Heitz, Dept. of Pathology, University of Basle, for the immunohistological examination of the adenomas, Miss V. Osterwalder, Dept. of Neurosurgery, University of Zürich, for technical assistance, Mrs. Susan Eastwood-Berry, B. A., Berkeley, California, USA, for editorial assistance, the Sandoz Foundation, Basle, and the EMDO Foundation Zürich, for financial support.

References

[1] Bilbao, J. M., F. Horvath, A. R. Hudson, et al.: Pituitary adenoma producing amyloid-like substance. Arch. Pathol. (Chicago) **100** (1975) 411–415.

[2] Chiodini, P. G., A. Liuzzi, R. Cozzi, et al.: Size reduction of macroprolactinomas by bromocriptine or lisuride treatment. J. Clin. Endocrinol. Metab. **53** (1981) 737–743.

[3] Crompton, M. R.: The pathology of pituitary tumours. In: Pituitary tumours (J. S. Jenkins, ed.), pp. 22–37. Butterworth, London 1973.

[4] Davies, C., J. Jacobi, H. M. Lloyd, et al.: DNA synthesis and the secretion of prolactin and growth hormone by the pituitary gland of the male rat: Effects of diaethylstilboestrol and 2-bromo-alpha-ergocryptine methanesulphonate. J. Endocrinol. **61** (1974) 411–417.

[5] Flückiger, E., E. del Pozo, K. v. Werder: Prolactin: Physiology, pharmacology and clinical findings. Springer-Verlag, Berlin 1982.

[6] Foncin, J. F.: Morphologie ultra-structurale de l'hypophyse humaine. Neurochirurgie **17**, Suppl. 1 (1971) 10–24.

[7] Fossati, P., G. Strauch, J. Tournaire: Etude de l'activitée de la bromocriptine dans les états d'hyperprolactinémie. Nouv. Presse Méd. **5** (1976) 1687–1691.

[8] Gen, M., T. Uozumi, S. Shinohara et al.: Does bromocriptine have a cytocidal effect on prolactinoma cells? Report of a case. Neurol. Med.-Chir. **23** (1983) 61–65.

[9] George, S. R., G. N. Burrow, B. Zinman, et al.: Regression of pituitary tumors, a possible effect of bromoergocryptine. Am. J. Med. **66** (1979) 697–702.

[10] Girod, C., M. Mazzuca, J. Trouillas, et al.: Light microscopy, fine structure and immunohistochemistry studies of 271 pituitary adenomas. In: Pituitary adenomas – biology, physiopathology and treatment (P. Derome, C. P. Jedynak, F. Peillon, eds.), pp. 3–18. Asclepios-Publishers, France 1980.

[11] Hachmeister, U.: Ultrastructural aspects of pituitary tumors. In: Modern aspects of neurosurgery, vol. 4 – Proceedings of the German Society of Neurosurgery (H. Kuhlendahl, M. Brock, D. Le Vay, T. J. Weston, eds.), pp. 108–115. Excerpta Medica, Amsterdam 1973.

[12] Hachmeister, U., R. Fahlbusch, K. v. Werder: Ultrastructural identity of pituitary adenoma cells in Forbes-Albright syndrome and of adenohypophyseal pregancy cells. Acta Endocrinol. (Kbh) Suppl. **152** (1972) 42.

[13] Hall, K., A. M. McGregor, M. F. Scanlon, et al.: Metrizamide cisternography in assessment of pituitary tumour size, with special reference to the demonstration of tumour (prolactinoma) shrinkage on bromocriptine therapy. Progr. Reprod. Biol. **6** (1979) 232–243.

[14] Horvath, E., K. Kovacs: Pathology of the pituitary gland. In: Pituitary diseases (C. Ezrin, E. Horvath, K. Kaufman, K. Kovacs, M. H. Weiss, eds.), pp. 1–83. CRC Press, Boca Raton, Florida 1980.

[15] Kuratsu, J.-I., Y. Matsukado, M. Miura: Prolactinoma of pituitary with amyloid-like substances. Case report. J. Neurosurg. **59** (1983) 1067–1070.

[16] Kurisaka, M., S. C. Tindall, Y. Takei: Cystic prolactinoma of the pituitary following surgery for polycystic ovaries. Neurol. Med.-Chir. (Tokyo) **23** (1983) 55–60.
[17] Landolt, A. M.: Ultrastructure of human sella tumors. Acta Neurochir. (Wien) Suppl. **22** (1975) 1–167.
[18] Landolt, A. M.: Progress in pituitary adenoma biology. In: H. Krayenbühl, (ed.): Advances and technical standards in neurosurgery **5** (1978) 3–49.
[19] Landolt, A. M.: Biology of pituitary microadenomas. In: Pituitary microadenoma (C. Faglia, M. A. Giovanelli, R. M. McLeod, eds.), pp. 107–122. Academic Press, London 1980.
[20] Landolt, A. M.: Surgical treatment of pituitary prolactinomas: postoperative prolactin and fertility in seventy patients. Fertil. Steril. **35** (1981) 620–625.
[21] Landolt, A. M.: Cerebrospinal fluid rhinorrhea: a complication of therapy for invasive prolactinomas. Neurosurgery **11** (1982) 395–400.
[22] Landolt, A. M.: Secreting pituitary adenomas: morphological and biological aspects. In: Pituitary hyperfunction: physiopathology and clinical aspects (F. Camanni, E. F. Müller, eds.), pp. 135–155. Raven Press, New York 1984.
[23] Landolt, A. M.: Morphology and natural course of prolactinomas. In: Proceedings of the 3rd european symposium on pituitary adenomas (S. W. J. Lamberts, J. Assies, F. J. H. Tilders, F. A. van der Veen, eds.). Blackwell Publishers, London 1984 (in press).
[24] Landolt, A. M.: Prolactinomas: Structure, ultrastructure and bromocriptine-induced changes. In: Functioning pituitary adenoma; proceedings of the fourth japanese workshop on pituitary tumors (T. Uozumi, ed.). Osaka 1984 (in press).
[25] Landolt, A. M., P. J. Keller, E. R. Froesch, et al.: Bromocriptine: does it jeopardise the result of later surgery for prolactinomas? Lancet **2** (1982) 657–658.
[26] Landolt, A. M., H. Minder, V. Osterwalder, et al.: Bromocriptine reduces the seize of cells in prolactin-secreting pituitary adenomas. Experientia **39** (1983) 625–626.
[27] Landolt, A. M., V. Osterwalder: Perivascular fibrosis in prolactinomas: is it enhanced by bromocriptine? Clin. Endocrinol. Metab. **58** (1984) 1179–1183.
[28] Landolt, A. M., V. Rothenbühler: Pituitary adenoma calcification. Arch. Pathol. Lab. Med. **101** (1977) 22–27.
[29] Landolt, A. M., V. Rothenbühler, G. S. Kistler: Morphology of the chromophobe adenoma. In: Treatment of pituitary adenomas (R. Fahlbusch, K. v. Werder, eds.), pp. 154–171. Georg Thieme Verlag, Stuttgart 1978.
[30] Landolt, A. M., R. Wüthrich, H. Fellmann: Regression of pituitary prolactinoma after treatment with bromocriptine. Lancet **1** (1979) 1082–1083.
[31] Le Beau, J., J. F. Foncin: Contribution à l'étude ultrastructurale des adénomes à prolactine. Ann. Endocr. (Paris) **33** (1972) 353–356.
[32] Lewis, P. D., S. van Noorden: "Nonfunctioning" pituitary tumors. Arch. Pathol. **97** (1974) 178–182.
[33] Matsumura, S., S. Mori, T. Uozumi: Size reduction of a large prolactinoma by bromoergocriptine (CB-154) treatment. In: Pituitary adenomas: biology, physiopathology and treatment (P. J. Derome, C. P. Jedynak, F. Peillon, eds.), pp. 336–339. Asclepios Publishers, France 1980.
[34] Maurer, R. A.: Dopaminergic inhibition of prolactin synthesis and prolactin messenger RNA accumulation in cultured pituitary cells. J. Biol. Chem. **255** (1980) 8092–8097.
[35] Maurer, R. A.: Transcriptional regulation of the prolactin gene by ergocryptine and cyclic AMP. Nature **294** (1981) 94–97.
[36] McGregor, A. M., M. F. Scanlon, K. Hall, et al.: Reduction in size of a pituitary tumor by bromocriptine therapy. N. Engl. J. Med. **300** (1979a) 291–293.

[37] McGregor, A. M., M. F. Scanlon, R. Hall, et al.: Effects of bromocriptine on pituitary tumour size. Br. Med. J. **2** (1979b) 700–703.

[38] Mirouze, J., C. Jaffiol, P. Mary, et al.: Deux syndromes originaux "Amenorrhée-Galactorrhée" par tumeur hypophysaire. Discussion anatomo-clinique. Etude ultrastructurale de l'un d'eux. Ann. Endocrinol. (Paris) **30** (1969) 810–821.

[39] Nurnberger, J. I., S. R. Korey: Pituitary chromophobe adenomas. Springer Publishing Comp., New York 1953.

[40] Pawlikowski, M., J. Kunert-Radek, H. Stepien: Direct antiproliferative effect of dopamine agonists on the anterior pituitary gland in organ culture. J. Endocrinol. **79** (1978) 245–246.

[41] Peake, G. T., D. W. McKeel, H. L. Jarett, et al.: Ultrastructural, histologic and hormonal characterization of a prolactin-rich human pituitary tumor. J. Clin. Endocrinol. Metab. **29** (1969) 1385–1393.

[42] Peillon, F., J. Racadot, D. Moussy, et al.: Prolactin-secreting adenomas. A correlative study of morphological and clinical data. In: Treatment of pituitary adenomas (R. Fahlbusch, K. v. Werder, eds.), pp. 114–122. Georg Thieme Verlag, Stuttgart 1978.

[43] Peillon, F., E. Vila-Porcile, L. Olivier, et al.: L'action des œstrogènes sur les adénomes hypophysaires chez l'homme. Documents histopathologiques en microscopie optique et électronique et àpport à l'expérimentation. Ann. Endocr. (Paris) **31** (1970) 259–270.

[44] Quadri, S. K., K. H. Lu, J. Meites: Ergot-induced inhibition of pituitary tumor growth in rats. Science **176** (1972) 417–418.

[45] Racadot, J., F. Vila-Porcile, F. Peillon, et al.: Adénomes hypophysaires à cellules à prolactine: étude structurale et ultrastructurale, corrélations anatomo-cliniques. Ann. Endocr. (Paris) **32** (1971) 298–305.

[46] Rengachari, S. S., T. Tomita, B. F. Jeffries, et al.: Structural changes in human pituitary tumor after bromocriptine therapy. Neurosurgery **10** (1982) 242–251.

[47] Robert, F.: Le prolactinome – aspects pathologiques. Neurochirurgie **27**, Suppl. 1 (1981) 61–73.

[48] Robert, F., J. Hardy: Prolactin-secreting adenomas: A light and electron microscopical study. Arch. Pathol. **99** (1975) 625–633.

[49] Saeger, W.: Hypophyse, In: Spezielle, pathologische Anatomie (W. Doerr, G. Seifert, eds.), vol. 14/I, pp. 2–226. Springer-Verlag, Berlin 1981.

[50] Scanarini, M., R. Giordano, S. Mingrino, et al.: Fine structure of prolactin pituitary adenoma with special reference to annulate lamellae. Acta Neuropath. (Berl.) **46** (1979) 163–166.

[51] Schnitker, M. T., E. C. Cutler, O. T. Bailey, et al.: The chromphobe adenomas of the pituitary: pathologic features and response to irridiation based on a study of 81 verified cases. Am. J. Roentgenol. **40** (1938) 645–659.

[52] Shucart, W. A.: Implications of very high serum prolactin levels associated with pituitary tumors. J. Neurosurg. **52** (1980) 226–228.

[53] Thorner, M. C., A. S. McNeilly, C. Hagan, et al.: Long-term treatment of galactorrhea and hypogonadism with bromocriptine. Br. Med. J. **2** (1974) 419–422.

[54] Thorner, M. O., R. C. Perryman, A. D. Rogul, et al.: Rapid changes of prolactinoma volume after withdrawal and reinstitution of bromocriptine. J. Clin. Endocrinol. Metab. **53** (1981) 480–483.

[55] Tindall, G. T., K. Kovacs, E. Horvath, et al.: Human prolactin-producing adenomas and bromocriptine: a histological, immunocytochemical, ultrastructural, and morphometric study. J. Clin. Endocrinol. Metab. **55** (1982) 1178–1183.

[56] Tournaire, J. P. Guinet, I. Bachelot, et al.: Les adénome à prolactine. Oto-Neuro-Ophth. **47** (1974) 303–320.
[57] Trouillas, J., M. Curé, M. Lheritier, et al.: Les adénomenes hypophysaires avec aménorrhée-galactorrhée ou galactorrhée isolée. Lyon Méd. **236** (1976) 359–375.
[58] Wass, J. A. H., P. J. H. Moult, M. O. Thorner, et al.: Reduction of pituitary tumour size in patients with prolactinomas and acromegaly treated with bromocriptine with or without radiotherapy. Lancet **2** (1979) 66–69.
[59] Weiss, M. H., R. R. Wycoff, R. Yadley, et al.: Bromocriptine treatment of prolactin-secreting tumors: surgical implications. Neurosurgery **12** (1983) 640–642.
[60] Woodhouse, N. J. Y., F. Khouqueer, J. O. Sieck: Prolactinomas and optic nerve compression: Disappearance of a suprasellar extension and visual recovery after two weeks bromocriptine treatment. Hormone Res. **14** (1981) 141–147.
[61] Yaghmai, F.: Clinical pathological correlation of pituitary adenomas. In: The pituitary – a current review (M. B. Allen, V. B. Mahesh, eds.), pp. 373–386. Academic Press, New York 1977.

Prolactinomas and mixed adenomas with prolactin cells: an immunohistochemical study of the subcellular localization of hormones

G. Jautzke, J. Iglesias

Introduction

Since the introduction of immunocytochemical investigations it has been known that, in most cases, pituitary adenomas are prolactinomas [3]. Increased prolactin values in serum in the case of a pituitary adenoma may either be due to a prolactinoma or to a disinhibition mechanism [5]. Therefore, only the immunohistochemical detection of prolactin production in the adenoma cells can provide evidence for the presence of a prolactinoma.

Materials and methods

In a retrospective study, we examined the surgical biopsies of 98 patients, who had been operated in Berlin between 1969 and 1983 mostly because of large pituitary adenomas. The material which was routinely fixed in formalin and embedded in paraffin, was examined by light microscopy using the PAP method [7], and more recently predominantly using the avidin-biotin-complex method [2]. From the paraffin blocks, suitable tissue specimens were re-embedded in resin (Epon). Several methods can be used for material embedded in resin:

1. After removal of the resin [4], the immune reaction can be performed in the semithin section, and, in addition, semithin serial sections can be examined for different hormones.

2. In the semithin section, the immunocytochemical reaction can be performed, and in the contrasted thin section, which follows immediately thereafter, the ultrastructure can be analyzed.

3. Immunohistochemistry can be performed in thin sections using either the PAP method or the protein A gold method [6].

The following antisera were used:
anti-human prolactin (Radioassay Systems Cab. Cal.), anti-porcine ACTH (1−39) (Immuno Nuclear Corporation), anti-human-GH (Serono), anti-TSH (Serono), monoclonal anti-alpha subunit (Medix). The bridge antiserum and the PAP-complex were obtained from Dako. The ABC-method was performed using a kit from Vector.

Results

In 36 of 98 pituitary adenomas, we found prolactin cells. In 17 cases, only prolactin was found, in 14 cases, prolactin and growth hormone (GH), and in 5 cases, prolactin and hormones other than GH.

Prolactinomas

In the 17 cases of "pure" prolactinomas, the ratio of men to women was 8:9, the age distribution in men was 15 to 69 years with an average of 40 years, in women it was 22 to 65 years with an average of 36 years. Clinically, and most adenomas were large and involved visual disorders, and in the women they also involved concomitant secondary amenorrhoea. Light-microscopically, all the adenomas were chromophobic. In immunohistochemistry, most tumour cells were labelled. In the semithin section, the prolactin immune reactivity manifested itself in the form of partly arched, partly ring-shaped bands near the nuclei. Only in one case, there were also individual cells (less than 5% of the adenoma cells) in which the cytoplasm showed a positive reaction along the cell membrane. The semithin-thin section technique, in which the immune reaction was performed in the semithin section and the subsequent thin section was contrasted with uranyl acetate, yielded the following results (fig. 1a, b, c):

The prolactin-positive areas corresponded to the cytoplasmic zones in the thin section which

1. were free from rough endoplasmic reticulum,
2. contained immature secretory granules, and
3. yielded indications of Golgi's membranes that were barely discernible due to the absence of contrast with osmium oxide.

The protein A gold method yielded a picture in the thin section which corresponded to the results already mentioned (fig. 2). Gold particles, which label the prolactin, were never found in the rough endoplasmic reticulum but only in the Golgi field, with the immature granules being densely labelled and the granula-free

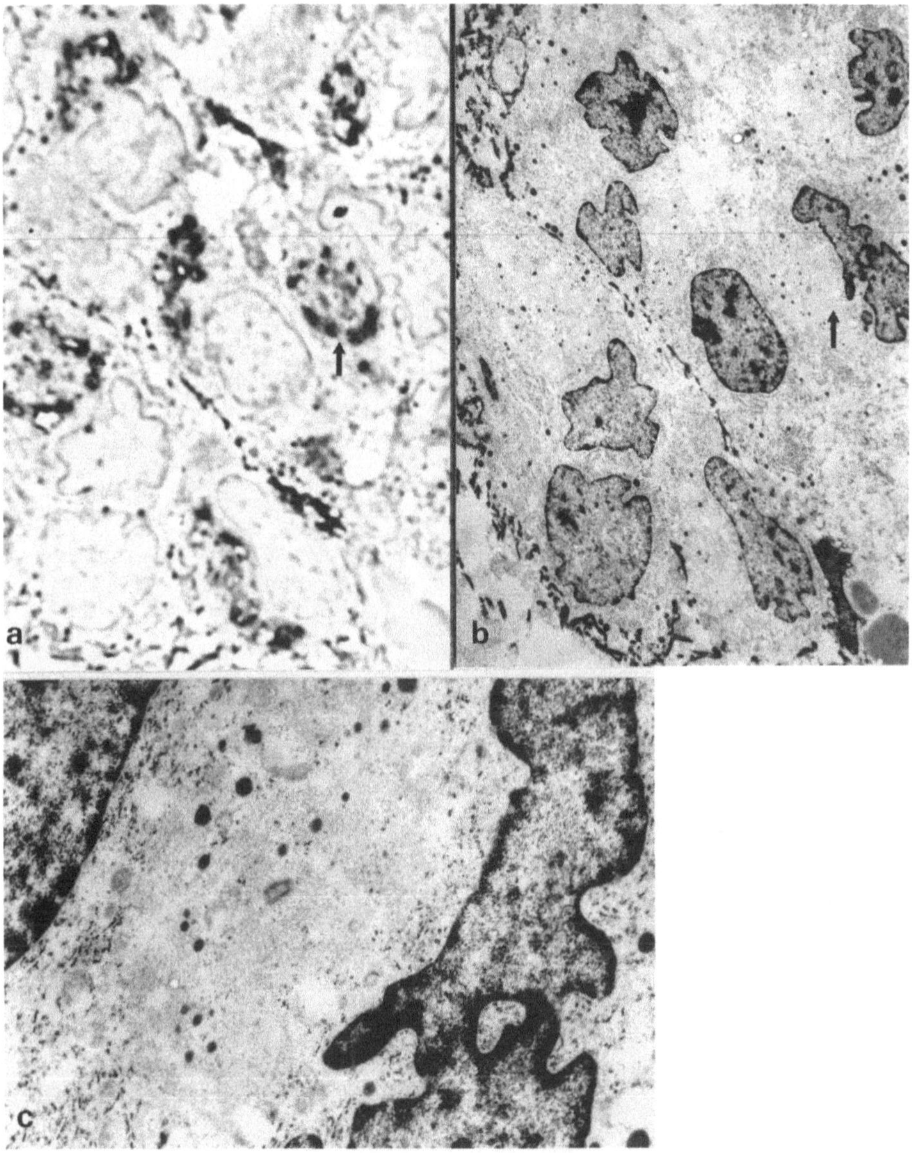

Fig. 1 a) Semithin section of a sparsely granulated prolactinoma immunostained for prolactin, which is found in circumscribed areas near the nucleus as dark deposits (arrow), (3600×). b) Thin section adjacent to the one shown in Figure 1a, contrasted with uranyl acetate. The immunostaining in Figure 1a corresponds to areas that are free of RER and contain immature granules (arrow), (3600×). c) Same section as Figure 1b at higher magnification shows barely discernible Golgi's membranes surrounding the immature secretory granules and a centriole (15000×).

areas of the Golgi fields being more weakly labelled. The labelled secretory granules were also found to be fused with the cell membrane (fig. 3). Some single granules had been released into the extracellular space, a process that has been designated as "misplaced exocytosis" [1].

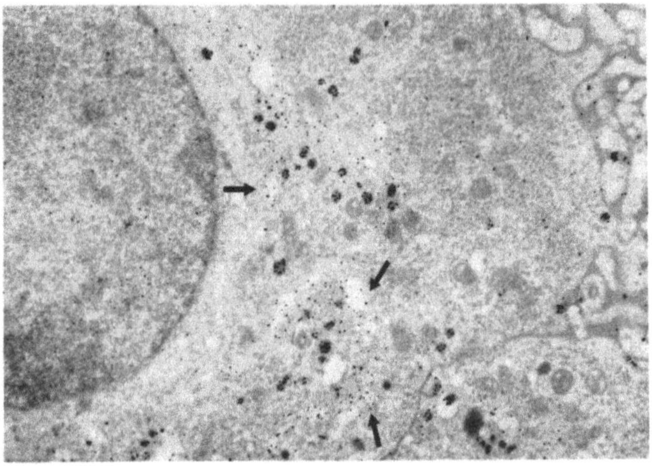

Fig. 2 Sparsely granulated prolactinoma immunostained for prolactin with the protein A gold method. Immature granules are densely labelled. Weak labelling of granule-free areas of the Golgi field (arrows), (12000×).

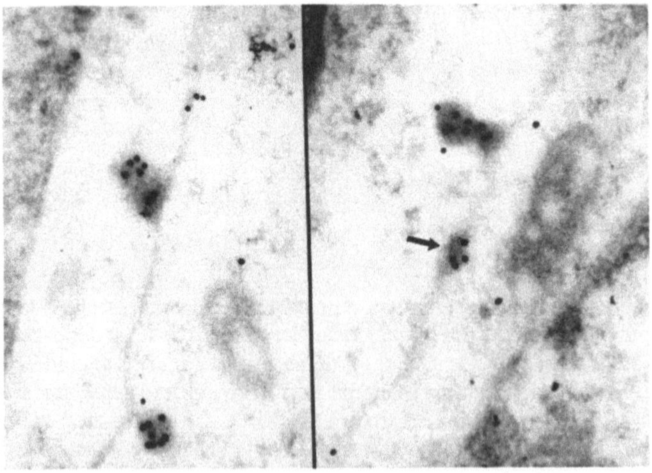

Fig. 3 Same section as in figure 2. Labelled secretory granules fuse with the cell membrane, some of which are released into the extracellular space (arrow), (25000×).

Adenomas with immunohistochemically detectable prolactin and GH-cells

In 14 cases, we found pituitary tumours which contained both prolactin and GH-immunoreactive cells (tab. 1). The majority of these cases (10 cases) showed a predominance of growth hormone cells. 4 of them were densely granulated, 6 were sparsely granulated. Only those cases with a predominance of GH-cells in pituitary adenoma clinically showed an acromegaly. In the densely granulated adenoma, the number of labelled growth hormone cells was between 60% and 100%; that of the

Table 1 Adenomas with prolactin cells and GH-cells

1. Predominance of prolactin cells	((?) densely granulated)	0 cases
	sparsely granulated	4 cases
2. Predominance of GH-cells	densely granulated	4 cases
	sparsely granulated	6 cases

prolactin-immunoreactive cells ranged from about 10% to 30% of adenoma cells. In semithin serial sections (fig. 4c and d), it became evident that the granula-containing positive prolactin cells were also positively labelled with growth hormone. However, there were also a few poorly granulated cells which were exclusively prolactin-labelled. In thin sections, in which double labelling was performed with prior visualization of prolactin by the protein A gold method and subsequent localization of growth hormone by the PAP method, it became evident that, apart from the gold labelling within the granules, the prolactin-positive cells showed concomitant labelling with the PAP complexes (figs. 5a and 6). The exclusively prolactin-labelled cells showed immune reactivity in the Golgi field (fig. 5c). Methodologically, this double-labelling does, of course, present a problem, since protein A, which labels prolactin, could also bind the antisera of the second incubation, although between these two incubations, incubation with a strong excess of normal serum was performed. Therefore, we only assess those places as double-stained, in which the PAP complexes and the gold labelling are recognizable as being spatially separated above the granules. Though the method of double-labelling in the present form must be treated with caution, our other results also indicate that the granules of these cells contain both hormones:

1. In the semithin serial sections, all granula-containing prolactin cells showed concomitant labelling with growth hormone.

2. The cells that were exclusively growth-hormone-positive showed the same intensity of immune reactions as the cells containing both growth hormone and prolactin: the majority of the granules could thus be assumed to be growth-hormone-labelled.

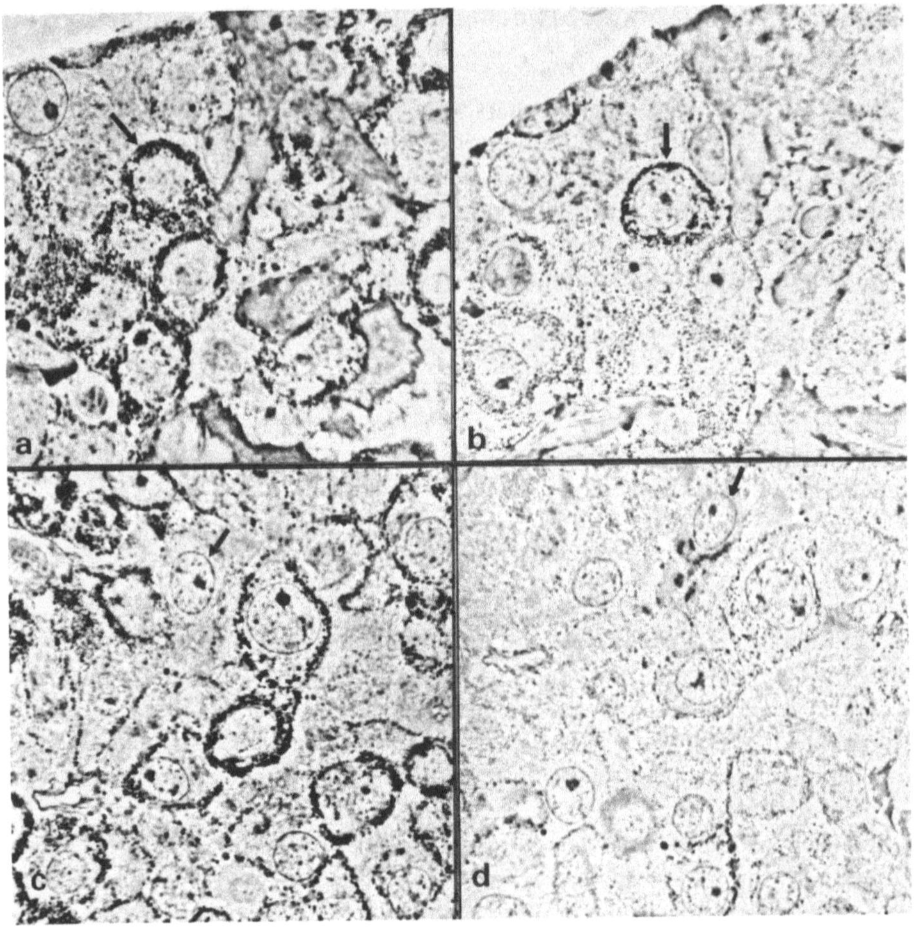

Fig. 4 Densely granulated mixed growth hormone cell and prolactin cell adenoma. a) Semithin section immunostained for growth hormone. Most cells are stained (1600×). b) Semithin section adjacent to the one shown in figure 4a immunostained for prolactin. The only cell stained is a double-stained cell, since the same cell is stained in Figure 4a for growth hormone (arrows) (1600×). c) Semithin section immunostained for growth hormone (1600×). d) Semithin section adjacent to the one shown in figure 4c immunostained for prolactin. One sparsely granulated cell is stained in the Golgi region. This cell is not stained with growth hormone in figure 4c (arrows) (1600×).

▶

Fig. 5 Densely granulated mixed growth hormone cell and prolactin cell adenoma. Thin section with double immunolabelling. Prolactin is visualized using the protein A gold technique in a first step. In a second step, growth hormone is stained with the PAP method. a) Double-stained cell. All granules contain prolactin-labelling gold particles and growth-hormone-labelling PAP-complexes (16500×). b) Double-stained granules at higher magnification (47500×). c) A few cells are solely prolactin-stained with gold particles over the Golgi region (arrows) (16500×).

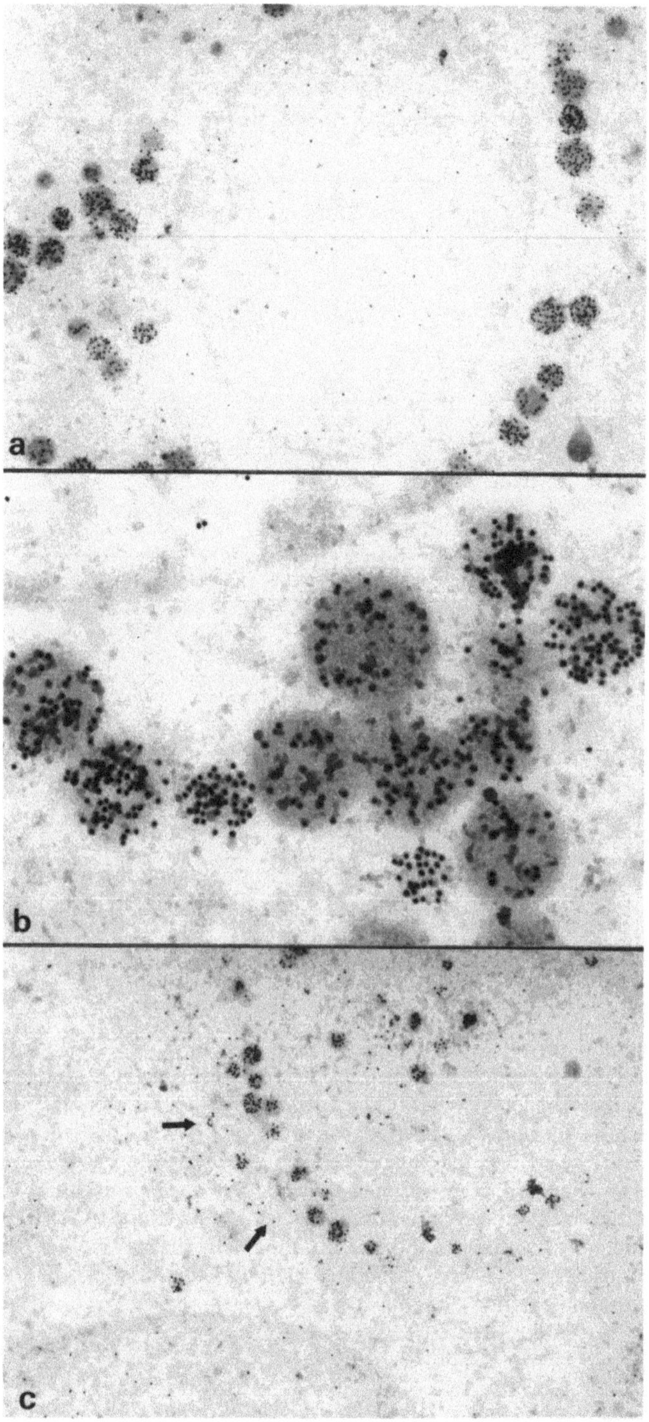

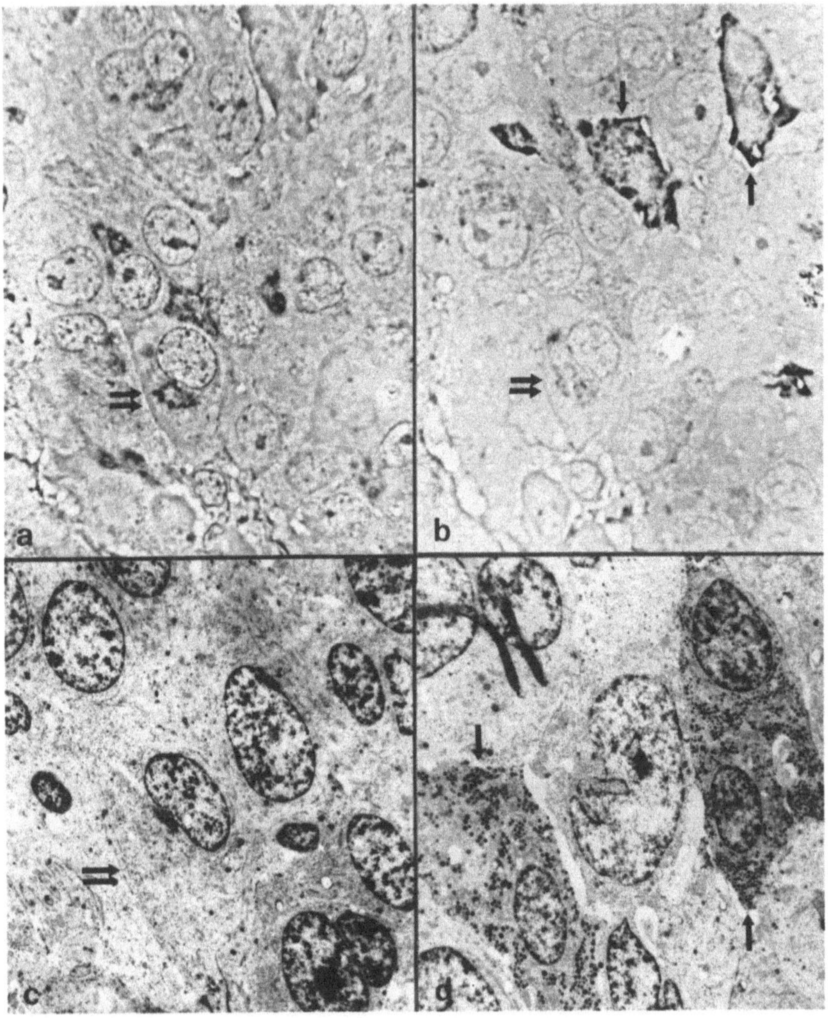

Fig. 6 Sparsely granulated mixed growth-hormone cell and prolactin cell adenoma. a) Semithin section immunostained for prolactin, which is found only in sparsely granulated cells over the Golgi region (1600×). b) Semithin section adjacent to the one shown in Figure 6a immunostained for growth hormone. Two densely granulated cells (arrows) and one sparsely granulated cell (double arrows) are labelled. The latter is a double-labelled cell, since this cell is also labelled for prolactin in figure 6a (1600×). c) Adjacent thin section contrasted with uranyl acetate. The double-labelled cell (double arrows) does not differ from the cells that are only prolactin-labelled (3600×). d) Same section as in Figure 6c. Densely granulated cells containing only growth hormone (arrows), (3600×).

3. In the thin section, the protein A gold method showed that nearly all granules were also labelled for prolactin in the double-stained cells.

In the sparsely granulated adenomas, the fraction of growth-hormone-positive cells amounted to 10% in one case and nearly 100% in 2 cases with values varying between these two in the other cases. The number of prolactin-immunoreactive cells ranged between 5% and 40% of the adenoma cells. In semithin serial sections (fig. 6a, b, c, d), it became evident that the few granula-containing cells were exclusively GH-labelled; in the ultrathin section, these cells contained granules ranging in size between 130 and 220 nm. The Golgi-field-labelled adenoma cells were largely prolactin-positive cells, though there were some cells that showed both prolactin and growth hormone in the Golgi region. These cells did not differ electron-microscopically from the cells that were only prolactin-labelled.

Similar results were observed in the 4 adenomas which showed a clear predominance of the prolactin cells. In these cases as well, there were some cells that were granulated and contained only growth hormone and a few cells that contained both growth hormone and prolactin in the Golgi region.

Mixed adenomas with immunostainable prolactin cells and hormones other than GH

We found two cases in which, in addition to prolactin, the alpha-chain of the glycoprotein hormones was also detectable. These adenomas did not differ clinically from the "pure" prolactinomas. They showed cells with concomitant prolactin and alpha-chain-labelling and identical distribution in the cytoplasm.

Furthermore, we found 3 adenomas in which prolactin appeared together with other hormones (tab. 2). One case contained ACTH-immunoreactive cells concomitantly labelled with prolactin. This adenoma was large and endocrinologically silent. A further adenoma contained prolactin, growth-hormone and the alpha-chain of the glycoprotein hormones. Some cells were concomitantly labelled with all 3 hormones (fig. 7a, b, c). Another adenoma contained prolactin in 30% of cells,

Table 2 Other mixed adenomas with prolactin cells

Hormones	Number of cases	Double-stained cells found	not found
Prolactin + α-chain	2	+	
Prolactin + ACTH (clinically silent)	1	+	
Prolactin + GH + α-chain	1	+ (3-fold)	
Prolactin + GH + TSH + α-chain (clinical hyperthyroidism)	1		+

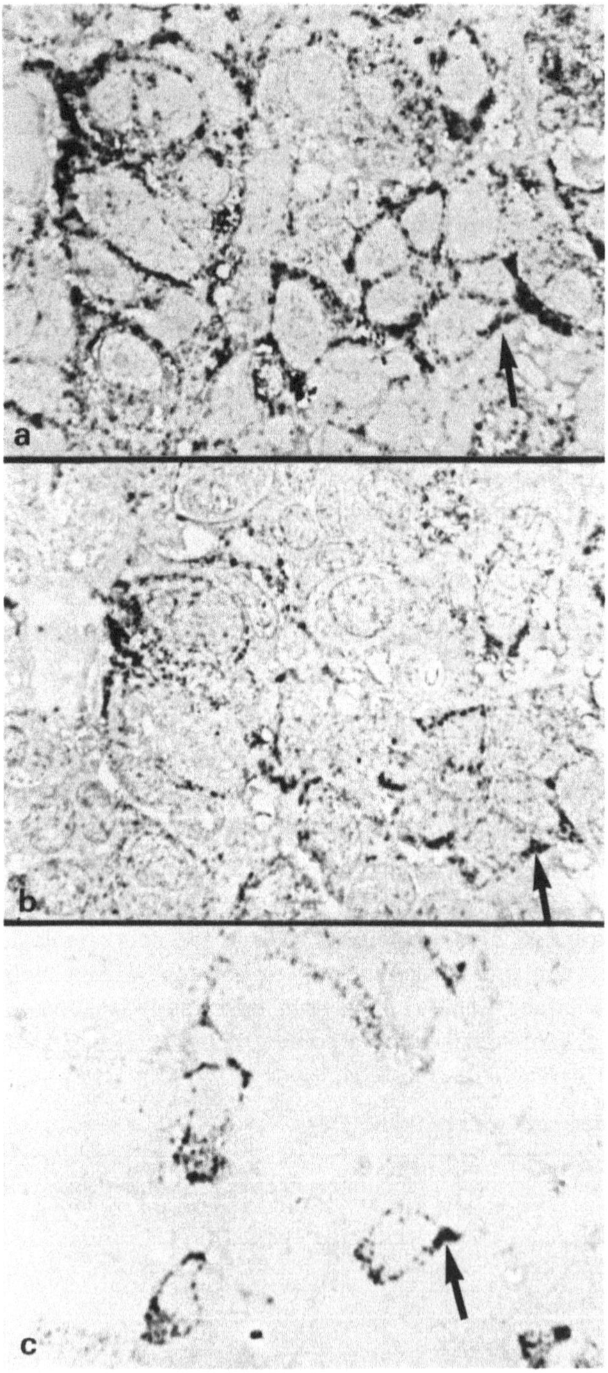

Fig. 7 Serial semithin sections of a mixed adenoma immunostained for alpha-chain (7a), prolactin (7b) and growth hormone (7c). One cell produces all three hormones (arrows).

growth-hormone in 10%, alpha chain in 30%, and TSH in 10% of cells. Nevertheless, the adenoma corresponded clinically to a TSH-producing adenoma with increased TSH-values in the blood.

Conclusions

1. The "pure" prolactinomas were all sparsely granulated in our material. Densely granulated prolactin cells were only found in mixed adenomas.

2. Prolactin- and GH-producing mixed adenomas are frequent. In addition to cells that only form one hormone, double-labelled cells also occur. If these are densely granulated, both hormones are found in one granule in the Golgi field in sparsely granulated cells. Only the cases in which the GH-cells predominate were clinically associated with acromegaly.

3. Mixed adenomas that form prolactin and ACTH or prolactin and alpha-chain are rarely found. Both hormones can also be formed in one cell in these adenomas.

4. In one adenoma, we found prolactin, GH and alpha-chains, in which these 3 hormones occasionally occurred in one cell. This means that, in cases of mixed pituitary adenomas, the thesis "one hormone, one cell" must be revised.

5. In one adenoma, we found prolactin, GH, alpha chain and TSH. Since this patient presented endocrinologically with hyperthyroidism, only the TSH-cell fraction was clinically active. This suggests that plurihormonal adenomas must be classified not only by immunohistochemical methods but by clinical parameters as well.

References

[1] Horvath, E., K. Kovacs: Misplaced exocytosis: Distinct ultrastructural feature in some pituitary adenomas. Arch. Pathol. **97** (1974) 221.

[2] Hsu, S. M., L. Raine, H. Fanger: Use of Avidin-Biotin-Peroxidase Complex (ABC). In: Immunoperoxidase Techniques. J. Histochem. Cytochem. **29** (1981) 577–580.

[3] Kovacs, K., E. Horvath, N. Ryan: Immunocytology of the human pituitary. In: Diagnostic Immunohistochemistry Masson Monographs in Diagnostic Pathology (A. Delellis, ed.), pp. 17–35. Masson, New York–Paris 1981.

[4] Mayor, H. D., J. C. Hampton, B. Rosario: A simple method for removing the resin from epoxy-embedded tissue. J. Biophys. Biochem. Cytol. **9** (1961) 909–910.

[5] Reichlin, S.: The prolactinoma problem. N. Engl. J. Med. **300** (1979) 313–315.

[6] Roth, J., M. Bendagan, L. Orci: Ultrastructural localization of intracellular Antigens by the use of Protein A Gold Complex. J. Histochem. Cytochem. **26** (1978) 1074–1081.

[7] Sternberger, L. A., P. H. Hardy, J. J. Cuculis et al.: The unlabelled antibody enzyme method of immunohistochemistry: Preparation and properties of soluble antigen-antibody complex (horseradish peroxydase – antihorseradish peroxydase) and its use in identification of spirochetes. J. Histochem. Cytochem. **18** (1970) 315–333.

Immunocytochemical, chemical and nuclear-DNA studies of pituitary tumours*

P. O. Lundberg, C. Muhr, L. Grimelius, Y. Olsson, R. Hugosson, J. Stahle, L. Wide, K. Bergström

Introduction

The introduction in recent years of immunocytochemical and chemical techniques in the diagnosis of pituitary adenomas have made it clearly evident that the previously used classification into chromophobe and chromophile types of these tumours is inadequate. Newer classification systems have been proposed in which adenomas are grouped on the basis of a combination of clinical symptoms, blood hormone activity, immunocytochemistry and electron microscopy (e.g. [4]). In other studies, however, considerable variability has been found in the characteristics of adenomas as revealed by the above methods [7, 10, 13, 14, 16].

DNA studies of tumour cells have contributed greatly towards solving problems of differentiation between different tumour types in many endocrine organs, for example the parathyroid gland [3] and the pituitary [1, 2].

The aim of the present investigation was to gain a more thorough knowledge of the characteristics of pituitary adenomas, in the hope of making possibly more accurate prognostic evaluations and of providing better grounds for the choice between different treatment alternatives.

Patients

Patients who had undergone surgery for a pituitary adenoma in the Department of Neurosurgery (29 cases) or the Department of Oto-Rhino-Laryngology (17 cases) at the University Hospital of Uppsala during the last 6-year period were studied. There were 31 females and 15 males. Their age at the time of operation ranged from 17–72 years (mean 46.8 years).

The patients were divided into three groups on the basis of clinical symptoms and determinations of serum growth hormone and serum prolactin. Group A consisted

* This work was supported by a grant from the Swedish Medical Research Council (project no. 102).

of 16 patients with acromegaly (basal serum growth hormone 6.8–156 μg/l). Twelve of them were females and four males. Eight of the females and one male had slight hyperprolactinaemia (serum prolactin 32–75 μg/l).

Group B consisted of 20 further patients with hyperprolactinaemia – 15 females and 5 males. All the males and 12 of the females had slight or moderate hyperprolactinaemia, with serum prolactin values between 23 and 124 μg/l. In three females the serum prolactin concentrations were 410, 419 and 1100 μg/l, respectively. In none of these patients was the serum level of growth hormone elevated.

Group C comprised 10 patients, 4 females and 6 males, with presumably functionless pituitary adenomas. None of them had any clinical symptoms or signs, or blood hormone values, indicating endocrine hyperfunction.

The indication for surgery in the group A was acromegaly and in groups B and C progressive tumour growth with compression of the optic chiasm and visual defects.

All patients had an asymmetrical or enlarged sella turcica on plain sellar films. Computed tomography showed a pituitary adenoma with higher attenuation after injection of contrast medium in all cases. The case material thus did not include any patients with so called microadenomas (a pituitary adenoma with a diameter of less than 10 mm). Nor were any cases of invasive pituitary adenoma included.

Methods

Surgery

Transfrontal surgery was performed with an osteoplastic bone flap in the right frontal region of the skull. The adenoma was reached by traction of the frontal lobes to the rear and by splitting the arachnoidea in the chiasmatic cistern. In all cases the adenoma was protruding from the midline in between the optic nerves. The adenoma tissue was removed in pieces. Necrotic or cystically transformed tumour tissue was not saved. The biopsy material thus examined represented the more solid parts of the adenoma.

In the transsphenoidal approach an orbital incision was made and the sphenoidal sinus was reached via the right ethmoid. The posterior part of the nasal septum was removed. The frontal inferior sella wall was then excised and a cruciate incision was made through the dura to expose the pituitary gland. The tumour tissue was removed with pituitary forceps.

After both procedures all tumour tissue was immediately taking care of in accordance with a predetermined scheme for further specialized preparation.

Tumour tissue examination

1. The major tissue portion was fixed in 10% buffered formalin or Bouin's fluid at room temperature for 24 hours. After dehydration, the specimens were embedded in paraffin. Sections 5 μ thick were then stained with haematoxylin-eosin, van Gieson's stain and immunostained with the peroxidase-antiperoxidase (PAP) method of Steinberger [17] for GH, prolactin, ACTH, TSH, β-endorphin and leu- and methenkephalin. The controls were those recommended by Goldman [6] including exposure to respective antisera in excess (100–200 μg/ml diluted antisera). The following antisera and dilutions were used: ACTH (1:400) and TSH (1:1600) from Dakopatts; GH (1:1600) and prolactin (1:400) from L Wide, Uppsala; β-endorphin (1:3200) and leu- and methenkephalin (1:400) a gift from L Terenius, Uppsala.

2. Tissue imprints were prepared before fixation by pressing glass slides against the tissue. The imprints were immediately fixed in acetone/absolute alcohol (1:1) at room temperature. The imprints were then incubated at 37 °C in 0.5 mg/ml ribonuclease solution and stained with buffered ethidium bromide solution. The DNA content of the cells was measured by a fluoroscence cytophotometric method [3]. Lymphocytes were used as reference cells.

3. Very small tissue specimens were fixed by immersion in 3% buffered glutaraldehyde, pH 7.4, at +4 °C. After post fixation for one hour in 1% osmium tetroxide the specimens were dehydrated and embedded in Epon. Semithin sections were cut and stained with toluidine blue for orientation. From selected areas ultrathin sections were cut and counterstained with uranyl acatate and lead citrate and examined in a JEOL −100 C transmission electron microscope.

4. In 18 of the 46 cases some tumour tissue specimens could be stored frozen in liquid nitrogen at −65 °C. GH, prolactin, TSH, FSH and LH in the tumour tissue were extracted in phosphate buffer, pH 5.7 followed by extraction with glycine buffer, pH 9.8. A radioimmunoassay technique [19] was used for determination of hormones in the tumour tissue extracts as well as in serum.

Results

Routine histopathology and electron microscopy

The histopathological characteristics and the ultrastructural features were in accordance with the morphology as described earlier in the literature. The details will be published elsewhere.

DNA measurements

DNA measurements showed a normal DNA content in 26 of the 46 patients (tab. 1). In 13 of these 26 patients tetraploidy was observed in 1–4% of the cells, but this finding is apparently not of pathological significance and can be made in normal pituitary tissue [5].

Twenty patients had a pathological DNA content. In 12 of these patients tetraploidy was found in 5 to 12% of the cells, and occasionally octaploid cells were also found. Eight further patients had grave DNA abnormalities with an aneuploid DNA content.

Table 1 Nuclear DNA-content in pituitary tumours

	DNA	
	normal	pathological
Acromegaly	5 (31%)	11 (69%)
Hyperprolactinaemia	14 (70%)	6 (30%)
Functionless	7 (70%)	3 (30%)

DNA abnormalities were much more common among the 16 acromegalic patients compared with the other two groups. In five of them more than 5% of the cells were tetraploid. Aneuploidy was found in six further cases. The DNA content was normal in only five (31%) of the acromegalic patients. Among the 20 patients with hyperprolactinaemia the DNA content was normal in 14 (70%); aneuploidy was found in two patients and increased tetraploidy in a further four patients. The DNA content was pathological in two of the three patients with high serum prolactin values. Among the 10 patients with functionless pituitary tumours, DNA abnormality in the form of increased tetraploidy was found in only three (70%) and in the other seven patients the DNA content was entirely normal.

Two of the 46 patients were operated on because of tumour recurrency. In both of these cases the DNA content was normal. During the rather short period of observation after surgery (less than 4 years), five patients have displayed clinical and roentgenological signs of tumour recurrency. In three of these patients the DNA content was definitely abnormal at the first operation.

Immunocytochemistry

Cells containing immunoreactive growth hormone were found in tumours from 11 of the 16 acromegalic patients. In three adenomas no GH immunoreactive cells could be found and in two adenomas the staining reaction was unsuccessful due to less well preserved tissue. Of the 11 tumours in which GH immunoreactive cells were found, eight also contained immunoreactive prolactin. In eight of the patients the prolactin reaction was negative. There was no correlation between the intensity of the immunoreactive staining for growth hormone or prolactin and the serum levels of these hormones.

Of the adenomas from the 20 patients with hyperprolactinaemia nine contained prolactin immunoreactive cells and five contained GH immunoreactive cells. In one patient the staining reaction was unsuccessful for technical reasons. In some further patients the specimens also contained normal pituitary tissue with GH and prolactin immunoreactive cells. There was no apparent correlation between the intensity of the staining and the serum prolactin values. Two of the three patients with high serum prolactin values had tumours containing both prolactin immunoreactive cells and GH immunoreactive cells. In the third case the reaction was negative to both prolactin and GH.

Among the 10 patients with functionless pituitary adenomas only two had tumours containing prolactin immunoreactive cells. In none of the adenomas from these patients were any GH immunoreactive cells found.

In 44 of the 46 cases minor cell populations were immunostained with antisera against ACTH, TSH, endorphin and enkephalin (tab. 2). Eight of the tumours contained ACTH immunoreactive cells, 16 TSH immunoreactive cells, eight endorphin immunoreactive cells and 15 enkephalin immunoreactive cells. The frequency of tumours containing ACTH, TSH, endorphin and enkephalin immunoreactive cells did not differ significantly between the three groups. It has not been possible so far to correlate the occurrence of ACTH, TSH, endorphin or enkephalin immunoreactive cells with the clinical picture or blood hormone levels in any of the three groups of patients.

Table 2 Number of patients with positive immunoreactivity in adenoma cells

	n	ACT	TSH	Endorphin	Enkephalin
Acromegaly	15	1 (7%)	6 (40%)	2 (13%)	4 (27%)
Hyperprolactinaemia	19	4 (21%)	6 (32%)	4 (21%)	7 (37%)
Functionless adenomas	10	3 (30%)	2 (20%)	2 (20%)	4 (40%)

Hormonal extraction from tumour tissue

Unfortunately it was only possible to obtain specimens large enough for hormonal extraction procedures in 18 of the 46 patients. Evaluation of the results is difficult because of the insufficient knowledge of values for non-tumourous pituitary tissue

[18]. Very high GH extraction values (more than 1000 ng/mg wet weight) were found in specimens from three of the acromegalic patients but in none of the patients in groups B and C. High prolactin extraction values (more than 100 ng/mg wet weight) were noted in five of the acromegalic patients and in two of the patients with hyperprolactinaemia in group B, and in one of the patients with a functionless pituitary adenoma. In five of the patients with hyperprolactinaemia the tissue extraction values for prolactin were low.

Discussion

DNA measurements have gained increasing interest in the last years. In several studies an abnormal DNA content has been demonstrated in tumours. The knowledge concerning the DNA content in normal human pituitary tissue and pituitary tumours is limited. However, a low percentage of tetraploidy seems to be common even in normal pituitary tissue [5]. If a tetraploidy frequency of up to 4 per cent is accepted as normal, then 20 of 46 patients (43.5%) in the present series had tumours with a pathological DNA content. This frequency is similar to that reported by Anniko et al. [2], who found aneuploidy in nine out of 24 patients (35.5%) with pituitary adenomas of different types, using a flow-cytofluorometric method.

It has generally been considered that an abnormal, and especially an aneuploid DNA content implies malignancy [5]. Pituitary adenomas expressing malignancy in the form of metastasis are extremely rare. However, invasive tumour growth, that is tumours growing in an infiltrative and destructive manner, destroying bone structures cranial nerves and the brain, are not uncommon [11, 15]. No such tumour was included in the present series, as we do not consider them suitable for surgery. In the present series routine histopathology did not reveal any indication of malignancy in any of the adenomas.

It is extremely difficult to evaluate the rate of tumour growth in such a series of patients as this, since the development of symptoms is often vague. Two patients operated on because of recurrency did not show an abnormal DNA content in the tumour tissue. On the other hand, three out of five patients who had already developed a recurrency after the DNA determination were included among those who had an abnormal DNA content. This might represent a tendency, but the question whether an abnormal DNA content carries an increased risk of recurrency can only be judged after a long period of follow-up.

The most conspicuous finding was that a pathological DNA content was much more common among patients with acromegaly (69%) than among those with hyperprolactinaemia or a functionless pituitary adenoma (30%).

In a recent study of 55 adenomas from patients with acromegaly, it was found that all of them contained GH immunoreactive cells and 25 (45%) contained prolactin immunoreactive cells [8]. Our findings of 78% and 50%, respectively, are in good accordance with these figures.

Hyperprolactinaemia in patients with a pituitary adenoma does not necessarily mean that the adenoma is actively producing hormone, i.e. that it is a prolactinoma. Serum prolactin values of up to 100 μg/l, or according to some authors even somewhat higher, may occur in patients with other types of tumours such as meningeomas, metastastic carcinomas and so on ([12] and others). This may be caused by impingement on the pituitary stalk. Suprasellar extension of a purely GH-secreting adenoma or a functionless pituitary adenoma may also give rise to hyperprolactinaemia in this way [8, 9].

Three patients in the present series had a hyperprolactinaemia of 410, 490 and 1100 μg/l, respectively. However, only in the latter two prolactin immunoreactive cells were found. The correlation between tissue extraction values of prolactin, the occurrence of prolactin immunoreactive cells and the level of serum prolactin was also poor both in the nine acromegalic patients with hyperprolactinaemia and in the other 20 patients with hyperprolactinaemia. One should bear in mind, however, that the techniques were employed on different tissue specimens.

The results from this series of patients shed no light on the clinical importance of the presence of ACTH, TSH, enkephalin and endorphin immunoreactive cells.

Conclusion

1. Pathological DNA content is much more common in pituitary adenomas from acromegaly patients than in those from patients with hyperprolactinaemia or functionless pituitary adenomas.

2. There is good correlation between GH immunoreactive cells in pituitary adenomas and increased serum GH levels.

3. Pituitary adenomas with moderately increased serum prolactin levels probably do not actively produce hormone, i.e. they are not prolactinomas.

References

[1] Anniko, M., L.-E. Holm, B. Tribukait, et al.: DNA characteristics of human pituitary tumours. Acta Otolaryngol. Suppl. 379 (1981a) 5.

[2] Anniko, M., L.-E. Holm, C. Silfverswärd, et al.: Cellular DNA content of pituitary tumours: Its relationship to morphology and hormonal type of tumour. Acta Otolaryngol. Suppl. **379** (1981b) 13.

[3] Bengtsson, A., L. Grimelius, H. Johansson, et al.: Nuclear DNA-content of parathyroid cells in adenomas, hyperplastic and normal glands. Acta Pathol. Microbiol. Scand., Sect A **85** (1977) 455.

[4] Berry, R. C., H. J. Caplan: An overview of pituitary tumours. Ann. Clin. Lab. Science **9** (1979) 94.
[5] Böhm, N., W. Sandritter: DNA in human tumours. A cytophotometric study. Curr. Top. Pathol. **60** (1975) 151.
[6] Goldman, M.: Fluorescent antibody methods, p. 159. Academic Press, New York 1968.
[7] Horwath, E., K. Kovacs: Ultrastructural classification of pituitary adenomas. J. Can. Sci. Neurol. Feb. (1976) 9.
[8] Kanie, N., N. Kageyama, A. Kuwayama, et al.: Pituitary adenomas in acromegalic patients: An immunohistochemical and endocrinological study with special reference to prolactin-secreting adenoma. J. Clin. Endocrinol. Metab. **57** (1983) 1093.
[9] Kruseman, A. C. N., G. Th. A. M. Bots, F. Roelfsma, et al.: Immunocytochemical growth hormone and prolactin in pituitary adenomas causing acromegaly and their relationship to basal serum hormone levels and the growth response to thyrotropin releasing hormone. Clin. Endocrinol. **19** (1983) 1.
[10] Landolt, A. M.: Praktische Bedeutung neuer Erkentnisse über Struktur und Funktion von Hypophysenadenomen. Schw. Med. Wschr. **108** (1978) 1521.
[11] Lundberg, P. O., B. Drettner, A. Hemmingsson et al.: The invasive pituitary adenoma. Arch. Neurol. **34** (1977) 742.
[12] Lundberg, P. O., P. O. Osterman, L. Wide: Serum prolactin in patients with hypothalamus and pituitary disorders. J. Neurosurg. **55** (1981) 194.
[13] Martinez, A. J., A. Lee, J. Moossy, et al.: Pituitary adenomas: Clinicopathological and immunohistochemical study. Ann. Neurol. **7** (1980) 24.
[14] McCormick, W. F., N. S. Halmi: Absence of chromophobe adenomas from a large series of pituitary tumours. Arch. Pathol. **92** (1971) 231.
[15] Robert, F.: Morphology of human prolactinomas: A study of invasive prolactin-secreting adenomas. In: Prolactin and Prolactinomas (G. Tolis et al., eds.), pp. 339–349. Raven Press, New York 1983.
[16] Saeger, W.: Modern concepts of pituitary morphology and pathology of pituitary adenomas. Per. Biol. **85**, Suppl. 1 (1983) 9.
[17] Sternberger, L. A.: Immunohistochemistry, pp 143–144. Prentice-Hall, Englewood Cliffs, NJ, 1974.
[18] Trouillas, J., C. Girod, G. Sassolas, et al.: A human β-endorphin pituitary adenoma. J. Clin. Endocrinol. Metab. **58** (1984) 242.
[19] Wide, L.: Radioimmunoassays employing immunosorbents. Acta Endocrinol. **142**, Suppl. (1969) 207.

Hyperplasia of prolactin pituitary cells with or without microadenoma

M. Scanarini, S. Mingrino, I. Mastrogiacomo, E. Serafini, D. Cervesato

Introduction

Among the various types of pituitary adenomas more and more interest has been focussed on prolactinomas, since many questions need to be answered concerning their biology and the therapeutic indications for these tumours [1, 2]. The aim with the present study was to correlate the clinical course and surgical results in a series of 58 prolactin-pituitary adenomas with the morphological findings and to assess the value and reliability of the immunocytochemical methods in the clinicopathological investigations of pituitary tumours.

Materials and methods

During the last three years 1981–1983, fifty-eight patients with prolactin-secreting pituitary adenomas were operated in the Department of Neurosurgery of Padua University. The clinical features of these cases are summarized in table 1. All patients underwent a formal protocol of testing for pituitary function before and one month after surgery. Endocrinological evaluation included, beside basal PRL levels, prolactin serum level variations after TRH. The radiological investigation consisted of anteroposterior and lateral hypocycloidal polytomography and thin-section computerized tomography (CT). Twenty-two patients had microadenomas,

Table 1 Clinical features of immunocytochemically defined PRL-pituitary adenomas (58 patients)

Sex	f = 49; m = 9
Age (average)	17–54 years
Amenorrhoea	30
Amenorrhoea – Galactorrhoea	19
Hypogonadism	7 (m)
Gynecomastia	2 (m)
PRL (average)	70–3500 ng/ml

24 had intrasellar macroadenomas and 12 patients presented with extrasellar macroadenomas.

In the 22 patients with microadenomas, abnormalities of the sella turcica were seen in 18 cases, while in the remaining 4 cases the sella turcica was normal. Only in 9 cases the CT scan showed an intrasellar focal area of decreased attenuation confirmed later as a tumour at surgery. In all these cases the unilateral transseptal, transsphenoidal microsurgical approach was performed; in all 22 patients it was possible to perform a selective removal of the microadenoma while saving the normal pituitary tissue. A soft tumour was found in all cases with a diameter of less than 10 mm (in 5 cases the diameter was less than 5 mm).

Histological verification of a pituitary adenoma was obtained in 19 cases while in 3 cases hyperplastic cell nests without microadenoma were found. Only in 6 cases it was possible to examine the surrounding peri-adenomatous tissue (tab. 2). The immunoperoxidase method was performed on serial sections of the formalin-fixed, paraffin-embedded tissue.

Sternberger's peroxidase-antiperoxidase (PAP)-method was used for detection of human prolactin hormone (PRL), human growth (GH) and human adrenocorticotropic hormone (ACTH) [3].

The tumours in 19 patients were classified as acidophil or chromophobe adenomas by light microscopy.

On immunoperoxidase staining all 19 tumours were immunoreactive for PRL; in 3 cases of this group up to 10% of the tumour cells were immunoreactive for GH. The immunoperoxidase staining on peri-adenomatous tissue showed prolactin po-

Table 2 Histological findings (22 patients)

Adenoma	Periadenomatous tissue	Adenohypophyseal cell hyperplasia
19	6	3

Table 3 Immunoperoxidase staining on adenohypophyseal cell hyperplasia

Hormones detected	No.
PRL	3
PRL-GH	0
PRL-ACTH	0
Negative	0
Total	3

sitivity only in 3 cases, while the others three cases were negative for PRL. The 3 cases presenting focal or diffuse adenohypophyseal hyperplasia without microadenoma revealed cells with characteristics of lactotroph and immunoreactivity for PRL (tab. 3).

The 6 patients, all women, with PRL-cell-hyperplasia with or without microadenoma, presented the classic symptoms and had radiological evidence of sellar abnormalities.

The prolactin levels returned the normal range after surgery in only one case (diffuse hyperplasia without microadenoma): this patient also becames pregnant.

In the other cases the PRL levels remained unchanged and medical therapy with bromocriptine was started (tabs. 4 and 5).

Table 4 Clinical data from 3 patients with prolactin cell hyperplasia

Cases	Sex	Age	Pituitary fossa	Mean PRL level (ng/ml)	Results
1	f	17	grade I	80	unchanged
2	f	20	grade I	100	unchanged
3	f	22	grade II	85	normalized

Table 5 Clinical data from 3 patients with prolactin periadenomatous hyperplasia

Cases	Sex	Age	Pituitary fossa	Mean PRL level (ng/ml)	Results
1	f	24	grade I	95	unchanged
2	f	33	grade I	105	unchanged
3	f	36	grade 0	120	unchanged

Discussion

Both the biological complexity and technical problems associated with surgery for human pituitary diseases result in frequent failures to do precise diagnostic and prognostic correlations with pituitary tumours, especially with prolactinomas. For this reason it is very difficult to draw conclusions about the existence and significance of "true" prolactin-cell-hyperplasia without the presence of microadenoma. Nevertheless, in our opinion, hyperplasia of cell type identical to those found in the tumour is often present in the surrounding non tumorous adenohypophysis. This concerns only the pituitary tissue studies in the vicinity of the microadenoma. This could not be verified for the more distant parts of the pituitary gland because of lack of information [4].

In spite of the difficulty in distinguishing hyperplasia of pituitary cells from adenoma in small fragments, focal or diffuse hyperplasia of prolactin-secreting cells with no circumscribed microadenoma may occur, and it may be functionally active.

The existence of PRL-cell-hyperplasia with or without microadenoma seems to indicate an impaired regulation at the hypothalamic level and the "so-called" functional hyperprolactinaemia could be related to these morphological findings in the pituitary gland.

Summary

The results of conventional histological staining, ultrastructural studies and immunoperoxidase methods were compared in a study of 58 prolactin-secreting pituitary adenomas and correlated with clinical features and with the surgical outcomes.

Three cases of prolactin-cell-hyperplasia without microadenoma and three cases of microadenoma with periadenomatous prolactin-cell-hyperplasia were found. The subjects, all women, showing such morphological findings, failed to respond to surgery (except for one patient) and the normalization of the prolactin levels was achieved only by medical treatment.

The real existence of prolactin-cell-hyperplasia without microadenoma and pathophysiology of related so-called "functional" hyperprolactinaemia are discussed.

References

[1] Molinatti, G. M.: A clinical problem: microprolactinoma. Proceedings of an Intern. Workshop, Saint Vincent, 22. April 1982. Excerpta Medica, Amsterdam–Oxford–Princeton.

[2] Martinez, A. J., A. Lee, et al.: Pituitary Adenomas Clinicophathological and Immunohistochemical Study. Ann. Neurol. **7** (1980) 24–36.

[3] Steernberger, L. A., P. H. Hardy Jr., J. J. Cuculis, et al.: The unlabeled antibody enzyme method of immunohistochemistry. Preparation and properties of soluble antigen-antibody complex and its use in identification of spirochetes. J. Histochem. Cytochem. **18** (1970) 315–333.

[4] Girod, C., M. Mazzuca, J. Trouillas, et al.: Light Microscopy, fine structure and immunohystochemistry studies of 278 Pituitary Adenomas. In: Pituitary Adenomas (P. J. Derome, C. P. Jedynak, F. Peillon, eds.). II. Europ. Workshop, Paris. Asclepios Ed., Paris 1980.

Hormone-secretion in cell culture of microprolactinomas, periadenomatous tissue and capsules

U. Schrell, M. Buchfelder, R. Fahlbusch, K. Mashiter

Introduction

Histological examinations of pituitary tumours combined with immunocytochemistry are able to differentiate between the normal pituitary and a hormone-producing adenoma in a reliable manner [5]. Up to now there have been difficulties in the differential diagnosis between adenomatous hyperplasia (which is assumed to be a central hypothalamic regulatory disorder) and the adenoma (microprolactinoma) itself [4]. Even scanning electron microscopy cannot distinguish conclusively between adenomatous and non-tumorous normal pituitary cells [1]. The explant culture seems to be a method with a grade of reliability to differentiate the tumour from the normal pituitary (periadenomatous tissue) by their secretion patterns [3].

This study summarizes the results of 23 patients suffering from microprolactinoma. Pseudocapsules were removed in 7 patients. In 5 patients the microadenoma seemed to consist of two different tumour types. The different types of intrasellar tissue were placed into the cell-culture-medium immediately after operation in the operating theatre and sent by air mail to London, Hammersmith Hospital.

Materials and methods

For the culture experiments, aseptic conditions were employed. The adenoma tissue was cut into tiny cubes of approximately 1 mm^3 and distributed in culture tubes containing 2 ml culture-medium and incubated at 37 °C. The amount of tissue obtained and cultured from each patient was not standardized. The experiments were started on the third day after setting up the cultures and after a complete medium change and wash of the tissue in order to reduce failures due to hormone leakage from damaged cells. The short term culture experiments were then carried out over two consecutive periods of 3 days, always with a complete medium change at the end of each period. Then the culture medium was stored at −20°C for further investigations by radioimmunoassay for PRL, GH, LH, FSH, TSH [3].

Results

The hormone-secretion of a typical microprolactinoma is documented by high amounts of prolactin sometimes accompanied by small amounts of human-growth hormone (hGH). In the periadenomatous tissue all the anterior lobe hormones could be detected in the culture medium: GH, PRL, FSH, LH, TSH, and ACTH, giving evidence of normal pituitary gland function [3].

Secretion patterns of 23 microprolactinomas removed by transsphenoidal microsurgery

In cell culture, each of the adenomas secreted prolactin accompanied in 90% of these cases by small amounts of human-growth hormone. The other hormones secreted by the anterior pituitary lobe could not be detected in the culture medium. From these negative findings we can conclude that this incubated tissue (described by the Neurosurgeon as the specific tumour tissue), represented the microprolactinoma itself.

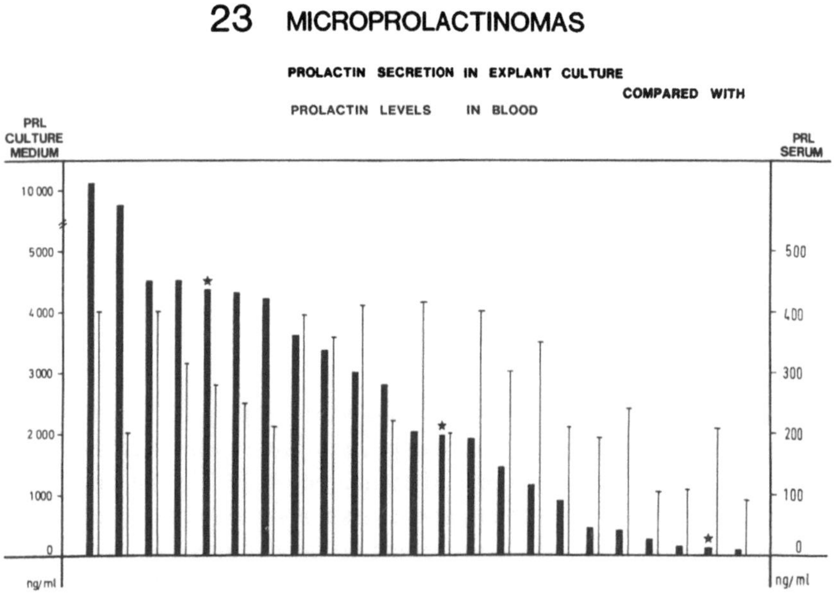

Fig. 1 The black bars represent the concentration of prolactin levels secreted into the culture medium (ng/ml on the left side).
The lines represent prolactin concentration of the blood (ng/ml on the right side). One bar and one line together are the results of one patient. Three microadenomas marked with asterisks show all of the anterior lobe hormones in the culture medium.

Three operatively removed adenomas marked by asterisks (fig. 1) secreted other anterior pituitary lobe hormones as well, indicating that there were some adjacent normal pituitary cells present.

When the hormone levels secreted in cell culture are compared with the hormone levels measured in the sera of the patients, it is obvious that the hormone levels do not correlate (fig. 1).

The conclusion is that the different hormone levels in explant cultures give no information of prognostic value. We only obtain information about the kind of tumour the patients have (in our cases, prolactinomas).

Secretion patterns of the capsules compared with the adenoma

In our series 7 (pseudo)capsules surrounding the adenoma had been removed in order to study their secretion patterns. This so-called capsule is generally thought to consist of normal pituitary tissue. Indeed the secretion patterns showed all the pituitary hormones but especially high levels of PRL and GH, similar to the secretion patterns of the adenoma.

Secretion patterns of the two types of adenomas

In five cases the surgeon had the impression that there were two parts to the adenoma.

Type I is a typical grey tumour of soft consistency and type II a yellow tumour of firm consistency. Both tissues could be clearly differentiated under higher magnification from the periadenomatous tissue. But only in one of the 5 cases did the hormone secretion activity of the tumour type I correlate well with the tumour type II. Both types secreted only PRL accompanied by hGH, and both tumour parts could be well distinguished by their secretion patterns from the periadenomatous tissue.

In contrast to these findings, there were no differences between the adenoma type II and the periadenomatous tissue in the other cases (fig. 2).

Discussion

1. The explant culture is of great value in differentiating between the prolactin-producing adenoma and the normal pituitary tissue. In only 3 cases out of 23 patients, did we find not only prolactin but also other pituitary hormones in the medium. The interpretation of these presence of multiple hormones measured by radio-

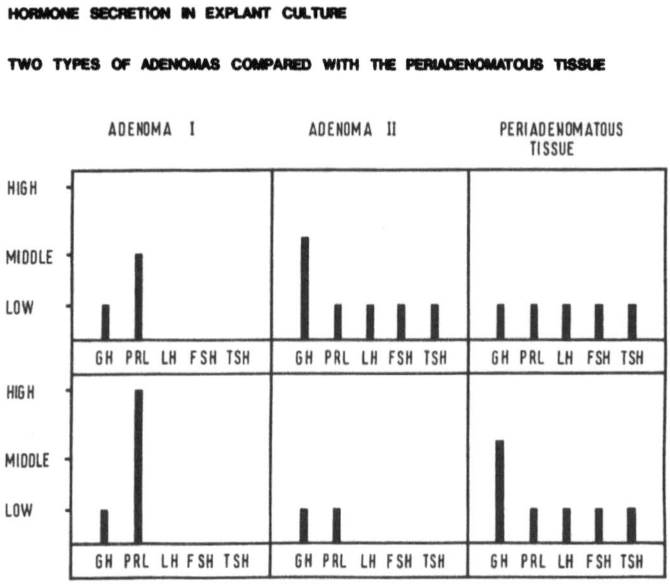

Fig. 2 The black bars represent the anterior pituitary lobe hormones, which were secreted in culture medium by adenomatous and periadenomatous tissue after transsphenoidal microsurgery.

immunoassay, suggested that specimens were not always homogenous and contained both the adenoma and also tiny parts of the adjacent normal pituitary tissue. In order to obtain representative results, the neurosurgeon has to distinguish exactly between the specific neoplastic tumour tissue (the adenoma) and other tissues of the pituitary gland [2].

2. Incubation of capsular tissue showed considerable amounts of prolactin and hGH, and smaller amounts of other pituitary hormones. Since it is not clear, whether the capsule has a tumorous or proliferative tendency, we decided to resect the capsule in all cases, hoping that this resection may improve surgical results in some patients.

3. Finally it is open to discussion whether there is a real practical significance of our observation that there are different types of cells in some tumours. Perhaps further investigations will demonstrate that the tissue type II corresponds to hyperplastic alterations of the pituitary gland.

References

[1] Kovacs, K., E. Horvath, D. J. McComb: The fine structure of pituitary tumors. In: Ultrastructure of endocrine cells and tissues (P. M. Motta, ed.). Martinus Nijhoff Publishers, Boston–The Hague–Dordrecht–Lancaster 1984.

[2] Lipson, L. G., I. Z. Beitins, P. D. Kornblith, et. al.: Tissue culture studies on human pituitary tumours: radioimmunoassayable anterior pituitary hormones in the culture medium. Acta Endocrinologica **88** (1978) 239–249.
[3] Mashiter, K., S. van Noorden, L. De Marco, et. al.: Hormone secretion by human somatotropic, lactotrophic, and mixed pituitary adenomas in culture. J. Clin. Endocrinol. Metab. **48** (1979) 108–113.
[4] Schwesinger, G., R. Warzok: Hyperplasien und Adenome der Hypophyse im unselektierten Sektionsgut. Zbl. allg. Pathol. u. pathol. Anat. **126** (1982) 495–498.
[5] Zimmerman, E. A., R. Defendi, A. G. Frantz: Prolactin and growth hormone in patients with pituitary adenomas: a correlative study of hormone in tumor and plasma by immunoperoxidase technique and radioimmunoassay. J. Clin. Endocrinol. Metab. **38** (1974) 577.

Immunocytochemical, ultrastructural and culture characteristics of prolactin-secreting pituitary adenomas

K. Bálint, L. Gazsó, F. Slowik, E. Pásztor

Introduction

With the combined use of modern methods such as electronmicroscopy-immunocytochemistry, cell culture, the number of studies published on pituitary tumours is rapidly increasing [1, 5, 8–14]. The most common tumour of the human adenohypophysis, the sparsely granulated prolactin cell adenoma has been extensively studied [2, 3, 4, 6, 7]. This paper records our clinicopathological analysis of 52 surgically removed sparsely granulated prolactinomas.

Materials and methods

The tumours were removed by the transsphenoidal approach. Tumour grade was determined by our own classification, based on Hardy's [1], into three groups: microadenomas, macroadenomas without suprasellar extensions and macroadenomas with suprasellar extensions. Hyperprolactinaemia was determined with radioimmunoassay. For light microscopy formalin fixed-paraffin embedded material was used. Sections were stained by haematoxylin-eosin and by Mallory techniques. For electron microscopy tumour tissue was fixed in 4% glutaraldehyde in 0,2 M phosphate buffer, postfixed in 2% osmium tetroxide and embedded in durcupan ACM. The technique has already been described [9]. For immunocytochemistry we used formalin fixed material embedded in paraplast. Sections of 4–6 micron thickness were prepared for the immunoperoxidase technique [15, 16]. In control experiments the primary antiserum was replaced by normal rabbit serum. For comparison, normal pituitary glands from necropsy cases were immunostained. We used rabbit antihuman PRL/1 : 800, rabbit antihuman GH/1 : 800, rabbit antihuman ACTH/1 : 500, rabbit antihuman TSH beta/1 : 800, rabbit antihuman LH beta/1 : 1000 and rabbit antihuman FSH beta/1 : 1000 hormones generously donated by the National Pituitary Agency, Baltimore, USA, Dr. A. F. Parlow. For evaluation the immunostained samples were divided into three groups. One + was used to indicate the reaction if the number of immunostained cells were few, mostly scattered, but large in size; two ++ were used, if more positively stained cells could be seen forming clusters of various sizes; three +++ when the reaction showed numerous immunostained cells to be found throughout the sections. In these latter cases the immunostaining was generally located spherically or in a crescent shape around the nuclei. For cell culture tumour specimens were explanted immediately after surgery. Techniques of cell culture have been described in a previous report [17].

Results

Clinical findings from 33 woman and 19 men aged between 20 and 67 years are summarized in table 1. Ninety-one percent of the females suffered from galactorrhoea-amenorrhoea and infertility. Only 31% of the males had impotency, hypogonadism or gynecomastia. Among them visual disturbances and headaches were frequently observed, associated with large tumours. Microadenomas occurred only in females. Each measured case had varying degrees of hyperprolactinaemia preoperatively. At light microscopic level using conventional staining, tumours corresponded to typical chromophobe adenomas. Ultrastructurally the tumours removed proved to be sparsely granulated prolactin cell adenomas according to the classification by Horvath and Kovacs [5]. These adenomas showed a characteristic ultrastructure (fig. 1). The adenoma cells were polyhedral and closely apposed with irregular nuclei and abundant cytoplasm. The rough-surfaced endoplasmic reticulum was very prominent, the Golgi apparatus was conspicuous. The secretory granules were sparse, spherical, oval or irregular, electron-dense and measured 150–500 nanometers with an average of 200–300 nm. One of the main cytoplasmic features was the misplaced exocytosis [2]. Growth hormone-producing cells could not be observed ultrastructurally. Immunocytochemical examinations revealed prolactin-producing activity in the cytoplasm of adenoma cells in all cases. The evaluation of immunopositivity can be seen in table 2. Out of 52 prolactinomas there were 3 tumours with positivity marked with +, 13 adenomas marked with

Table 1 Prolactinomas (52 cases) – preoperative clinical and serum hormone findings

Sex	Females	Males
Avarage age	31 years	37 years
Hormonal disturbances	91%	31%
Visual disturbances	32%	65%
Headaches	50%	68%
Average basal serum PRL level	405 ng/ml	696 ng/ml

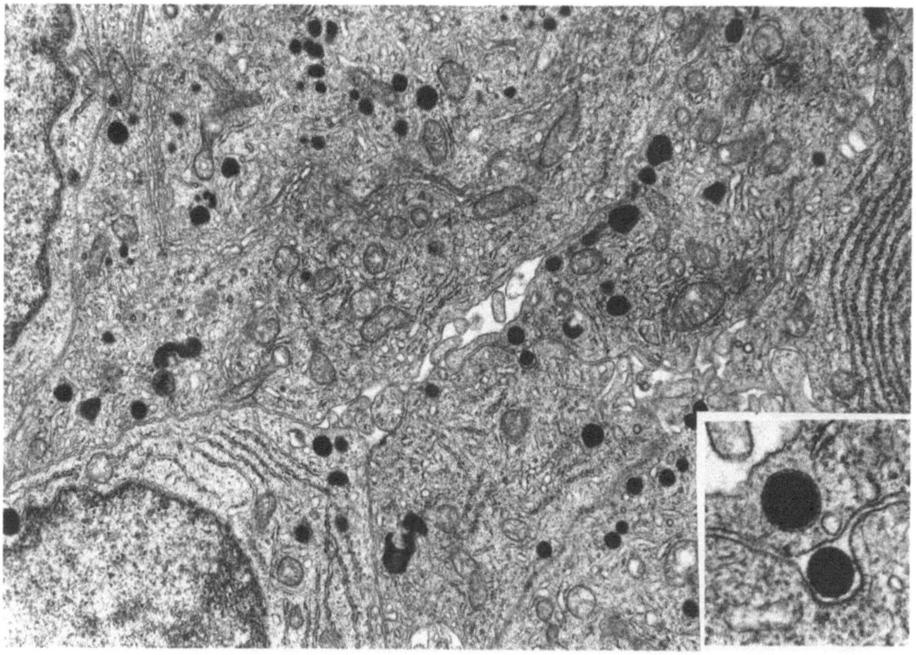

Fig. 1. Electron micrograph showing portions of adenoma cells with abundant rough-surfaced endoplasmic reticulum, a prominent Golgi complex and misplaced exocytosis X 6000.
Inset: misplaced exocytosis.

Table 2 Grading of immunopositivity for prolactin in 52 prolactinomas according to the number of immunostained cells

Case number	immunopositivity for PRL		
	+	++	+++
52	3 (6%)	13 (25%)	36 (69%)

\+ few, scattered cells;
\+ more cells forming clusters;
+++ majority of cells are positive.

++, and 36 prolactinomas were marked with +++ (fig. 2 a, b, c). Fifty four percent of these latter cases had high blood PRL values, and 57% of them belonged to the large tumours with suprasellar extensions (tab. 3). In 9 of all prolactinomas a few tumour cells appeared positive for GH and in the following 3 for TSH beta antisera. Of the GH positive cases 3 patients had an elevated blood GH level and two showed acromegaly. Only one tumour removed from a pregnant patient

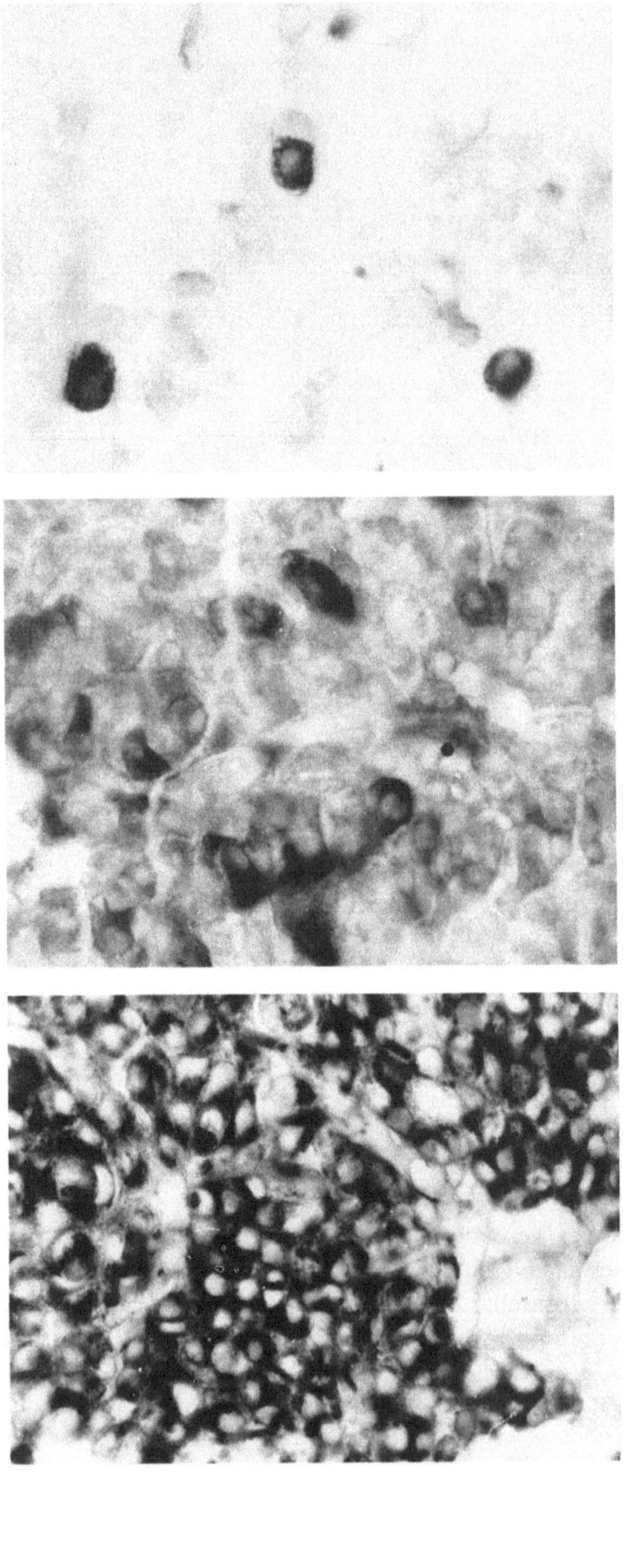

a

b

c

Table 3 Immunocytochemical findings in 52 prolactinomas

Immunopositivity for	Case number	%
PRL only	40	77
PRL and GH	8	15
PRL and TSH	3	6
PRL and GH and TSH	1	2
Total	52	100

Table 4 Growing characteristics of cultivated prolactinomas

- Prolactinomas 52 cases
  - not cultivated 5 cases
  - cultivated 47 cases
    - cells died 11 cases
    - cells alive 36 cases
      - survival only 14 cases
      - cell growth 22 cases

showed immunopositivity for three hormones. She had a moderately elevated serum PRL and GH level, with acromegaly. It was impossible to make a differentiation with immunocytochemistry in the light microscopic level between hyperplastic "pregnancy cells" [22] and true "heterogenous" [24] neoplastic cells. In all cases immunostaining for LH beta for FSH beta and for ACTH hormones were negative. Comparing the clinical data with the results of morphological investigations, we could establish relationships between the tumour size and basal serum PRL level (tab. 5); between tumour size and immunocytochemical findings (tab. 6); and between basal serum PRL level and immunocytochemical positivity (tab. 7). Out of 52 prolactinomas, in 47 cases tissue culture was carried out (tab. 4). In 11 cases the

◄

Fig. 2 a, b, c Light micrographs showing the presence of immunoreactive prolactin in the cytoplasm of adenoma cells. a) Reaction marked +; immunopositivity only in few, scattered cells. b) Reaction marked ++: more positively stained cells formed into clusters. c) Reaction marked +++: majority of tumour cells show immunopositivity, located around the nuclei, for PRL. Immunoperoxidase technique. X 400.

Table 5 Relationship between tumour and basal serum PRL level

Grading of tumour size	Case number	Average basal serum PRL level (ng/ml)
Microadenomas	11	200 (680–50)
Microadenomas without suprasellar extensions	9	180 (450–50)
Macroadenomas with suprasellar extensions	32	1000 (6800–100)

Table 6 Relationship between tumour size and immunocytochemical findings

Grading of tumour size	Case number	immunocytochemical positivity		
		+	++	+++
Microadenomas	11	1 (9%)	4 (36%)	6 (54%)
Macroadenomas without suprasellar extensions	9	–	2 (23%)	7 (77%)
Macroadenomas with suprasellar extensions	32	2 (6%)	7 (22%)	23 (72%)

\+ few, scattered cells;
++ more cells forming clusters;
+++ majority of cells are positive.

Table 7 Relationship between basal serum PRL values and immunocytochemical positivity – 11 basal PRL levels weren't measured

Basal serum PRL values (ng/ml)	immunocytochemical positivity		
	+	++	+++
30–100	2 (17%)	6 (50%)	4 (33%)
100–200	–	4 (33%)	8 (67%)
higher than 200	–	3 (9%)	14 (81%)

\+ few, scattered cells;
++ more cells forming clusters;
+++ majority of cells are positive.

explanted cells died after seeding, while from 36 biopsies viable cultures actually developed. From the latter, cells from only 14 biopsies survived, while in 22 cases an active growth started. No direct correlation could be demonstrated between the in vitro growth capacity of biopsies and serum PRL values of the patients involved. Cells of surviving biopsies ahowed practically no change during cultivation. The spherical cells arranged into clusters, the centrally located nuclei with dense chromatin content were surrounded by scanty cytoplasm. These cells retained their healthy condition for a long period. In actively growing samples however, the cells changed into cuboidal forms shortly after explantation. The loose chromatin was finely dispersed, therefore nucleoli were prominent. The closely arranged polygonal cells produced either confluent monolayers of mosaic structures or formed follicle-like colonies of various sizes (fig. 3). Mitoses could frequently be observed. A certain number of actively growing samples contained giant cells of irregular shapes, whose cytoplasms showed a pale staining and a ragged structure (fig. 4).

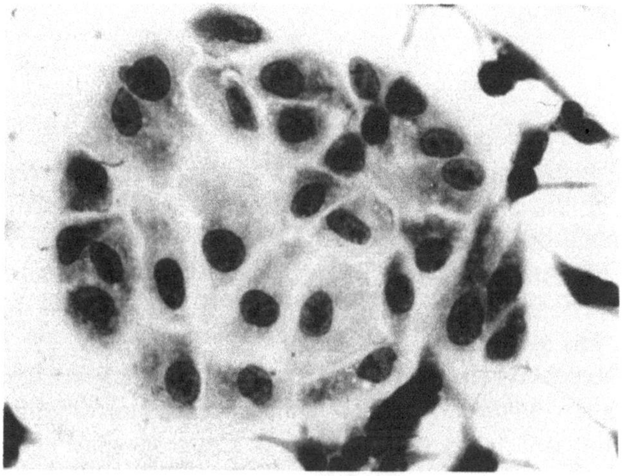

Fig. 3 Follicle-like arrangement of polygonal cells in 9-day-old culture of a prolactin producing pituitary adenoma. May-Grünwald-Giemsa. X 160.

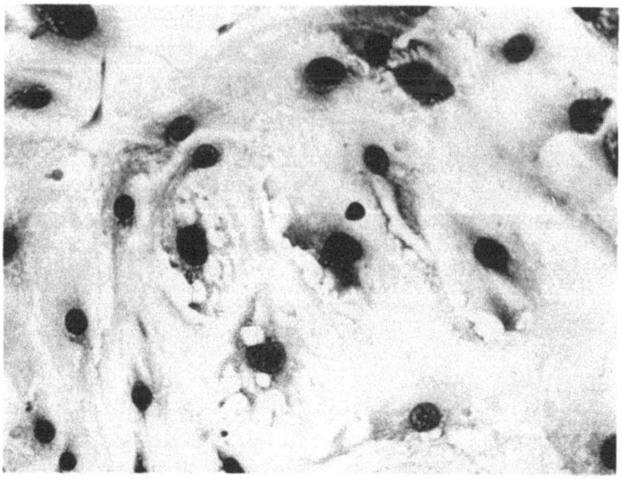

Fig. 4 Giant cells with faded outlines and ragged cytoplasm in a 6-day-old culture of a prolactinoma with extremely high hormone production. May-Grünwald-Giemsa. X 100.

These forms arranged into smaller or bigger fields discontinuing the confluency of the monolayers. In comparing the present culture findings with or previous experiences, we concluded that such forms are generally to be found in cultures of pituitary adenomas which are remarkable for their extremely high PRL production [18]. Adenomas of acromegalic patients with elevated serum GH levels display completely different cultural characteristics from prolactinomas [17]. Based on these striking morphological differences GH-producing cells could not be found.

Discussion

Of 250 unselected pituitary adenomas 52 (21%) sparsely granulated prolactinomas could be found, which are considered to be the most frequent pituitary tumours [8, 12, 19, 20, 21, 26, 27, 29]. They have a very typical ultrastructure previously described in numerous papers [2–6, 13, 14], with signs of intensive PRL secreting activity. The presence of immunoreactive PRL was detected in all cases in the cytoplasms of the adenoma cells in various amounts, but in 69% of the tumours the immunopositivity was widespread, marked with +++ [25, 28, 29, 30]. In 9 cases, besides the PRL positivity GH and TSH beta positivity for specific antisera could be observed in a low number of cells. It is an open question whether these cells are "normal pituitary cells" [23], or "heterogenous" true neoplastic cells [24]. Because GH and TSH producing cells could not be demonstrated either by our ultrastructural investigations or by cell culture, we supposed that normal pituitary cells could be occasionally intermingled with the adenomatous tissue. Several investigators have attempted to correlate the serum hormone levels with ultrastructural and immunocytochemical studies [25, 28, 29, 30]. A number of reports have published the relationship between the blood PRL values and the tumour size [26, 27]. In our material the number of positively immunostained prolactinoma cells showed correlation with the elevation of serum PRL level and with the tumour size. Our findings suggest that there are close connections between hormone-secreting activity and the ultrastructural-immunocytochemical and cultivation properties of sparsely granulated prolactinomas

Summary

Fifty-two pituitary adenomas were investigated ultrastructurally, immunocytochemically and in cell cultures. Ultrastructurally the tumour cells contained sparsely granulated prolactinomas. Immunocytochemical examinations verified only PRL secreting activity in 75% of cases, while 23% of tumours produced two hormones and in one case three hormones showed reactions with adequate antisera.

When cultured, adenomas revealed particular characteristics even at light microscopic level. Prolactin values were measured preoperatively in 80% of the patients and all of them had an elevated serum hormone level 40–6800 ng/ml. Out of 33 women 91% and out of 19 males only 31% had hormonal disturbances. Our material consisted of 11 microadenomas, occurring only in females. 9 were macroadenoma without suprasellar extensions and 32 macroadenomas with suprasellar extensions, which occurred mostly in males and caused visual disturbances. We found a positive correlation between serum PRL values and the tumour size. There seems to be a relationship between serum PRL level and the number of immunostained tumour cells. When cultured no direct correlation could be demonstrated between in vitro growth capacity and serum PRL values of the patients involved. On the other hand, giant cells of irregular shapes occurred in cultures only of those adenomas which showed in vivo an extremely high PRL production.

Acknowledgements

We thank Mrs Agnes Mizsei, Mrs Edit Kerekes and Mrs Márta Simon for their skillful technical assistance and Ms Klára Biró for her photographical work.

References

[1] Hardy, J., J. L. Vezina: Transsphenoidal neurosurgery of intracranial neoplasm. Adv. Neurol. **15** (1976) 261–274.
[2] Horvath, E., K. Kovacs: Misplaced Exocytosis. Distinct Ultrastructural Feature in Some Pituitary Adenomas. Arch. Pathol. **97** (1974) 221–224.
[3] Kovacs, K., E. Horvath, B. Corenblum, et. al.: Pituitary Chromophobe Adenomas Consisting of Prolactin Cells. Virchows Arch. A. Path. Anat. and Histol. **366** (1975) 113–123.
[4] Robert, F., J. Hardy: Prolactin-Secreting Adenomas. A Light and Electron Microscopical Study. Arch. Pathol. **99** (1975) 625–633.
[5] Horvath, E., K. Kovacs: Ultrastructural classification of pituitary adenomas. Canad. J. Neurol. Sci **3** (1976) 9–21.
[6] Kovacs, K., B. Corenblum, A. M. T. Sirek, et. al.: Localization of prolactin in chromophobe pituitary adenomas: study of human necropsy material by immunoperoxidase technique. J. of Clin. Pathol. **29** (1976) 250–258.
[7] Kovacs, K., N. Ryan, E. Horvath, et. al.: Prolactin Cell Adenomas of the Human Pituitary. Morphologic Features of Prolactin Cells in the Nontumorous Portions of the Anterior Lobe. Horm. Metab. Res. **10** (1978) 409–412.
[8] Ezrin, C., K. Kovacs, E. Horvath: Hyperprolactinemia. Morphologic and Clinical Considerations. Medical Clinics of North America **62**, No. 2 (1978) 393–408.
[9] Slowik, F., K. Lapis, J. Takács: The Ultrastructure of Human pituitary adenomas. Acta Morphol. Acad. Sci. Hung. **27** (1979) 235–249.
[10] Kovacs, K., E. Horvath: Pathology of Pituitary Adenomas, pp. 97–119. 1982 Year Book Medical Publishers, Inc.
[11] Esiri, M. M., C. B. T. Adams, C. Burke, et. al.: Pituitary Adenomas: Immunohistology and Ultrastructural Analysis of 118 Tumors. Acta Neuropathol. (Berl) **62** (1983) 1–14.

[12] Kovacs, K., E. Horvath: The pituitary. In: Principles and Practice of Surgical Pathology (S. G. Silverberg, ed.), pp. 1393–1414. John Wiley and Sons, Inc., 1983.
[13] Kovacs, K., E. Horvath, D. J. McComb: The fine structure of pituitary tumors. In: Ultrastructure of endocrine cells and tissues (P. M. Motta, ed.), chapter 8, pp. 89–113. Martius Nijhoff Publ., Boston–The Hague–Dordrecht–Lancaster 1984.
[14] Landolt, A. M.: Ultrastructure of human sella tumors. Acta Neurochir. (Wien) Suppl. **22** (1975) 1–167.
[15] Sternberger, L. A., P. H. Hardy, Jr., J. J. Cuculis, et. al.: The unlabeled antibody enzyme method of immunohistochemistry. Preparation and properties of soluble antigen-antibody complex (horseradish peroxidase-antihorseradish peroxidase) and its use in identification of spirochetes. J. of Histochem. and Cytochem. **18**, No. 5 (1970) 315–333.
[16] Kovacs, K., E. Horvath, N. Ryan: Immunocytology of the human pituitary. In: Diagnostic Immunohistochemistry (R. A. De Lellis, ed.), chapter 3, pp. 17–35. Masson, New York 1981.
[17] Gazsó, L., E. Pásztor: Growth characteristics of human pituitary adenomas in tissue and cell cultures. Acta Neuropathol. (Berl) **49** (1980) 225–230.
[18] Gazsó, L. E. Bácsy, E. Pásztor: Light- and electronmicroscopic features of an endocrinologically active pituitary adenoma cultured in vitro. Acta Neuropathol. (Berl) **56** (1982) 245–249.
[19] Robert, F.: Prolactinoma-aspects pathologiques. Neurochirurgie **27**, Suppl. 1 (1981) 61–73.
[20] Saeger, W.: Modern concepts of pituitary morphology and pathology of pituitary adenomas. Periodicum Biologorum. **85**, Suppl. 1 (1983) 9–28.
[21] Rnadall, R. V., E. R. Laws Jr., C. F. Abboud, et. al.: Transsphenoidal Microsurgical Treatment of Prolactin-Producing Pituitary Adenomas. Results in 100 patients. Mayo Clin. Proc. **58** (1983) 108–121.
[22] Halmi, N. S.: Immunostaining of growth hormone and prolactin in paraffin-embedded and stored or previously stained materials. J. of Histochem. and Cytochem. **26**, No. 7 (1978) 486–495.
[23] Girod, C., M. Mazzuca, J. Trouillas, et. al.: Light microscopy, fine structure and immunohistochemistry studies of 278 pituitary adenomas. In: II. European Workshop on pituitary adenomas (P. J. Derome, C. P. Jedynak, F. Peillon, eds.), pp. 3–18. Asclepios, Paris 1980.
[24] Martinez, D., D. Barthe: Heterogeneous Pituitary Adenomas. A light microscopic, immunohistochemical and electron microscopic study. Virchows Arch. (Pathol. Anat.) **394** (1982) 221–233.
[25] Zimmerman, E. A., R. Defendini, A. G. Frantz: Prolactin and Growth Hormone in Patients with Pituitary Adenomas; A Correlative Study of Hormone in Tumor and Plasma by Immunoperoxidase Technique and Radioimmunoassay. J. Clin. Endocrinol. Metab. **38** (1974) 577–584.
[26] McComb, D. J., K. Kovacs, E. Horvath, et. al.: Correlative Ultrastructural Morphometry of Human Prolactin-producing Adenomas. Acta Neurochirurgica **53** (1980) 217–225.
[27] Hardy, J.: Prolactinoma: Clinical, biological, radiological and pathological studies. Therapeutic results of transsphenoidal selective adenomectomy in 355 patients., Neurochirurgie **27**, Suppl. 1 (1981) 105–109.
[28] Cravioto, H., T. Fukaya, E. A. Zimmerman, et. al.: Immunohistochemical and Electron-microscopic Studies of Functional and Non-functional Pituitary Adenomas In-

cluding One TSH Secreting Tumor in a Thyrotoxic Patient. Acta Neuropathol. (Berl) **53** (1981) 281–292.

[29] Mukai, K.: Pituitary Adenomas. Immunocytochemical Study of 150 Tumors With Clinicopathologic Correlation. Cancer **52** (1983) 648–653.

[30] Lloyd, R. V., P. W. Gikas, W. F. Chandler: Prolactin and growth hormone-producing pituitary adenomas. An immunohistochemical and ultrastructural study. Am J. Surg. Pathol. **7** (1983) 251–260.

Immunohistochemical hormone determinations in pituitary adenomas in comparison with endocrinological findings in vivo

H. Schatz, M. Daun, H. Leicht, H. Stracke, W. Saeger, J. Zierski

Introduction

In patients with pituitary adenomas both the pre- and postoperative endocrinological evaluations [19, 22, 23] and the immunohistochemical hormone determinations in tissue specimens of the removed tumours [13, 18, 22] have been carried out in our endocrinological laboratory. Therefore, we were especially interested whether a correlation exists between the (quantitative) results obtained in serum and in the findings in the adenomatous tissue. Furthermore, we wanted to see if calcitonin might be detected in pituitary tumour cells since this hormone has been reported to be present in pituitary tissue [3].

Material and methods

From altogether 218 patients with tumours in the pituitary region tested by us in the last 6 years, complete pre- and postoperative data, including the whole spectrum of immunohistochemical determinations, were available in 62 cases with adenomas. The endocrinological evaluations comprised a combined stimulation test of anterior pituitary hormones [19, 23]. After the usual test procedures (X-ray plain and tomography, computerized tomography, visual field determination, angiography) the adenomas were removed mostly by the transnasal-transsphenoidal route. Specimens of the adenoma tissue were stained routinely with haematoxylin-eosin. Immunohistochemical determinations were carried out using the peroxidase-antiperoxidase method [21] with antisera against prolactin, growth hormone, LH, FSH, TSH, ACTH, β-endorphin and calcitonin at appropriate dilutions. A description of the procedures used by us has been given elsewhere [8, 13, 18].

In an attempt to quantitate the immunohistochemical results all the cells of the tissue specimens available from one tumour were considered for calculating the percentage of positive cells. These were at least 800 cells in the smallest tissue specimens of one tumour, mostly however many more. A special counting occular

Table 1

n	preoperative in vivo diagnosis	n	PRL	GH	LH	FSH	TSH	ACTH	β-E	CT
			immunohistochemical hormone content of adenoma tissue							
21	prolactinoma	12	PRL	–	–	–	–	–	–	–
		1	PRL	GH	–	–	–	–	β-E	–
		1	PRL	GH	LH	FSH	–	–	–	–
		1	PRL	GH	LH	FSH	–	ACTH	–	–
		2	PRL	–	LH	FSH	–	–	–	–
		1	PRL	–	–	–	TSH	–	–	–
		1	–	–	LH	FSH	–	–	–	–
		2	–	–	–	–	–	–	–	–
4	M. Cushing	1	–	GH	–	–	–	ACTH	β-E	–
		1	–	–	LH	–	–	ACTH	β-E	–
		1	PRL	–	–	–	–	ACTH	–	–
		1	–	–	–	–	–	–	–	–
17	acromegaly									
12	GH-cell-adenoma	4	–	GH	–	–	–	–	–	–
		4	PRL	GH	–	–	–	–	–	–
		1	PRL	GH	–	FSH	–	–	–	–
		1	PRL	GH	–	FSH	–	–	β-E	–
		1	PRL	GH	–	–	–	–	β-E	–
		1	–	–	–	–	–	–	–	–
5	GH + PRL-cell-adenoma	5	PRL	GH	–	–	–	–	–	–
19	inactive adenoma	3	PRL	–	–	–	–	–	–	–
		1	PRL	–	LH	FSH	–	–	–	–
		1	–	–	LH	FSH	–	–	–	–
		1	–	GH	–	–	–	–	β-E	–
		13	–	–	–	–	–	–	–	–
1	gonadotroph-cell-adenoma (in vivo: FSH-elevation)	1	–	–	LH	–	–	–	–	–

PRL: prolactin; GH: growth hormone; LH: luteinizing hormone; FSH: follicle stimulating hormone; TSH: thyrotrophic hormone; ACTH: adrenocorticotrophic hormone; β-E: β-endorphin; CT: calcitonin.

was used for this laborious procedure which was chosen because quite often an inhomogenous distribution of the positive cells or cell areas was seen which might have biased the results if only a few parts of the tumour tissue chosen at random would have been counted. The strength of the colour reaction in the positive cells although estimated by +, ++ and +++ in each case was not considered in the final evaluation.

In order to get information both about the size and consistency (regressive or necrotic parts etc.) of the tumorous process the protocols of the preoperative studies (X-ray, computer tomogram etc., see above) and also the neurosurgical reports

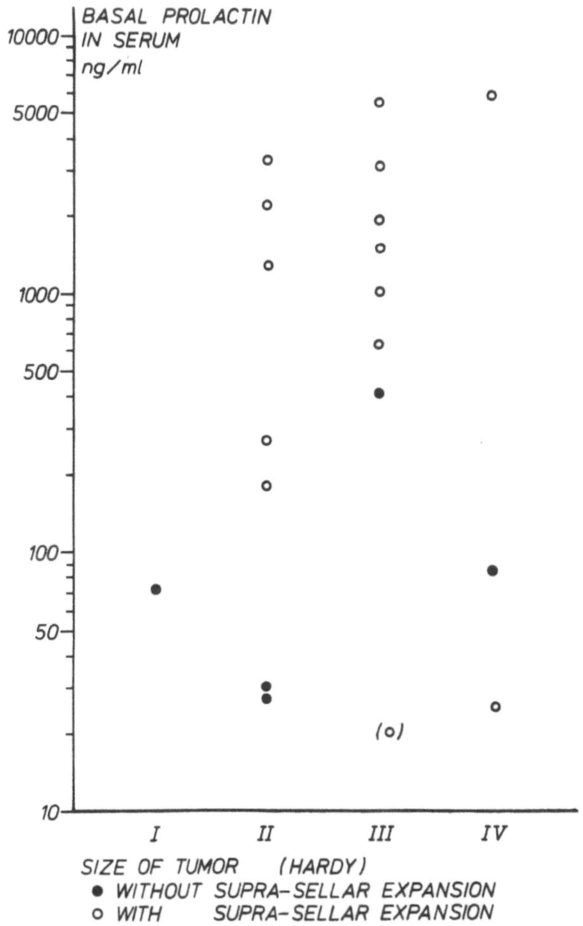

Fig. 1 Basal serum levels of prolactin in prolactin-producing pituitary tumours of different sizes (I to IV according to Hardy). The case within brackets was re-classified as "inactive adenoma". The increase in prolactin level with tumour size is apparent.

about the intraoperative findings were taken into consideration. The size of the tumorous process (groups I to IV, with or without suprasellar extension) was estimated according to Hardy [7].

Results

Table 1 shows the preoperative diagnosis and the *qualitative* findings by immunohistochemistry in the adenoma tissue. It can be seen that prolactin was detectable

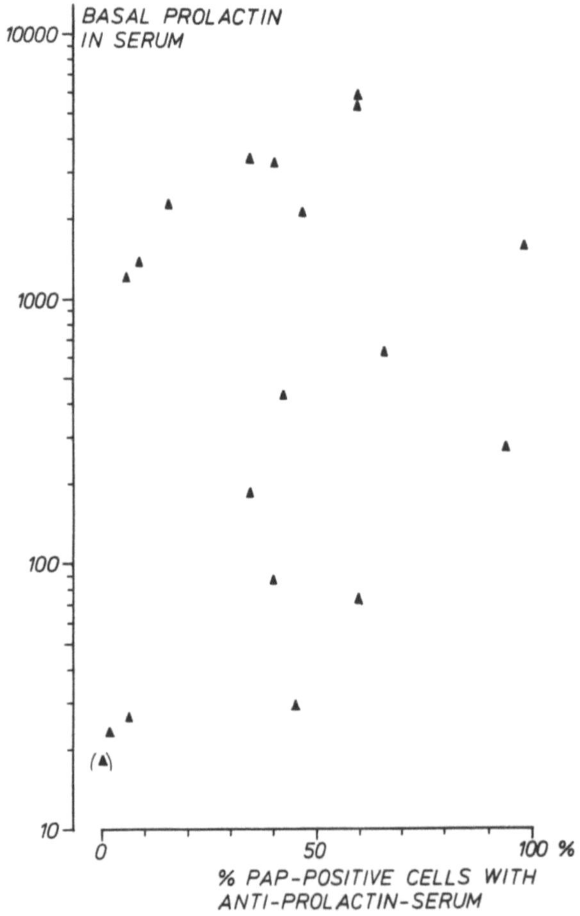

Fig. 2 Basal serum levels of prolactin and mean percentage of prolactin-positive cells by immunohistochemistry (PAP method) in the tissue of the removed tumour. The case within brackets was re-classified as "inactive adenoma". There was no correlation (r = 0.238, n.s.).

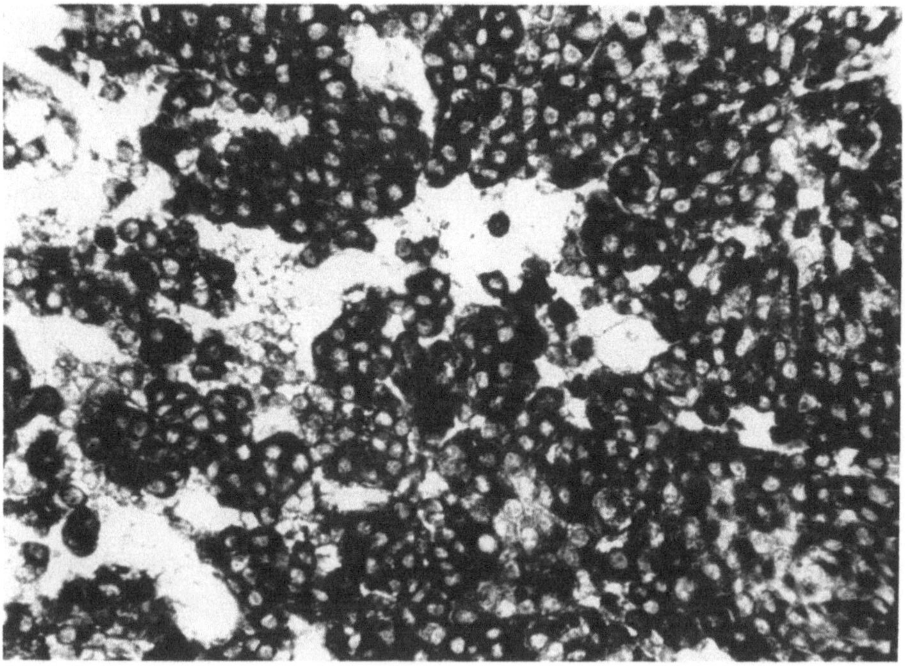

Fig. 3 Example for almost 100 per cent positivity for prolactin in immunohistochemistry of a prolactinoma tissue.

not only in tissue from most of the patients with (pronounced) hyperprolactinaemia but also in several other tumour forms, altogether in 35 of the 62 adenomas. Growth hormone (GH)-containing cells were found in 17 of the 62 tumours. Also cells positive for gonadotrophins and β-endorphin were not infrequently detected, in contrast to TSH which was present only in one adenoma (without elevation of this hormone in the serum). Calcitonin was never found in any adenoma. In the one patient with a gonadotrophic cell adenoma, a 50 fold elevation of FSH in the serum was measured preoperatively. However, only one of several anti-gonadotrophine antisera, an anti LH-antiserum, gave a positive staining. Qualitatively a fairly good correlation existed between the in vivo diagnosis and the immunohistochemical findings. Among the 21 patients with a preoperatively suspected prolactinoma, i.e. with hyperprolactinaemia and a pituitary tumour (tab. 1) a more pronounced hyperprolactinaemia was present in 18 cases. From the 3 remaining cases with only slight hyperprolactinaemia, one tumour was completely negative with our antiprolactin antiserum so that this case had to be re-classified as "inactive adenoma" with concomitant hyperprolactinaemia. The other two adenomas showed prolactin-positive cells in 5.7 and 1.2 per cent only. In 5 patients with pronounced hyperprolactinaemia and elevation of GH in the serum, both hormones were also present in the

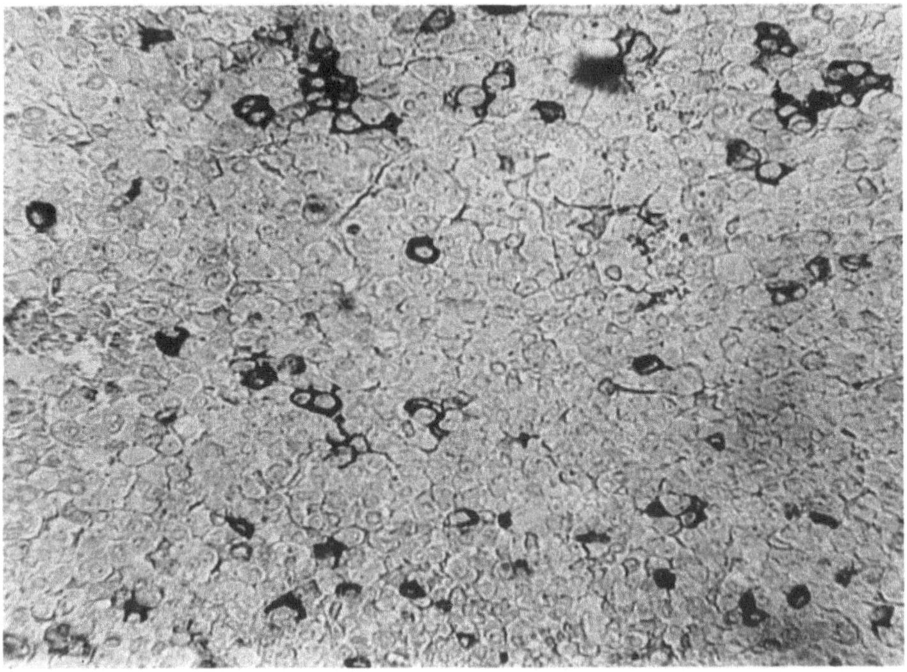

Fig. 4 Example of a low percentage of prolactin-positive cells in immunohistochemistry in tissue of another prolactinoma.

adenoma tissue. In altogether 17 acromegalics with enhanced GH-secretion in vivo, only one case was GH-negative in the immunohistochemical study of the tumour tissue. The number of positive cells for hormones which had not been found elevated preoperatively in vivo was always small. Such cells were only scattered over the tissue. On the other hand, the hormones elevated in vivo were detected in a mostly higher percentage of tumour cells, in prolactinomas in $42 \pm 6\%$, and in tumours with hyperprolactinaemia and associated with acromegaly in $31 \pm 9\%$ ($\bar{x} \pm$ SEM).

Figures 1, 2, 3 and 4 show the results of our *quantitative* studies concerning interrelations between the secretory activity as estimated by the height of the serum prolactin level and the morphological findings. It appears from figure 1 that a correlation exists between serum prolactin and the size of the pituitary process as judged by the criteria of Hardy [7]. On the other hand, there was no correlation ($r = 0.238$, n. s.) between prolactin in the serum and the percentage of prolactin-positive cells in the tumour (fig. 2), neither for our whole material (groups I–IV), nor separately for each of the 4 groups.

Calcitonin was undetectable in all 62 tumours tested by us.

Discussion

Our qualitative results of immunohistochemical hormone determination in tumour correspond quite well to the hormone which had been elevated in serum (cf. also [6, 9, 15, 20, 25]). The fact that no full congruence was found is in agreement with the results of other authors [9] and may be partly explained by differences, for example, in the specifities of the antisera used for radioimmunoassay or immunohistochemistry.

In many adenomas scattered cells containing other hormones than those increased in the serum have been detected. The lack of elevation of these hormones above the upper limit of the normal range in the serum might well be due to their small number and thus be a quantitative problem. On the other hand, it has also to be discussed that these cells are unable to release their hormonal content, at least in such a way that it reaches the circulating blood.

In 6 of our 19 adenomas diagnosed in vivo as "inactive", one or several hormones were detected in a few scattered cells. Similar findings have been described by Kovacs et al. [11] for the group of "null cell adenomas" and also "unclassified ade-

Table 2 Classification and incidence of pituitary adenomas according to Kovacs et al. [11]

	n = 490	100%
GH Cell adenoma, densely granulated	40	8
GH cell adenoma, sparsely granulated	47	10
PRL cell adenoma, densely granulated	1	<1
PRL cell adenoma, sparsely granulated	148	30
Mixed GH cell – PRL cell adenoma (2 cell types)	22	4
Acidophil stem cell adenoma (1 cell type, acromegaly seldom)	18	4
Mammosomatotroph cell adenoma (GH + PRL in 1 cell type, with acromegaly)	6	1
ACTH cell adenoma, with Cushin's syndrome	25	5
ACTH cell adenoma, with Nelson's syndrome	17	3
ACTH cell adenoma silent	34	7
Gonadotroph cell adenoma	10	2
TSH cell adenoma	2	<1
Null cell adenoma ("inactive adenoma")	82	17
Oncocytomas (non-functioning adenoma)	28	6
Unclassified adenoma	10	2
	n = 490	100%

nomas" according to their classification (tab. 2). Ultrastructural studies (including immunoelectron microscopy) would be needed for a further subdivision in these cases, and possibly also in some other adenomas, as in our group of prolactinomas, which might be classified, for example, as "acidophil stem cell adenomas" according to the classification of Kovacs et. al. [11].

Several publications in the last decade deal with the question whether the hormone levels in the serum are related to the morphological findings in endocrine active pituitary adenomas (tabs. 3–6).

In acromegaly (tab. 3) two ultrastructurally distinct tumour types exist with about the same frequency (see [11]), the densely and the sparsely granulated GH-cell

Table 3 Correlation of *serum GH* levels with tumour *morphology* in acromegaly?

Yes, inverse to granulation: well granulated: 88 ng/ml poorly granulated: 266 ng/ml	Lewis, v. Noorden [14]	(n = 78)
Yes, to activity signs	Saeger [17]	(n = 11)
No, no simple inverse relation to granule size	Landolt, Rothenbühler [12]	(n = 22)
Yes, to activity signs (light and el. micr.) No, not to granulation: densely granulated: 49 ng/ml sparsely granulated: 41 ng/ml (tissue content of GH related to granular appearance)	Trouillas et al. [24]	(n = 31, 22 + 9)

adenomas. Whereas some authors [14] described an inverse correlation of serum GH levels to granularity ("well" or "poorly granulated") others could not find a clear inverse correlation with the granules [12, 24]. (Ultra-)Structural signs of activity, on the other hand, appear to correlate with the serum GH levels [17, 24].

In contrast to GH-cell adenomas, the tumour cells of prolactinomas (tab. 4) are almost always sparsely granulated. In a large series of 149 prolactinomas only 1 densely granulated prolactin cell adenoma was found [11]. This might agree with the idea of prolactin being a "high turn-over hormone" (cf. [5]). Concerning the relationship between hormone levels in serum and (ultra-)structural morphometry, the reports are contradictory also for the prolactinomas. Some authors found no correlation [2, 10, 16], others described an inverse correlation of serum prolactin to granularity [4, 15] and a positive correlation both to the development of the rough endoplasmatic reticulum and the frequency of exocytosis [4]. Tissue content of prolactin was not related to serum levels in 2 reports [1, 10].

In most of these publications the size of the tumorous process has not been taken into consideration for the evaluations. However, a correlation appears to be well

Table 4 Correlation of *serum prolactin* levels with tumour *morphology* in prolactinomas?

Not	to activity signs (light micr.)	Child et al. [2]	(n = 8, 5 and 18)
Not	to granule size (but to sella size)		
Not	to ultrastructural morphometry (but to adenoma size)	McComb et al. [16]	(n = 24)
Not	to size or density of granulation (not to tissue content of PRL)	Kornfeld et al. [10]	(n = 9)
Yes,	inverse to granularity (el. micr.)	Martinez et al. [15]	(n = 25)
Yes,	inverse to granular density, to frequency of exocytosis, to development of RER	Dingemans et al. [4]	(n = 19)
	(not to tissue content of PRL)	Archer et al. [1]	(n = 10)

Table 5 Correlation of *serum GH* levels with tumour immunohistochemistry in acromegaly?

Qualitatively yes Semi-quantitatively not clearly (yes?)	Zimmerman et al. [25] (n = 8)
Qualitatively yes Semi-quantitatively not clearly (yes?)	Fukaya et al. [6] (n = 24, 15 + 9)
Qualitatively yes Quantitation done, no correlation with serum GH given	Martinez et al. [15] (n = 5, 4 + 1)

established between tumour cell mass (as estimated by indirect but also by direct parameters) and the serum levels of prolactin (for a review, see [5]). It has been found also in some of the studies [2, 16] cited above.

By immunohistochemistry, the hormone which was markedly elevated in the serum has been mostly detected also in the tumour tissue [6, 9, 15, 20, 25], apart from patients with slight (concomitant) hyperprolactinaemia in cases of inactive (big) adenomas. Semi-quantitation of the immunohistochemical results did not clearly correlate, or not correlate at all with the serum levels of GH (tab. 5) or prolactin (tab. 6) [6, 25]. In the study of Martinez et. al. [15] the percentage of cells positively stained with antiserum against GH or prolactin has been estimated, however, no evaluation was given concerning the relationship of these values to hormone levels in vivo.

From our quantitative data (figs. 1 and 2) it can be seen that the percentage of immunohistochemically positive prolactin cells in tumour tissue specimens does not reflect the total secretory activity of the whole adenoma even though at least 800 cells from one tumour were always investigated for calculating the percentage of positive cells. With the size of the tumorous process (I to IV) an increase of

Table 6 Correlation of *serum prolactin* levels with tumour *immunohistochemistry* in prolactinomas?

Qualitatively yes Semi-quantitatively not clearly	Zimmerman et al. [25] (n = 12, 8 + 4)
Qualitatively yes (no quantitation done)	Sherman et al. [20] (n = 35)
Qualitatively yes Quantitation done, no correlation to serum PRL given	Martinez et al. [15] (n = 25)
Qualitatively yes (no quantitation done)	Kameya et al. [9] (n = 14)
No (?)	Fukaya et al. [6] (n = 9, GH + PRL)

serum prolactin is also apparent in our patients (fig. 1). However, within each of the 4 groups (I–IV) there was no correlation when serum prolactin was compared with the percentage of hormone-positive cells. Our findings are plausible if one considers the microsurgical technique including removal of tumorous tissue by suction etc. and the protocols of the operation in which partly cystic, partly haemorrhagic, necrotic or liquid structures from the tumours have been frequently described. On the other hand the intracellular content of hormone – or granules – cannot reflect the secretory activity – or inactivity – of a cell. It may well be that different types, or different functional states, of prolactin-producing adenoma cells exist.

Finally, concerning calcitonin, it appears from our negative results in 62 pituitary adenomas that this hormone does not occur in pituitary adenoma cells. Our negative findings are not due to the antiserum against calcitonin used by us since this antiserum has proved to be very potent in tissue of thyroid C-cell carcinomas [8].

Acknowledgements

We would like to thank Prof. Kracht, Gießen, for his valuable suggestions and help in performing these studies.

References

[1] Archer, D. F., H. Salazar, J. C. Maroon, et. al.: Prolactin-secreting pituitary adenomas: Serum and tissue prolactin levels with ultrastructural correlation. Am. J. Obstet. Gynecol. **137** (1980) 646–652.

[2] Child, D. F., S. Nader, K. Mashiter, et. al.: Prolactin Studies in "Functionless" Pituitary Tumors. British Medical Journal **1** (1975) 604–606.

[3] Deftos, L. J., D. Burton, B. D. Catherwood, et. al.: Demonstration by Immunoperoxidase Histochemistry of Calcitonin in the Anterior Lobe of the Rat Pituitary. Journal of Clinical Endocrinology and Metabolism (1978) 457–460.
[4] Dingemans, K. P., J. Assies, N. Jansen, et. al.: Sparsely Granulated Prolactin Cell Adenomas of the Pituitary Gland. Virchows Arch. (Pathol. Anat.) **396** (1982) 167–186.
[5] Flückiger, E., E. Del Pozo, K. von Werder: Prolactin: Physiology, Pharmacology and Clinical Findings. (Monographs on Endocrinology, Vol. 23). Springer, Berlin–Heidelberg–New York 1982.
[6] Fukaya, T., N. Kageyama, A. Kuwayama, et. al.: Immunoenzymatic Study of Pituitary Adenomas in Acromegalic Patients. In: Pituitary Microadenomas (G. Faglia, M. A. Giovanelli, R. M. McLeod, eds.), pp. 205–210. Academic Press, London–New York–Sydney–Toronto–San Francisco 1980.
[7] Hardy, J.: Transsphenoidal surgery of hypersecreting pituitary tumors. In: Diagnosis and treatment of pituitary tumors, pp. 179–194. Excerpta Medica, Amsterdam 1973.
[8] Henninger, S., H. Stracke, U. Wagner, et. al.: Immunhistorischer Nachweis von Calcitonin, Samotostatin und Thyreoglobulin in C-Zellkarzinomen und undifferenzierten Karzinomen der Schilddrüse. Verh. Dtsch. Ges. Inn. Med. **90** (1984) 1297–1299.
[9] Kameya, T., M. Tsumuraya, I. Adachi, et. al.: Ultrastructure, Immunohistochemistry and Hormone Release of Pituitary Adenomas in Relation to Prolactin Production. Virchows Arch. A. Path. Anat. and Histol. **387** (1980) 31–46.
[10] Kornfeld, M., M. T. Buckmann, G. McClellan: Morphometric Analysis of Secretory Granules and Prolactin Levels in Chromophobe Pituitary Adenoma. Acta Neuropathol. (Berlin) **53** (1981) 1–5.
[11] Kovacs, K., E. Horvath, D. J. McComb: The fine structure of pituitary tumors. In: Ultrastructure of endocrine cells and tissues (R. M. Motta, ed.), pp. 89–113. Martius Nijhoff Publ., Boston–The Hague–Dordrecht–Lancaster 1984.
[12] Landolt, A. M., V. Rothenbühler: The size of growth hormone granules in pituitary adenomas producing acromegaly. Acta Endocrinology **84** (1977) 461–469.
[13] Leicht, R., O. Schröder, H. Stracke, et. al.: Immunhistochemischer Hormonnachweis im Tumorgewebe bei 37 Patienten mit Hypophysenadenomen. Therapiewoche **33** (1983) 6094–6100.
[14] Lewis, P. D., S. van Noorden: Pituitary Abnormalities in Acromegaly. Arch. Path. **94** (1972) 119–126.
[15] Martinez, A. J., A. Lee, J. Moossy, et. al.: Pituitary Adenomas: Clinicopathological and Immunohistochemical Study. Ann. Neurol. **7** (1980) 24–36.
[16] McComb, D. J., K. Kovacs, E. Horvath, et. al.: Correlative Ultrastructural Morphometry of Human Prolactinproducing Adenomas. Actas Neurochirurgica **53** (1980) 217–225.
[17] Saeger, W.: Licht- und elektronenmikroskopische Untersuchungen zur sekretorischen Aktivität von Hypophysenadenomen bei Akromegalie. Virchows Arch. Abt. A. Path. Anat. **358** (1973) 343–354.
[18] Schatz, H., R. Leicht, O. Schröder, et. al.: The significance of immunohistochemistry in the postoperative evaluation of patients with pituitary adenomas. Acta endocrin. (Kbh) **99** (1982) Suppl. 246, 160–161.
[19] Schatz, H., H. Stracke, O. Schröder: Hypophysenfunktionstestung. Untersuchungen zur Wertigkeit unmittelbar nach Hypophysenoperationen zur Beurteilung der Substitutionsbedürftigkeit. Therapiewoche **33** (1983) 6345–6349.
[20] Sherman, B. M., C. E. Harris, J. Schlechte, et. al.: Pathogenesis of Prolactin-Secreting Pituitary Adenomas. Lancet **II** (1978) 1019–1021.

[21] Sternberger, L. A., P. H. Hardy, J. J. Cuculis, et. al.: The unlabelled antibody enzyme method of immunocytochemistry: Preparation and properties of soluble antigen-antibody complex (horseradish peroxidase-antihorseradish peroxidase) and its use in identification of spirochetes. Histochem. Cytochem. **18** (1970) 315–333.
[22] Stracke, H., O. Schröder, R. Leicht, et al.: Immunhistochemische Klassifizierung, medikamentöse und operative Therapieergebnisse und Untersuchungen zur Evaluierung der postoperativen (Rest)-Hypophysenfunktion bei insgesamt über 100 Patienten mit Hypophysengeschwülsten. Verh. Dtsch. Ges. Inn. Med. **88** (1982) 1110–1114.
[23] Stracke, H., O. Schröder, H. Bleyl, et. al.: Assessment of Definitive Residual Pituitary-Adrenal Function and of Hydrocortisone Replacement Therapy 10 to 14 Days after Microsurgery for Pituitary Adenomas. Horm. metabol. Res. **16** (1984) 157–158.
[24] Trouillas, J., C. Girod, M. Lheritier, et. al.: Morphological and Biochemical Relationships in 31 Human Pituitary Adenomas with Acromegaly. Virchows Arch. A. Path. Anat. and Histol. **389** (1980) 127–142.
[25] Zimmerman, E. A., R. Defendini, A. G. Frantz: Prolactin and Growth Hormone in Patients with Pituitary Adenomas: A Correlative Study of Hormone in Tumor and Plasma by Immunoperoxidase Technique and Radioimmunoassay. J. Clin. Endocrinol. Metab. **38** (1974) 577–585.

New immunocytochemical observations in prolactinomas

H. Höfler, G. F. Walter, H. Denk

Introduction

In general, the immunocytochemical investigation of pituitary hormones in normal or tumorous pituitary tissue permits a clear pathological classification. In pituitary adenomas, problems may arise when (i) more than one hormone can be found (multihormonal adenomas) or when (ii) due to the applied microsurgical technique the tissue specimens are very small and fragmented. In both cases, the morphological differentiation between normal pituitary tissue and a pituitary adenoma may be almost impossible.

The differentiation between non-neoplastic pituitary tissue, eventually with a diffuse or nodular hyperplasia of prolactin-producing cells, and a microprolactinoma seems to be of great importance regarding the different therapeutic approaches such as surgery, radiation or pharmacotherapy with bromocriptine. In the present study, immunohistochemical criteria for the differentiation of pituitary adenomas and non-neoplastic pituitary tissue are demonstrated with regard to the distribution of folliculo-stellate cells [2, 3].

Materials and methods

7 normal pituitary glands (5 from adults and 2 from children) obtained at autopsy, 7 prolactinomas, one mixed prolactin-growth hormone-producing adenoma, 6 hormonally inactive pituitary adenomas, and 14 pituitary adenomas producing hormones other than prolactin were investigated.

The tissue specimens were fixed in 10% neutral formaldehyde and embedded in paraffin. For the demonstration of antigens the peroxidase-antiperoxidase or the biotin-avidin methods were used. The colour reaction was intensified by the addition of cobalt chloride (1%) and nickel ammonium sulfate (1%) to the DAB-solution [1]. Antisera to the following antibodies were used: pituitary hormones (prolactin, hGH, ACTH, β-FSH, β-LH, β-TSH, alpha subunit), S-100 protein, neuron specific enolase (NSE), and glial fibrillary acidic protein (GFAP). The simultaneous demonstration of two antigens was achieved by using different peroxidase-substrates, e.g. DAB with or without the addition of heavy metals in the first reaction and 4-chloro-1-naphthol or 3-amino-9-ethylcarbazol in the second. Using these modifications, S-100 protein/GFAP and S-100 protein/pituitary hormones were demonstrated simultaneously.

Results

The endocrine cells in all pituitary glands as well as in adenomas revealed NSE-reactivity and also reactivity with the respective pituitary hormones. They were negative with S-100 protein- and GFAP-antibodies. In all normal pituitary glands,

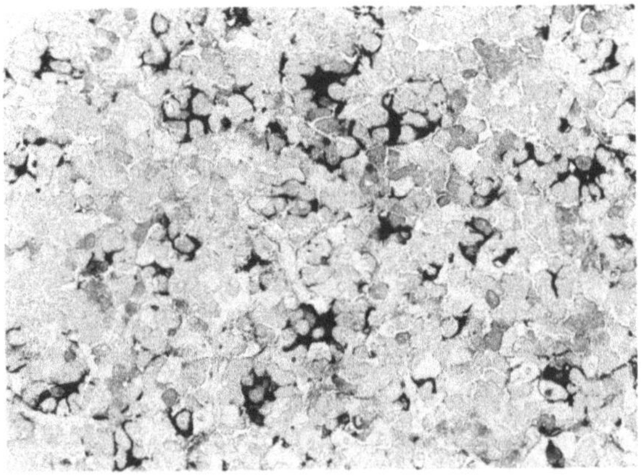

Fig. 1 S-100 protein-immunoreactivity of folliculo-stellate cells in normal human pituitary gland. 700×, PAP-technique.

folliculo-stellate cells were present (fig. 1). They were situated in close contact with endocrine cells and blood vessels. Folliculo-stellate cells were not reactive with antibodies to pituitary hormones or NSE, but were S-100 protein-positive. Approximately half of the S-100 protein-reactive folliculo-stellate cells reacted simultaneously with antibodies to GFAP, whereas only few GFAP-positive cells without S-100 protein-reactivity could be found (fig. 2).

In pituitary adenomas on the contrary, no S-100 protein-reactive folliculo-stellate cells and no GFAP-reactivity could be demonstrated. The border between adenomas and normal pituitary tissue was distinct. In the bordering normal tissue, always S-100 protein- and GFAP-positive folliculo-stellate cells were present, eventually even in increased numbers, probably due to a compression of the tissue bordering the tumour (fig. 3).

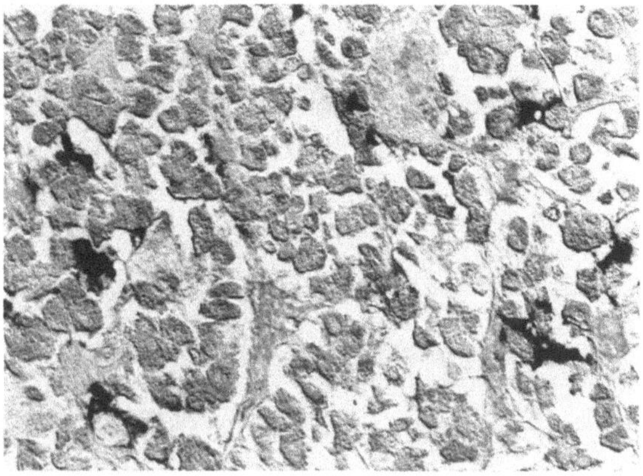

Fig. 2 GFAP-immunoreactivity of folliculo-stellate cells in normal human pituitary gland. 000×, PAP-technique.

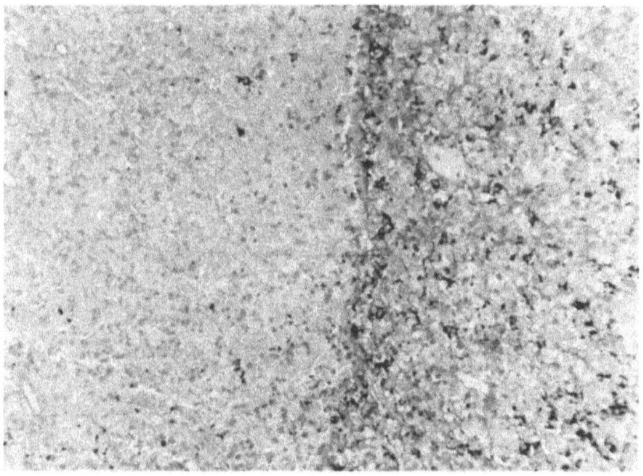

Fig. 3 Border-zone of an adenoma and non-neoplastic pituitary tissue: lack of S-100 protein-reactive folliculo-stellate cells within the adenoma and normal distribution in the normal tissue. 240×, PAP-technique.

Discussion

The immunohistochemical demonstration of S-100 protein is a reliable method to exhibit folliculo-stellate cells in normal pituitary tissue [4]. The lack of folliculo-stellate cells is of practical diagnostic importance in the differentiation between non-neoplastic pituitary tissue and adenoma. Bromocriptine-therapy seems to influence selectively the prolactin-producing cells whereas folliculo-stellate cells in the pituitary tissue bordering prolactinomas remain unaffected or show even a relative increase in number.

Further immunohistochemical investigations on larger groups of patients with hyperprolactinaemia could improve the knowledge on the hyperplasia- or adenoma-rate and simplify the decision for either surgical treatment, radiation therapy, pharmacotherapy or a combination-treatment.

References

[1] Adams, J. C.: Heavy metal intensification of DAB-based HRP reaction product. J. Histochem. Cytochem. **29** (1981) 775.
[2] Bergland, R. M., R. Torack: An ultrastructural study of follicular cells in the human anterior pituitary. Am. J. Pathol. **57** (1969) 273–297.
[3] Rinehard, J. F., M. G. Farquhar: Electron microscopic studies of the anterior pituitary gland. J. Histochem. Cytochem. **1** (1953) 93–113.
[4] Vila-Porcile, E., L. Olivier: The problem of folliculo-stellate cells in the pituitary gland. In: Ultrastructure of endocrine cells and tissue (P. M. Motta, ed.), pp. 64–76. Martinus Nijhoff Publ., Boston–The Hague–Dordrecht–Lancaster 1984.

Problematic divergencies between clinical and immunocytochemical findings in prolactinomas

H. Höfler, G. F. Walter, G. Leb, L. M. Auer, G. Clarici, G. Tscherne, W. Urdl, H. Warnkross, G. Schneider

Introduction

In most cases of pituitary adenomas including prolactinomas, the clinical symptoms and the immunocytochemical findings in the resected tumours tissue correlate quite well. However, uncertainties may arise when, in cases with a clinical expression of an exclusive endocrine disorder of only one pituitary hormone, a so-called "mixed" plurihormonal adenoma is diagnosed by immunocytochemical means seemingly exhibiting a positive immunoreactivity with more than one hormone. Another divergency exists in cases with a clearly elevated preoperative sPRL-level, if the resected adenoma tissue does not reveal any immunocytochemical PRL-reactivity.

Materials and methods

In 66 pituitary adenomas, the surgically resected tissue was fixed in 10% neutral formaldehyde and embedded in paraffin. The material was deparaffinized in xylene. For the demonstrations of antigens to the pituitary hormones the peroxidase-antiperoxidase method or the biotin-avidin method were employed (tab. 1). The

Table 1 List of antibodies used in the present study

ra-h prolactin	1:3000	NIAMDD* (USA)
mouse-h prolactin (monoclonal)	1:15000	Hybritech (USA)
ra-hGH	1:640	Milab (Sweden)
mouse-hGH (monoclonal)	1:10000	Hybritech
ra-porcine ACTH	1:320	Milab
	1:500	Immuno Nuclear Corp. (USA)
ra-h-β-FSH	1:1000	NIAMDD
ra-h-β-TSH	1:4000	NIAMDD
ra-alpha-hCG	1:7500	NIAMDD

* National Institute of Arthritis, Metabolism and Digestive Diseases.

DAB-based colour reaction was intensified by addition of 1% cobalt chloride and 1% nickel ammonium sulfate to the 3′,3′-diaminobenzidine solution [1]. Preimmune sera or sera from other animal species served as controls.

For ultrastructural studies small samples of prolactinomas were dewaxed and reembedded in Epon 812. They were alternately cut into semithin (1 μm) and ultrathin (60 nm) sections. Ultrathin sections were contrasted with uranyl acetate and lead citrate. In uncontrasted ultrathin sections, the immunoreactivity was localized using the immunogold technique [6] with a particle size of 20 nm.

Results

The general findings in all immunocytochemically investigated pituitary adenomas showed in accordance with the literature a predominance of prolactinomas (tab. 2). In the present study, only two plurihormonal adenomas were seen revealing immunoreactivity for PRL/hGH and PRL/alpha-hCG respectively.

Table 2 Immunocytochemical findings in 66 pituitary adenomas

PRL	19
hGH	10
ACTH	6
β-TSH	2
β-FSH/LH	1
plurihormonal	2
alpha-subunit only	2
immunocytochemically negative	24

The ultrastructural study of prolactinomas demonstrated the typical cytoplasmic hormone granules which were mainly sparsely distributed but also either densely or sparsely distributed even within the same tumour (fig. 1). In some cases the sparse granulation may not allow an unequivocal light microscopic identification of a positive PRL-reactivity. Then the immunogold technique enables one to make a correct immunocytochemical diagnosis at the ultrastructural level (fig. 2).

In three cases, the preoperative sPRL-levels were – in part even extremely – elevated, whereas the immunocytochemical examination for PRL-reactivity as well as for the other hormones was negative (tab. 3). In case 2, the negative outcome was confirmed after two separate operations. Interestingly, exactly those three cases did not respond to the postoperative treatment with bromocriptine. There was no long-term improvement of the clinical symptoms. In case 4 (tab. 3), a first immunocytochemical investigation gave a positive PRL-reactivity. One year later, the

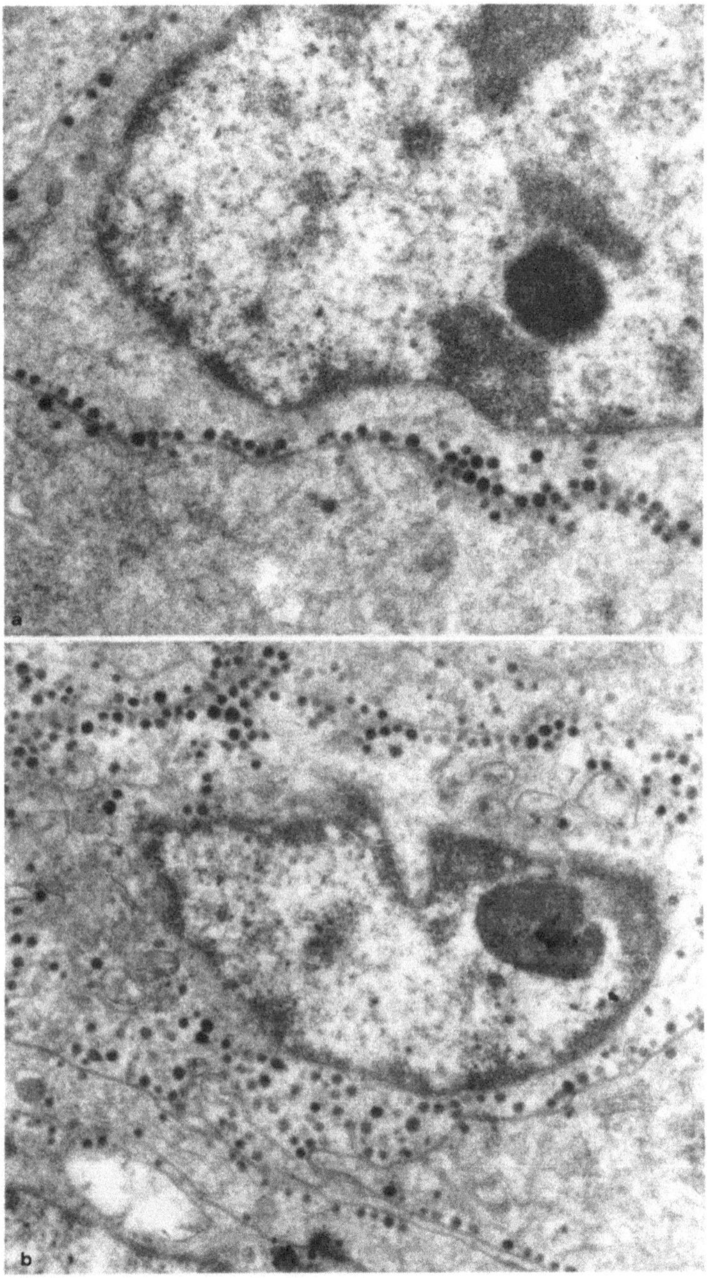

Fig. 1 Sparsely granulated (a) and densely granulated (b) prolactinoma cells. 18600×.

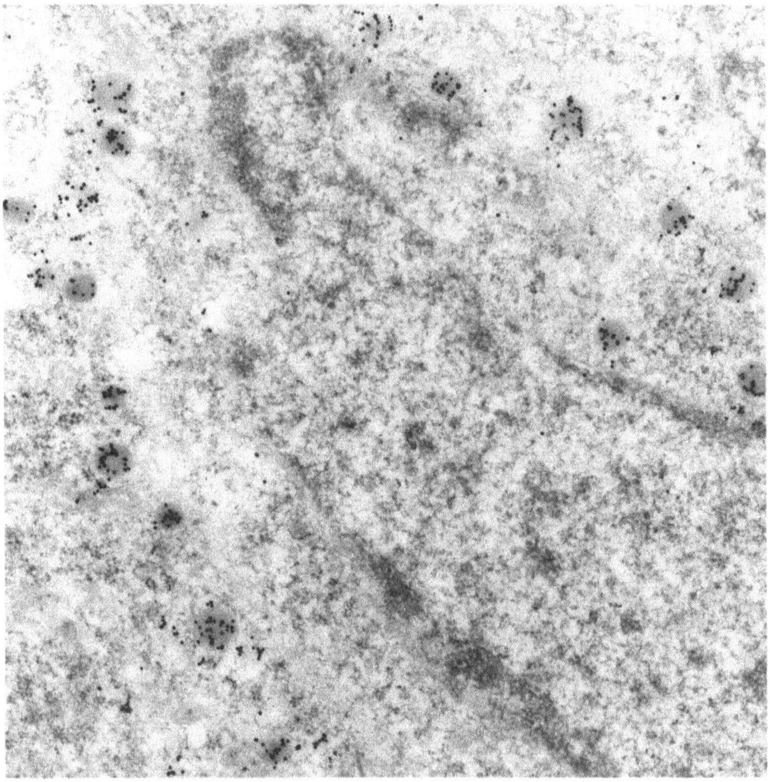

Fig. 2. PRL-reactive prolactinoma cell with sparse granulation. Immunogold technique, 30000×.

Table 3 Prolactinomas with negative immunocytochemical PRL-reactivity

Case	Symptoms	Age/Sex	preop. sPRL	postop. sPRL	Morphology
1	hyperprolactinaemia amenorrhaea	30 yrs, f	140 ng/ml	3 ng/ml	microadenoma chromophobic
2	hyperprolactinaemia amenorrhoea	29 yrs, f	2020 ng/ml	78 ng/ml 127 ng/ml	macroadenoma chromophobic
3	hyperprolactinaemia cephalea	27 yrs, m	4000 ng/ml	0 ng/ml [radiation]	macroadenoma chromophobic
4	hyperprolactinaemia	61 yrs, m	760 ng/ml	1527 ng/ml 356 ng/ml	macroadenoma chromophobic

tissue of a second operation revealed a negative PRL-reactivity despite a distinct hyperprolactinaemia. The light microscopical impression of the adenoma cells was that of "empty" cells.

Discussion

Plurihormonal pituitary adenomas which produce more than one hormone mainly consist of combinations of PRL and hGH. In a large study, Asa and Kovacs [2] found plurihormonal adenomas in 11% of 674 cases (8% with PRL- and hGH-reactivity). In our series of 66 cases, only two were plurihormonal. However, applying the widely used NIAMDD-ra-h prolactin antibody cross-reactions with hGH sometimes were seen in our material too, but the results could be corrected after the use of the monoclonal mouse-h prolactin. It seems necessary to pay attention to the methodological restrictions and not to overestimate the possibilities of immunocytochemical stainings. The avoidance of methodological failures such as cross-reactions by using the inappropriate antibodies, but also the critical interpretation of "ambiguous" findings [8] such as strong background-reactions – especially when clinical symptoms are missing – should reduce the high incidence of plurihormonal adenomas as reported in some studies [11]. The subcellular localization of the hormonal reactivity as shown in this study (fig. 2) or by Jautzke and Iglesias [7] might be very helpful for the correct classification of prolactinomas with very sparse granulation.

The interpretation of the negative immunocytochemical results in the above described four cases with hyperprolactinaemia and pituitary adenoma appears more difficult. Similar cases were reported by Barrow et al. [3]. The reason for the negative immunocytochemical results might be (i) an extremely sparse granulation after an enhanced extrusion of granules or (ii) a granular depletion after a "hormonal diarrhoea" [9]. A granule release occurs already normally along the entire cell circumference [10].

A hormonal diarrhoea could be responsible for the negative result in case 4. This might in part explain the high s-PRL-levels. Further, these cases can be non-responders to bromocriptine therapy [4, 5]. Whether they form a special subgroup within the prolactinomas at present remains unclear.

References

[1] Adams, J. C.: Heavy metal intensification of DAB-based HRP reaction product. J. Histochem. Cytochem. **29** (1981) 775.

[2] Asa, S. L., K. Kovacs: Histological classification of pituitary disease. Clin. Endocrinol. Metabol. **12** (1983) 567–596.

[3] Barrow, D. L., G. T. Tindall, K. Kovacs, et al.: Clinical and pathological effects of bromocriptine on prolactin-secreting and other pituitary tumors. J. Neurosurg. **60** (1984) 1–7.
[4] Bergh, T., S. J. Nillius, P. Enoksson, et al.: Bromocriptine-induced pregnancies in women with large prolactinomas. Clin. Endocrinol. **17** (1982) 625–631.
[5] Crosignani, P. G., C. Ferrari, A. Liuzzi, et al.: Treatment of hyperprolactinemic states with different drugs: A study with bromocriptine, metergoline, and lisuride. Fertil. Steril. **37** (1982) 61–67.
[6] De Mey, J.: Colloidal gold probes in immunocytochemistry. In: Immunocytochemistry. Practical applications in pathology and biology (J. M. Polak, S. van Noorden, eds.), pp. 82–112. Wright, Bristol–London–Boston 1983.
[7] Jautzke, G., J. Iglesias: Prolactinomas and mixed adenomas with prolactin cells: An immunohistochemical study of the subcellular localization of hormones. Proc. Int. Symp. on Prolactinomas, Graz 1984.
[8] Kameya, T., M. Tsumuraya, I. Adachi, et al.: Ultrastructure, immunohistochemistry and hormone release of pituitary adenomas in relation to prolactin production. Virchows Arch. A. Path. Anat. and Histol. **387** (1980) 31–46.
[9] Landolt, A. M.: Personal communication (1984).
[10] Robert, F.: Le prolactinome – aspects pathologiques. Neurochir. **27**, Suppl. 1 (1981) 61–73.
[11] Schatz, H., M. Daun, H. Leicht, et al.: Immunohistochemical hormone determination in pituitary adenomas in comparison to endocrinological findings in vivo. Proc. Int. Symp. on Prolactinomas, Graz 1984.

Necrosis of prolactinoma cells after bromocriptine treatment

M. Gen, T. Uozumi, M. Ohta, K. Sakoda, S. Shinohara, K. Mukada, A. Ito, M. Naito, H. Kajiwara, S. Mori

Introduction

This study was performed to examine if necrosis occurred in prolactinomas after bromocriptine therapy.

Materials and methods

Patients: Six patients with prolactinoma were studied. All were treated with bromocriptine first and then underwent transsphenoidal surgery. Bromocriptine was administered before surgery in an average daily dose of 3 to 23 mg/day for 14 to 36 weeks. Tumour size was estimated by CT scans. Pathology: For light microscopy, tissue was fixed in Bouin's solution. Paraffin sections were stained with HE and with the Azan-Mallory method. For the demonstration of PRL, the immunoperoxidase technique was used with the Dako pap kit system. For electron microscopy, the tissue was fixed in 2% glutaraldehyde and 1% paraformaldehyde. Epon sections were stained with uranyl acetate and lead.

Results

Blood PRL levels: Blood PRL levels in 6 patients before therapy ranged from 151 ng/ml to 13,886 ng/ml. After preoperative bromocriptine therapy they were decreased significantly. Reduction in tumour size by bromocriptine: A marked size reduction was observed in patient 1, while only a slight shrinkage was observed in patient 6. Pathology: 1. Light microscopy: In patients 1–5 compact shrunken tumour cell nests surrounded by acellular spaces were observed. The cells of these island-like cell nests had hyperchromatic nuclei and scanty cytoplasm (figs. 1–3). In the sections stained with the immunoperoxidase technique for PRL, the scanty cytoplasm of these cells was weakly stained. In the acellular spaces some degenerative and necrotic tumour cells were observed and inflammatory cell infiltration was

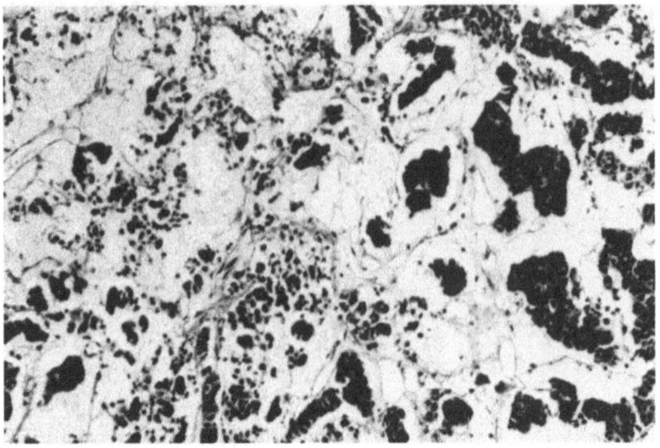

Fig. 1 Light photomicrograph of the pituitary tumour from patient 1. Compact shrunken tumour cell nests are surrounded by acellular spaces. In the acellular spaces fibrosis and hyaline substance are seen. HE stain, ×100.

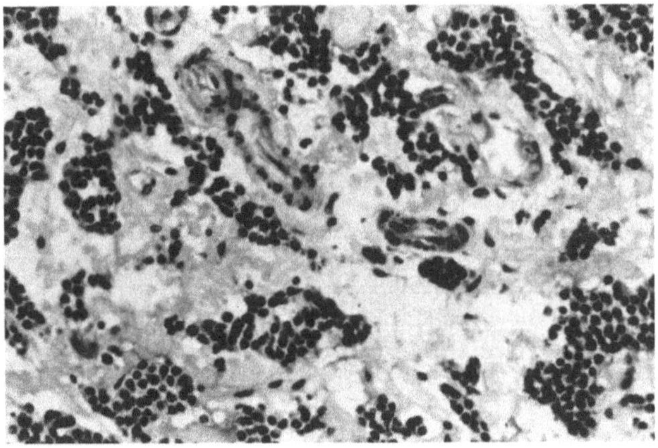

Fig. 2 Light photomicrograph of the pituitary tumour from patient 4. Acellular spaces are clearly seen among shrunken tumour cell nests. Hyaline substance, degenerative tumour cells are seen in these acellular spaces. HE stain, ×200.

seen among these damaged cells (fig. 2). Fibrosis and hyaline substance were also seen in these acellular spaces (figs. 1–3). In patient 6, few acellular spaces or fibrotic areas were observed. Most of the tumour cells had abundant cytoplasm, and some of them showed hydropic degeneration. Others were atrophic (fig. 4). 2. Electron microscopy: the island-like tumour cell nests had cells with scanty cytoplasm in which a few secretory granules 50 to 350 nm in size were seen and a rough endoplasmic reticula and Golgi apparatus which were poorly developed (fig. 5). In the degenerative and necrotic areas, pycnosis, karyorrhexis, and karyolysis of the

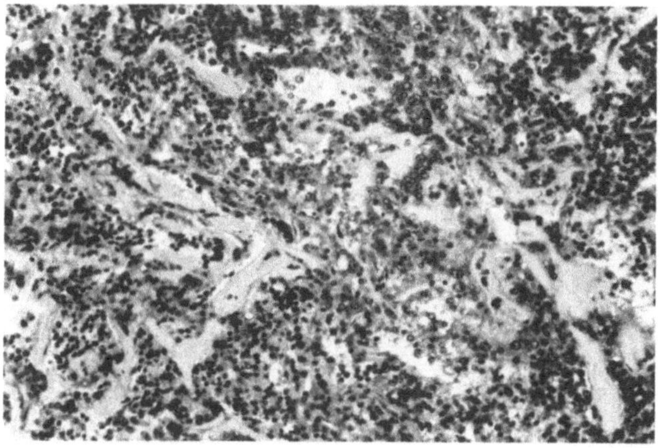

Fig. 3 Light photomicrograph of the pituitary tumour from patient 5. A considerable number of tumour cells are degenerated and necrotic. Fibrosis in the acellular spaces is seen. HE stain, ×100.

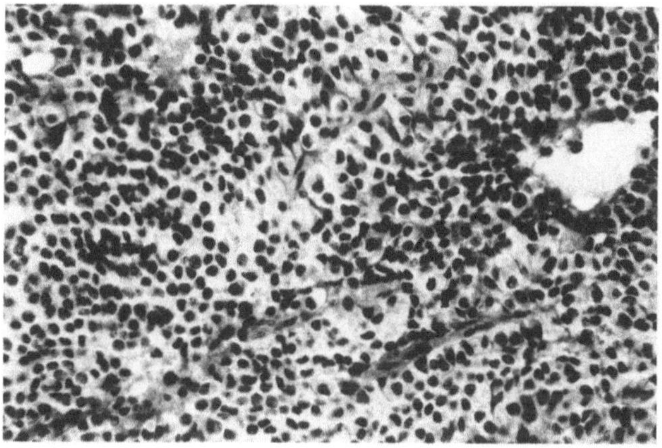

Fig. 4 Light photomicrograph of the pituitary tumour from patient 6. A mosaic mixture of cells with ample cytoplasm and scanty cytoplasm are seen. HE stain, ×200.

tumour cells were seen (fig. 6). These findings of tumour cell nests and degenerative or necrotic areas were observed in patients 1–5.

Discussion

Rengachary et al. [5] and Tindall et al. [6] reported that cytoplasmic atrophy of prolactinoma cells by bromocriptine treatment of 4 to 6 weeks caused a reduction in tumour size. However, we observed after bromocriptine therapy of 14 to 36

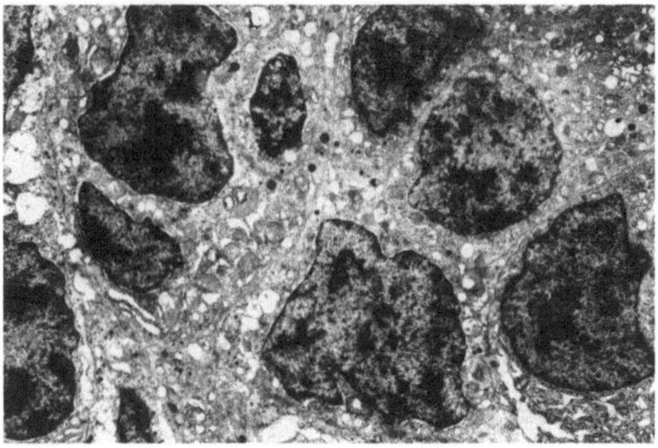

Fig. 5 Electron photomicrograph of the pituitary tumour from patient 3. Nuclear chromatin is clumped. Cell size is reduced and cell organelles such as RER and Golgi apparatus are poorly developed. ×6286.

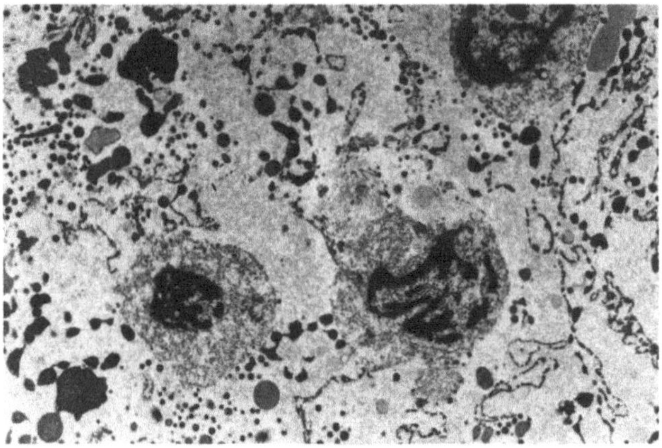

Fig. 6 Electron photomicrograph of the pituitary tumour from patient 1. Pycnosis, karyolysis and karyorrhexis of the tumour cells are seen. ×8100.

weeks not only shrunken tumour cell nests, identical with the observations of Rengachary et al. and Tindall et al., but also acellular spaces. At least some of these acellular spaces are considered to be the necrotic area, because necrotic tumour cells, fibrosis, hyaline substance and inflammatory cell infiltration were seen in them (figs. 1–3). Electron microscopic findings of pycnosis, karyorrhexis and karyolysis of tumour cells supported this consideration (fig. 6). As for morphometric analysis of tumour shrinkage, the nucleus to cytoplasm ratio is usually 1 to 2 in non-pretreated prolactinoma cells [3]. Therefore, it is considered that tumour shrinkage resulting in becoming much smaller than one-third of its original diameter, or tumour disappearance in the CT [4] cannot occur by cell shrinkage alone. Thus, it is suggested that the marked size reduction in large prolactinomas may be attributable not only to cytoplasmic atrophy but also death and disappearance of the tumour cells. Namely, bromocriptine may have a cytocidal effect on some prolactinoma cells and a cytostatic effect on others. In patient 6, blood PRL level did not decrease to the normal range and only a slight reduction in tumour size was observed. The histological findings (fig. 4) show that the majority of the tumour cells received only a cytostatic effect. Therefore, it can be considered that the proportion of cell populations which receive the cytocidal effect of bromocriptine varies from tumour to tumour. A rapid increase in blood PRL levels after discontinuation of bromocriptine [1, 2] may be explained by the rapid restoration of PRL secretion by the surviving tumour cells during bromocriptine treatment.

Abstract

Six prolactinomas were examined histologically after bromocriptine therapy. In patient 1, a marked size reduction and remarkable decrease in the elevated blood PRL level were observed with bromocriptine treatment for eight months. The histological findings consisted of acellular spaces and shrunken island-like cell nests. Some degenerative and necrotic tumour cells were observed in these acellular spaces. Island-like cell nests consisted of atrophic cells with scanty cytoplasm. The same histological findings were observed in 4 other patients (2–5). However in patient 6 whose tumour showed only a slight shrinkage after bromocriptine, the specimen was found to have few acellular spaces. Thus, it was shown that bromocriptine treatment of prolactinoma patients may result in necrosis of some adenoma cells in some patients.

References

[1] Eversman, et al.: Persisting suppression of prolactin secretion after long-term treatment with bromocriptine in patients with prolactinomas. Acta Endocrinol. (Kbh) **87** (1979) 687.

[2] Gen, et al.: Does bromocriptine have a cytocidal effect on prolactinoma cells? Neurol. Med. Chir. (Tokyo) **23** (1983) 61.

[3] Landolt, et al.: Bromocriptine reduces the size of cells in prolactin-secreting pituitary adenomas. Experimentia **39** (1983) 625.

[4] Matsumara, et al.: Size reduction of a large prolactinoma by bromocriptine treatment. Report of a case. Neurol. Med. Chir. (Tokyo) **21** (1981) 127.

[5] Rengachary, et al.: Structural changes in human pituitary tumour after bromocriptine therapy. Neurosurgery **10** (1982) 242.

[6] Tindall, et al.: Human prolactin-producing adenomas and bromocriptine: A histological, immunocytochemical, ultrastructural, and morphometric study. J. Clin. Endoclinol. Metab. **55** (1982) 1178.

Spontaneous pituitary lesions and plasma prolactin levels in rats

J. H. J. van Nesselrooij, C. F. Kuper, M. C. Bosland, J. P. Bruyntjes, R. Kroes

Introduction

Proliferative and hypertrophic pituitary lesions occur frequently in ageing rats [1, 4, 5, 11]. Most of these lesions consist of prolactin (PRL) containing cells as assessed by immunohistochemical methods [1]. Preliminary findings from studies in this laboratory showed a clear relationship between specific types of pituitary lesions and elevated plasma PRL levels in male rats [10]. In the present study, these findings in male rats were compared with those in female rats.

Materials and methods

From 40 male and 38 female Wistar rats (Cpb:WU) pituitary glands were collected at 30 months of age. At the same time, blood samples were taken to measure PRL levels by radioimmunoassay (RIA) [6]. Blood samples were taken between 9 and 12 a.m. from animals killed by decapitation without anaesthesia. The pituitary glands were fixed in a 4% buffered formaldehyde solution and embedded in paraplast. Step sections were stained with haematoxylin and eosin. In addition, immunoperoxidase staining for PRL was carried out [9], using antisera obtained through the courtesy of Dr. S. Riati (National Institute of Arthritis, Metabolism and Digestive Diseases, Bethesda, MD, USA).

Results

Pituitary lesions observed were morphologically classified as haemorrhagic tumours, spongiocytic tumours or pleomorphic tumours [1] and foci of hyperplasia [7] or foci of hypertrophic cells. Foci of hypertrophic cells consist of enlarged cells with clear cytoplasm and distinct eosinophilic cell boundaries when stained with haematoxylin and eosin. The incidences of spontaneous pituitary lesions found in 30-month old Wistar rats are presented in table 1. Most tumours were haemorrhagic tumours. Only one spongiocytic tumour was found and pleomorphic tumours were only occasionally observed. More male than female rats had foci of hypertrophic cells. Many animals had more than one type of lesion.

Foci of hyperplasia and haemorrhagic tumours were all immunohistochemically positive for PRL, while all foci of hypertrophic cells were negative. In general, plasma PRL levels were higher in females than in males. In males, haemorrhagic tumours and, to a lesser extent, foci of hyperplasia were associated with elevated plasma PRL levels (tab. 1). In females, plasma PRL levels above the normal range were always found in animals with haemorrhagic tumours or foci of hyperplasia (tab. 1). These associations only held when the most severe lesion per animal was taken into consideration. The presence of these proliferative pituitary gland lesions did, however, not entirely explain the individual variation in plasma PRL levels.

Table 1 The incidence of spontaneous pituitary lesions and plasma PRL levels in 30-month old Wistar rats

	Males			Females		
	number of lesions[1]	incidence[2]	plasma PRL levels[3]	number of lesions[1]	incidence[2]	plasma PRL levels[3]
Number of animals examined	40			38		
No abnormalities	2	2	3.0 1.5–4.5)	8	8	17.9 8.7–28.1)
Number of animals with tumours	13	13		22	22	22
Haemorrhagic tumours	12	12	53.6 3.7–394.0)	18	18	90.6 (30.6–253.0)
Spongiocytic tumours	1	1	40.0 (40.0)	0	0	
Pleomorphic tumours	5	0		7	4	54.6 (36.2–83.7)
Foci of hypertrophic cells	25	12	2.1 1.5–2.8)	7	1	38.5 (38.5)
Foci of hyperplasia	15	13	4.2 1.5–7.9)	12	7	44.3 (15.8–59.7)

[1] Many animals had more than one type of lesion.
[2] The most severe lesion per animal was taken into consideration.
[3] Mean plasma PRL concentrations; the range is given in brackets.

Discussion

Foci of hyperplasia were PRL positive and were associated with elevated plasma PRL levels. This supports a precursor role of this lesion in the pathogenesis of haemorrhagic tumours in rats as suggested for men by Landolt [7]. The present data do not clarify the significance of foci of hypertrophic cells for the development of proliferative pituitary gland lesions in rats.

The presence of haemorrhagic tumours and, to a lesser degree, foci of hyperplasia were associated with elevated plasma PRL levels. However, the observed pituitary lesions could not entirely explain the differences in plasma PRL levels. Therefore, these levels are probably influenced by other factors as well. Gonadal activity and perhaps the presence of lesions such as mammary gland tumours may influence plasma PRL levels [2, 3, 5, 8]. Nevertheless, from the present study it appears that elevated PRL levels are indicative of the presence of proliferative lesions consisting of PRL-containing cells in rat pituitaries.

References

[1] Berkvens, J. M., J. H. J. van Nesselrooij, R. Kroes: Spontaneous tumours in the pituitary gland of old Wistar rats. A morphological and immunocytochemical study. J. Path., vol. **130** (1980) 179–191.

[2] Burack, E., J. M. Wolfe, W. Lansing, et al.: The effect of age upon the connective tissue of uterus, cervix and vagina of the rat. Cancer res. **1** (1941) 227.

[3] Fainstat, T.: Endocrine influences on collagen bundle deposition and maintenance in rat endometrium, p. 549. Proc. 1st Int. Congr. Endocrin. Copenhagen 1960.

[4] Furth, J., P. Nakana, J. L. Pasteels: Tumours of the pituitary gland. In: Pathology of tumours in laboratory animals, vol. 1; Tumours of the rat, Part 2 (V. S. Turosov, ed.), p. 201. Larc, Lyon 1976.

[5] Kroes, R., J. M. Berkvens, T. de Vries, et al.: Histopathological profile of a Wistar rat stock including a survey of the literature. J. of Geront., vol. 36, no. **3** (1981) 259–279.

[6] Kwa, H. G., A. A. van der Gugten, F. Verhofstad, et al.: Radio immuno assay of rat prolactin. Prolactin levels in plasma of rats with spontaneous pituitary tumours, primary oestrone-induced pituitary tumours or pituitary tumour transplants. Europ. J. Cancer **5** (1969) 571.

[7] Landolt, A. M.: Biology of pituitary microadenomas. In: Pituitary microadenomas (G. Faglia, M. A. Giovanelli, R. M. MacLeod, eds.), pp. 105–122. Academic Press, London 1980.

[8] Mandl, A. M.: Clinical changes in the vaginal smears of senile nuuliparous and multiparous rats. J. Endocrin. **22** (1961) 257.

[9] Nakana, P. K., G. B. Pierce: Enzyme-labeled antibodies for the light and electron microscopic localisation of tissue antigens. J. Cell. Biol. **33** (1967) 307.

[10] Nesselrooij, J. H. J. van, H. van de Berg, R. Kroes: Interactions between morphological changes in the pituitary gland and plasma prolactin levels in rats, p. 17. 3rd European workshop on pituitary adenomas 7.–10. 9. 1983.

[11] Trouillas, J., C. Girod, B. Claustrat, et al.: Spontaneous pituitary tumours in the Wistar/Furth/Ico rat strain. An animal model of human prolactin adenoma. Am. J. Pathol. **109** (1982) 57–70.

II Radiology

CT-findings in pituitary adenomas

G. H. Schneider

Introduction

In cases of endocrine disturbances such as acromegaly or amenorrhoea and galactorrhoea, a hormone-secreting pituitary adenoma is suspected first. As a result of an improvement in hormonal assays, a clinical diagnosis can be etablished earlier and therefore the tumours responsible for the disease are small. Because of improved operating techniques the detection of pituitary microadenomas is of increasing importance; therefore, the neuroradiological examination of the pituitary gland has undergone development in the last few year.

Of the various radiological modalities, such as coned-down lateral and antero-posterior (p.a.) plain films of the sella, thin-section tomography, angiography, and computed tomography, computed tomography has the highest sensitivity in the diagnosis of pituitary tumours.

Ambrose [1] pointed out, in the first paper on clinical applications of CT, that examinations involving the skull base and pituitary fossa are not satisfactory in many cases. The basal cistern could be shown in only about 85% of cases with first-generation CT equipment, with this equipment exclusively intrasellar pituitary adenomas could not be visualized in the CT scan due to artifacts arising from petrous bones.

With the further development of CT scanners and the introduction of high-resolution computed tomography, intrasellar scanning became possible and the normal pituitary gland and stalk could be made directly visible. This step from the second to third generation of CT scanners has led to a greater sensitivity in detecting microadenomas within the pituitary gland. On the other hand, technical factors may affect the appearance of the sella contents on the scanner, and the results may therefore differ between the two generations of scanners.

Materials and methods

The material on which this paper is based consists of data from 103 patients. All patients had been referred to the Radiological Departments from the Departments of Neurology and Neurosurgery at the University hospital in Graz during the period from 1977 to 1983. The decision to carry out a CT examination of the sella was based on sellar enlargement, visual field defects or endocrine disturbances.

The pituitary tumour was removed in each case using the transsphenoidal approach.

About 90% of the CT scans were obtained on an EMI 1010 or EMI 5005, using 5 or 10 mm sections parallel to the canthomeatal plane. There was no overlapping of scans. The contrast medium was Meglumindiatrizoate 65%. After the plain scan, 1 ml/kg body weight of contrast medium was injected before scanning. About 10% of the studies were performed using a Siemens Somatom DR 2 or DR 3, using 2 mm sections. In macroadenomas, axial scanning with reformatting into the coronal and sagittal planes was performed.

In microadenomas without sellar enlargement, the examination was performed in the following manner: the patient was placed supine and a lateral digital localizer image (Topogramm) was obtained. The optimal gantry angle was determined, so that the petrous bones were avoided by the axial scans in order to diminish artifacts within the sellar fossa. After the plain scan a series of contrast scans during bolus injection were obtained. In equivocal cases direct coronal scanning with the patient's head hyperextended was performed after the series with contrast medium. Usually 60 ml to 90 ml of 65% Meglumindiatrizoate contrast medium was given. When direct coronal scanning was necessary, another bolus of 60 ml was administered. In every patient, at least one preoperative and one postoperative CT examination were performed, including a plain series and a contrast enhanced series of scars. For this retrospective study CT scans were assessed for the following:

1. In the plain scan tumour density was compared with normal brain tissue.

2. The degree of enhancement after contrast injection was assessed.

3. Focal areas of low density in the lesion and ring-shaped enhancement of the tumour were estimated, as was cystic degeneration.

4. Calcification was evaluated.

These data were correlated with the biological activity of the adenomas.

Results

The pathological findings in 103 patients are listed in table 1. In 91 adenomas there were 65 macroadenomas and 26 microadenomas. Craniopharyngiomas occurred in 4 cases. There was one meningioma. In one case there was involvement of the pituitary by Hodgkin's disease, and in one patient an abscess was found. Twice the operation showed a cyst and in three cases an empty sella. With the exception of microadenomas, the space-occupying lesions were diagnosed in each case. The

Table 1 Results (n = 103)

Adenomas	91
Macroadenomas	65
Microadenomas	26
Craniopharyngiomas	4
Meningiomas	1
Mb. Hodgkin	1
Abscess	1
Cyst	2
Empty-sella	3

Table 2 Pituitary adenomas (n = 91)

adenomas	nonsecreting	secreting	total
males	24	20	44 (48%)
females	10	37	47 (52%)
total	34 (37%)	57 (63%)	91 (100%)

Table 3 Secreting adenomas (n = 57)

	males	females	total
Prolactin	11	23	34 (60%)
HGH	8	12	20 (35%)
ACTH	1	2	3 (5%)
total	20	37	57 (100%)

Table 4 Prolactin producing adenomas (n = 34)

	microadenomas	macroadenomas	total	%
males	2	9	11	32
females	16	7	23	68
total	18 (53%)	16 (47%)	34	100

group of microadenomas includes the false negative results from this material. 39% of prolactin-producing microadenomas and 57% of growth-hormone-producing microadenomas were missed.

The sex distribution of patients with pituitary adenomas was nearly equal (tab. 2): 48% males and 52% females. 63% of these lesions of the adenomas were hormone-secreting adenomas. In the males 45% and in the females 78% were secreting adenomas. In those cases with secreting adenomas (tab. 3), prolactinomas were seen in 60%, acromegaly in 35% and Cushing adenomas in 5%. The sex distribution of prolactinomas (tab. 4) shows that about two thirds of the cases occurred in females and 32% in males. The ratio between microadenomas and macroadenomas is of importance. In the total group of prolactin producing tumours 53% were found to be microadenomas. But in the male patients only 18% of the tumours

Table 5 Prolactin producing adenomas (n = 34)

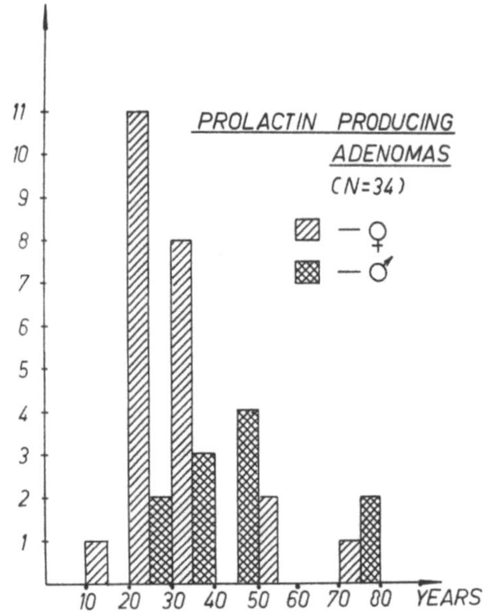

Table 6 HGH producing adenomas (n = 20)

	microadenomas	macroadenomas	total	%
males	–	8	8	40
females	7	5	12	60
total	7 (35%)	13 (65%)	20	100

were microadenomas, whereas in the female patients the amenorrhoea-galactorrhoea-syndrome was caused in 68% of the cases by a microadenoma.

The age distribution of prolactinomas (tab. 5) demonstrates a high incidence in women of childbearing age. The peak of incidence in men in our material is later than in women in the fifth decade of life. The sex distribution in patients with acromegaly (tab. 6) showed 60% females and 40% males. Microadenomas were detected in 58% of the females; in males no microadenomas were seen. The age distribution of growth-hormone secreting adenomas (tab. 7) shows the first occurrances in women of childbearing age and a peak of incidence in the sixth decade in both sexes. A similar age distribution is seen in nonsecreting adenomas (tab. 8). The peak of incidence is in the sixth and seventh decades in both sexes. In the three cases of Cushing adenoma (tab. 9), one macroadenoma was found in a male patient and one macro- and one microadenoma in the two female patients. The CT findings are listed in tables 10 and 11.

Table 7 HGH producing adenomas

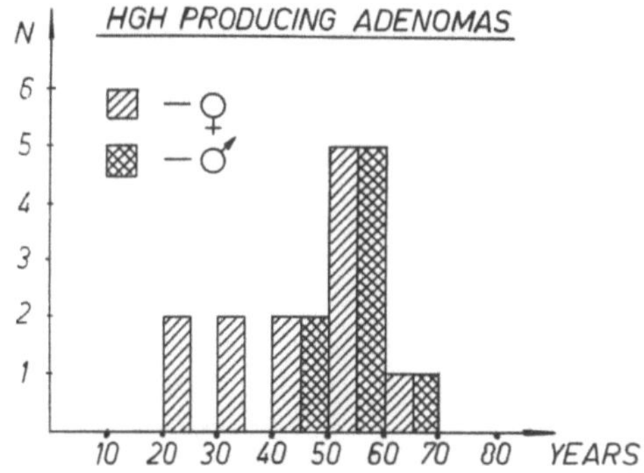

Table 8 Nonsecreting adenomas

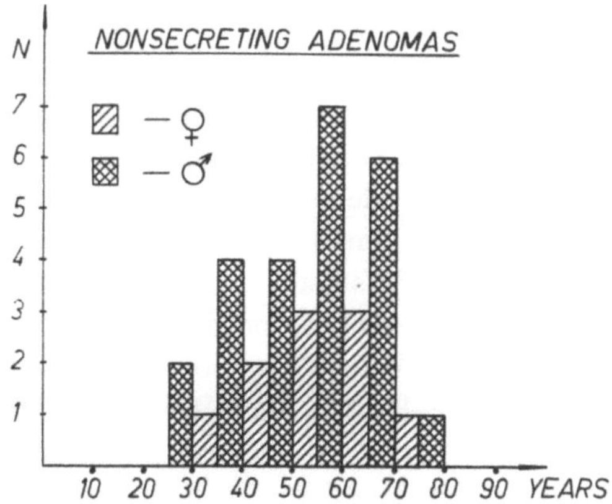

Table 9 ACTH producing adenomas (n = 3)

	microadenomas	macroadenomas	total
males	–	1	1
females	1	1	2
total	1	2	3

Table 10 CT-findings (%)

	plain scan			contrast enhancement		cyst	calci-fication
	hyper	iso	hypo	+	O		
macroadenomas nonsecreting	47.1	38.2	14.7	79.4	20.6	17.6	7.3
macroadenomas PRL	37.5	50.0	12.5	75.0	25.0	6.2	6.2
microadenomas PRL (n = 11)	–	63.6	36.4	54.6	45.4	27.2	–

Table 11 CT-findings (%)

	plain scan			contrast enhancement		cyst	calci-fication
	hyper	iso	hypo	+	O		
macroadenomas HGH	38.5	46.1	15.4	46.1	53.9	23	7.7
microadenomas HGH (n = 3)	–	100.0	–	33.3	66.7	–	–
adenomas ACTH (n = 3)	33.3	66.7	–	66.7	33.3	–	–

Discussion

The introduction of high-resolution computed tomography has altered the choice of means of investigation for patients with suspected pituitary tumours [29, 40]. The radiological evaluation of a pituitary adenoma includes preliminary skull radiographs or a coned-down lateral and p. a. films of the sella. This is not expected to be used as a screening method because this is done by endocrinologic examinations and, in any case plain films are inadequate [34] for indicating the presence of a pituitary microadenoma. Rather, the diagnostic CT approach differentiates as to whether or not the sella is enlarged. In an enlarged sella in which a big tumour may be suspected, axial scans using 2 mm or 4 mm continuous sections with reformatting into coronal and sagittal images suffice. Besides the magnitude of the tumour, the increased volume of the pituitary fossa decreases the relative size of the potential intrasellar artifact [15]. In a normal-sized sella the pituitary gland [7, 9] and microadenomas are best demonstrated by direct coronal scanning, or indirectly by scanning in the axial plane with coronal and sagittal reformation using 1 mm or 2 mm sections [10]. The advantage of direct coronal scanning is the better spatial resolution and the elimination of low density artifacts associated with the bones of the skull base [15].

In a patient who cannot be positioned with the head hyperextended for direct coronal scanning, an optimal choice of scanning plane is mandatory. With the lateral digital localizer image, the scanning plane through the orbits above the petrous ridges is chosen and the avoidance of the petrous bones minimizes the low attenuation artifacts within the sella [15].

Indirect signs of intrasellar masses are, on the one hand, bony changes in the sellar floor. These are seen as a ballooning of the whole sella in large tumours and a localized bulging of the sella, with depression of the sellar floor and cortical thinning in small intrasellar tumours. But the normal configuration of the sella and sella floor varies considerably [4, 26, 27, 28, 32] and the pathological significance of minor bony changes of the sella turcica is controversial [2, 5, 17, 22, 25, 28, 33, 34, 39, 44, 45]. On the other hand, the bony structures of the pituitary fossa can be evaluated with the soft tissue structures of sellar contents simultaneously by CT. The low accuracy, extra irradiation and costs have displaced pluri-directional thin-section tomography. Carotid angiography is essential to rule out vascular lesions within the pituitary fossa [23]. CT examination after metrizamide cisternography shows the basal cistern and may be necessary for differentiation between cystic intrasellar lesions and the empty sella syndrome. The statistically analysed data of the CT findings in macro-adenomas are comparable with those mentioned in the literature [3, 13, 19, 30, 43]. In the plain scans the density values of the pituitary masses were hyper-, iso- and hypodense with respect to normal brain tissue. Contrast enhancement was noted in about three-quarters of these cases with nonsecreting and prolactin producing macroadenomas. In acromegaly the causative macroadenomas enhanced in 46% of cases. Enhancing adenomas show the same dynamic contrast behaviour as meningeomas [42], with an early peak of the time-density curve after the injection of contrast medium, followed by a rapid decrease in density. Therefore, the way in which the contrast medium is introduced (whether by an infusion, a bolus-injection) before a scan is an important point, because the findings concerning the contrast behaviour of the pituitary tumours may differ when using different techniques. On the other hand the results are influenced if for logistic reasons there is a delay between the injection of the contrast medium and the CT examination. Cystic degeneration occurred in 23% of the tumours in acromegaly, in 18% in nonsecreting macroadenomas and in 6% in macroprolactinomas. A marked increase in the absorption values within a pituitary adenoma as seen in the plain scan may be caused by calcification. The frequency of calcification was almost evenly distributed in those three groups. High absorption values within the pituitary adenoma with sudden enlargement of the adenoma, which is often followed by deterioration of clinical findings, is due to haemorrhage into the tumour (fig. 1). Nonsecreting macroadenomas resemble macroadenomas of the prolactin- and HGH-producing types and the CT appearance is not specific for one of these adenomas (fig. 2).

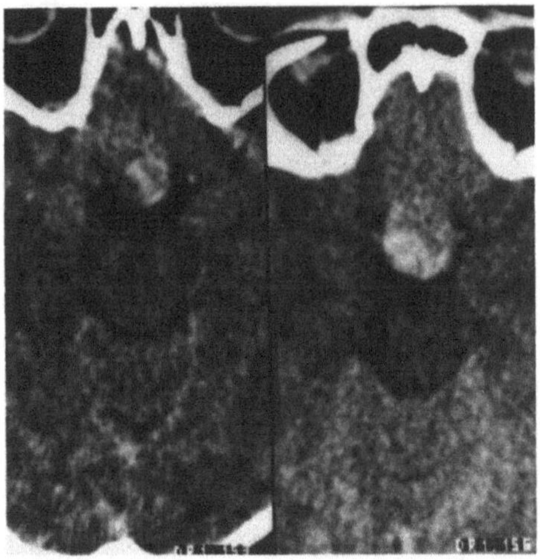

Fig. 1 Pituitary apoplexy: Enlargement and patchy hyperdensity of the gland.

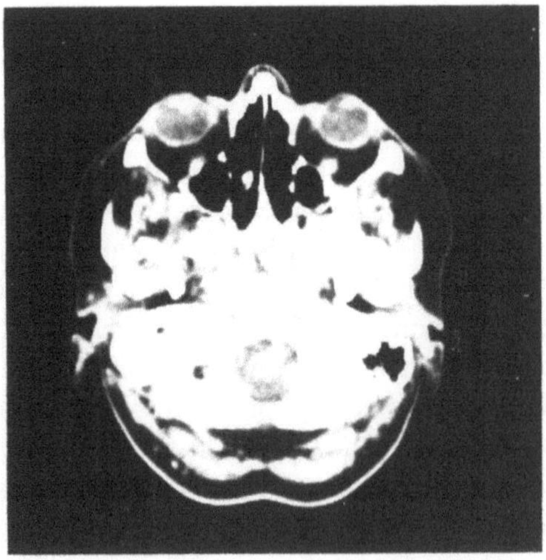

Fig. 2 Macroprolactinoma: Large tumour with osseous destruction of the skull base.

The diagnosis of pituitary microadenomas is based on an increase in the height of the gland and an alteration in the configuration, with convex bulging of the gland surface [41]. The microadenoma itself usually appears as a region of low density in the contrast-enhanced pituitary gland [6, 10, 12, 21, 43, 46] (figs. 3–5). Because about 90% of our patients were examined with a second generation scanner, there was a high percentage of false negative results in the group of microadenomas. But the percentage of false negative results differed between the prolactin and the

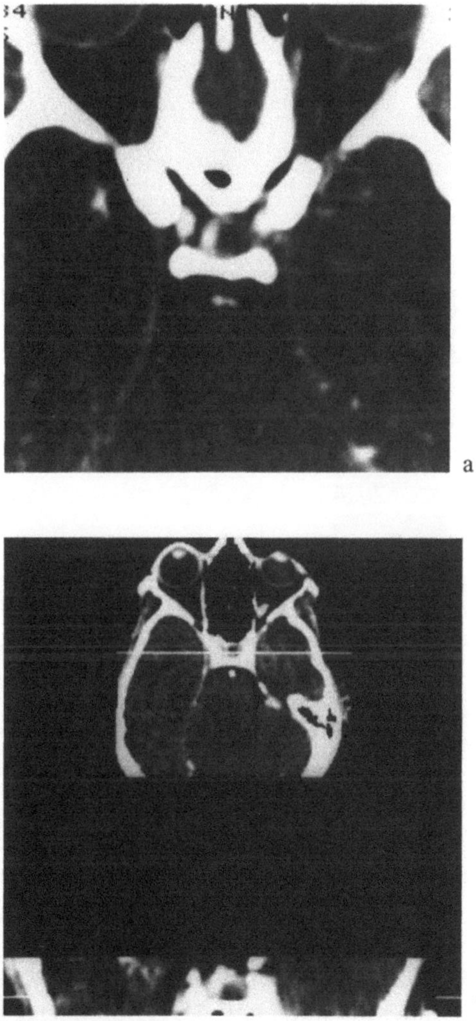

a

b

Fig. 3 Microprolactinoma in
a) axial and
b) reformatted coronal plane.

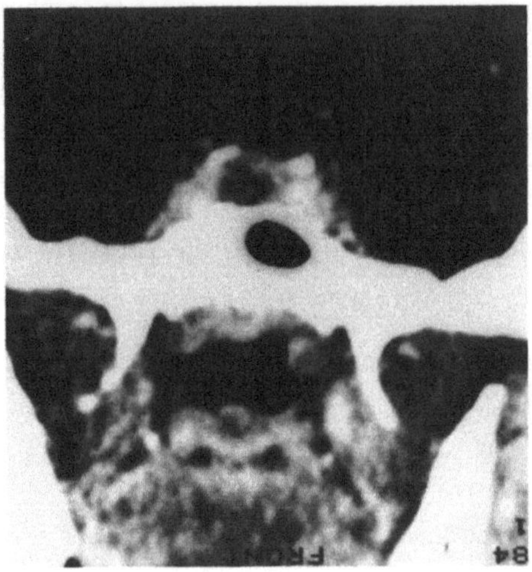

Fig. 4 Microprolactinoma; coronal scan.

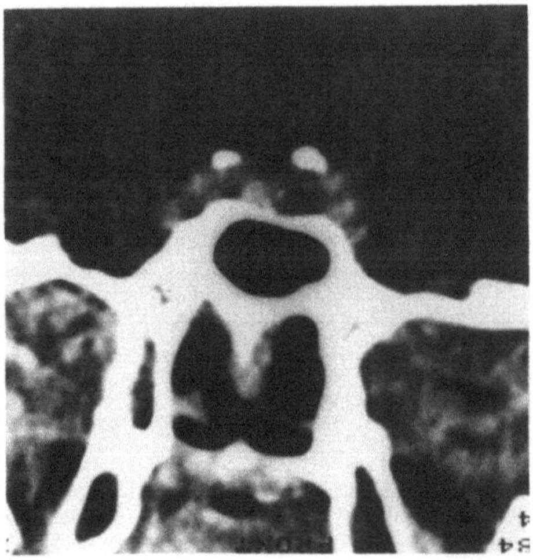

Fig. 5 HGH-secreting microadenoma; coronal scan.

growth hormone producing microadenomas. 39% of prolactin producing microadenomas were missed in comparison with 57% of growth hormone producing microadenomas. Hypodense lesions and enlargement of the pituitary are less reliable criteria for the diagnosis of ACTH- or HGH-secreting microadenomas [21]. The lack of difference of absorption values in HGH- and ACTH-producing microadenomas, the homogeneous enhancement pattern and the mass effect being minimal or absent can make detection of these microadenomas very difficult or even impossible. Therefore, a negative CT study of the sella does not exclude such a tumour [21]. The low-density region caused by microadenoma in the contrast-enhanced pituitary is due to differences in the enhancement patterns of normal and adenomatous tissue. The normal pituitary enhances rapidly, with an early peak in the time-density curve, because of high vascularity and the lack of blood brain barrier. Pituitary adenomas show various degrees of contrast enhancement from minimal or absent enhancement to homogeneous enhancement with normal pituitary tissue, but the adenomas seem to enhance more slowly [21] with a delayed peak in the time density curve. So the largest density differences are seen immediately after contrast injection. Later, while the density of the pituitary diminishes the adenoma enhances slowly. Therefore, the appearance of pituitary adenomas is highly dependent on the type of contrast administration and the time interval between contrast-injection and the CT examination. The results may be influenced further by low density artifacts in the sella region caused by bony structures of the base of the skull [15], and by partial volume artifacts of sella contents with air in the sphenoid sinus and cerebrospinal fluid in the basal cistern. Partial volume effects between enhanced normal glandular tissue and less- or not enhanced adenomatous tissue may obscure the hypodense region, and the resulting appearance may be isodense or hyperdense. Low-density areas in the contrast-enhanced pituitary can be due also to pathological conditions other than microadenomas. Chambers found in 100 autopsy specimens from patients with no known pituitary disease abnormalities in 24% of them (10). 54% of these findings showed disease processes other than microadenomas. These abnormalities included pars intermedia cysts, which can be seen in 13% to 22% of the postmortem studies [14, 28, 37, 38]. Metastases and infarcts, epidermoidal cysts and abscesses may also one rise focal low density areas in the pituitary. In the differential diagnosis an empty sella giving a low density appearance to the sella is also to be excluded [20, 35]. The incidence of asymptomatic pituitary microadenomas found incidentally upon postmortem examination is between 8.5% and 27% [8, 11, 12, 24, 31]. In conclusion, it is to be stressed that focal low-density lesions in the contrast-enhanced pituitary represent ambiguous findings. For a correct interpretation both the clinical and endocrinological data must be correlated carefully.

References

[1] Ambrose, J.: Computerized transverse axial scanning (tomography). Part 2: Clinical application. Brit. J. Radiol. **47** (1973) 1023–1047.

[2] Banna, M., W. Nicholas, M. McLachlan: The borderline pituitary fossa in patients with amenorrhoea and/or galactorrhoea. Neuroradiology **16** (1978) 440–442.

[3] Banna, M., H. L. Baker jr., O. W. Houser: Pituitary and parapituitary tumours on compted tomography. Brit. J. of Radiol. **53** (1980) 1123–1143.

[4] Bergland, R. M., B. S. Ray, R. M. Torack: Anatomical variations in the pituitary gland and adjacent structures in 225 human autopsy cases. J. Neurosurg. **28** (1968) 93–99.

[5] Besser, G. M.: The pituitary fossa: normal or abnormal. Brit. J. Radiol. **49** (1976) 652–653.

[6] Bonafe, A., D. Sobel, C. Manelfe: Relative value of computed tomography and hypocycloidal tomography in the diagnosis of pituitary microadenoma. A radiosurgical correlative study. Neuroradiology **22** (1981) 133–137.
[7] Brown, S. B., I. K. Murphy, D. R. Enzmann: CT Characteristics of the Normal Pituitary Gland. Neuroradiology **24** (1983) 259–262.
[8] Burrow, G. N., G. Worthman, N. B. Rewcastle, et al.: Microadenomas of the pituitary and abnormal sellar tomograms in an unselected autopsy series. N. Engl. J. Med. **304** (1981) 156–158.
[9] Chakeres, D. W.: Computed Tomography demonstration of a hypothalamic metastasis. Neuroradiology **25** (1983) 103–104.
[10] Chambers, E. F., P. A. Turski, D. LaMasters, et al.: Regions of Low Density in the Contrast-Enhanced Pituitary Gland: Normal and Pathologic Processes. Radiology **144** (1982) 109–113.
[11] Costello, R. T.: Subclinical adenoma of the pituitary gland. Am. J. Pathol. **12** (1936) 205–216.
[12] Cusick, J. F., V. M. Haughton, T. C. Hagen: Radiological assessment of intrasellar prolactin-secreting tumours. Neurosugery **6** (1980) 376–379.
[13] Daniels, D. L., A. L. Williams, R. S. Thornton, et al.: Differential Diagnosis of Intrasellar Tumors by Computed Tomography. Radiology **141** (1981) 697–701.
[14] Dietemann, J. L., J. F. Bonneville, F. Buchheit, et al.: CT Findings in Symptomatic Rathke's Cleft Cysts of the Pituitary Gland. Neuroradiology **24** (1983) 263–267.
[15] Earnest, IV, F., E. C. McCullough, D. A. Frank: Fact of Artifact: An Analysis of Artifact in High-Resolution Computed Tomographic Scanning of the Sella. Radiology **140** (July 1981) 109–113.
[16] Fitz, Ch. R., G. Wortzman, D. C. Harwood-Nash, et al.: Computed Tomography in Craniopharyngiomas. Radiology **127** (1978) 687–691.
[17] Geehr, R. B., W. E. Allen, S. G. L. Rothman: Pluridirectional tomography in the evaluation of pituitary tumors. AJR **130** (1978) 105–109.
[18] Hashimoto, N., H. Handa, J. Takeuchi, et al.: Collection of Gas Within a Huge Chromophobe Adenoma. Neuroradiology **23** (1982) 289–290.
[19] Hatam, A., M. Bergström, T. Greitz: Diagnosis of Sellar and Parasellar Lesions by Computed Tomography. Neuroradiology **18** (1979) 249–258.
[20] Haughton, V. M., A. E. Rosenbaum, A. L. Williams, et al.: Recognizing the Empty Sella by CT: The Infundibulum Sign. AJR **136** (1981) 293–295.
[21] Hemminghytt, S., R. K. Kalkhoff, D. L. Daniels: Computed tomographic study of hormone-secreting microadenomas. Radiology **146** (1983) 65–69.
[22] Kricheff, J. J.: The radiologic diagnosis of pituitary adenoma. Radiology **131** (1979) 263–265.
[23] MacPherson, P., D. E. Anderson: Radiological Differentiation of Intrasellar Aneurysms from Pituitary Tumours. Neuroradiology **21** (1981) 177–183.
[24] McCormick, W. F., N. S. Halmi: Absence of chromophobe adenomas from a large series of pituitary tumors. Arch. Pathol. **92** (1971) 231–238.
[25] McLachlan, M. S., A. D. Wright, F. H. Doyle: Plain film and tomographic assessment of pituitary fossa in 140 acromegalic patients. Br. J. Radiol. **43** (1970) 360–369.
[26] McLachlan, M. S., E. D. Williams, R. W. Fortt, et al.: Estimation of pituitary gland dimensions from radiographs of the sella turcica. A post mortem study. Br. J. Radiol. **41** (1968) 323–330.
[27] Muhr, C., K. Bergström, P. Enoksson, et al.: Follow-up study with compouterized tomography and clinical evaluation 5 to 10 years after surgery for pituitary adenoma. J. Neurosurg. **53** (1980) 144–148.

[28] Muhr, C., K. Bergström, L. Grimelius, et al.: A Parallel Study of the Roentgen Anatomy of the Sella Turcica and the Histopathology of the Pituitary Gland in 205 Autopsy Specimens. Neuroradiology **21** (1981) 55–65.
[29] Naidich, Th. P., R. S. Pinto, M. J. Kushner, et al.: Evaluation of Sellar and Parasellar Masses by Computed Tomography. Radiology **120** (1976) 91–99.
[30] Numaguchi, Y., T. Kishikawa, J. Ikeda, et al.: Neuroradiological Manifestations of Suprasellar Pituitary Adenomas, Menangiomas and Craniopharyngiomas. Neuroradiology **21** (1981) 67–74.
[31] Parent, A. D., J. Bebin, R. R. Smith: Incidental pituitary adenomas. J. Neurosurg. **54** (1981) 228–231.
[32] Renn, W. H., A. L. Thoton: Microsurgical anatomy of the sellar region. J. Neurosurg. **43** (1975) 288–298.
[33] Richmond, I. L., Th. Newton, C. B. Wilson: Prolactin-secreting pituitary adenomas: Correlation of radiographic and surgical findings. AJR **134** (1980) 707–710.
[34] Robertson, W. D., Th. Newton: Radiologic Assessment of Pituitary Microadenomas. Am. J. Roentgenol. **131** (1978) 489–492.
[35] Sage, M. R., P. C. Blumbergs, B. P. Mulligan, et al.: The Diaphragma Sellae: Its Relationship to the Configuration of the Pituitary Gland. Radiology **145** (1982) 703–708.
[36] Scotti, G., G. Scialfa, S. Pieralli, et al.: Macroprolactinomas: CT Evaluation of Reduction of Tumor Size After Medical Treatment. Neuroradiology **23** (1982) 123–126.
[37] Shanklin, W. M.: The incidence and distribution of cilia in the human pituitary with a description of micro-follicular cysts derived from Rathke's cleft. Acta Anat. **11** (1951) 361–381.
[38] Shuangshoti, S., M. G. Netsky, B. S. Nashold jr.: Epithelial cysts related to sella turcica: proposed origin from neuroepithelium. Arch. Pathol. **90** (1970) 444–450.
[39] Swanson, H. A., G. du Boulay: Borderline variants of the normal pituitary fossa. Br. J. Radiol. **48** (1975) 366–369.
[40] Swartz, J. D., K. B. Russell, B. A. Basile, et al.: High-Resolution Computed Tomographic Appearance of the Intrasellar Contents in Women of Childbearing Age. Radiology **147** (1983) 115–117.
[41] Syvertsen, A., V. Haughton, A. L. Williams, et al.: The Computed Tomographic Appearance of the Normal Pituitary Gland and Pituitary Microadenomas. Radiology **133** (1979) 385–391.
[42] Steinhoff, H., Ch. Aviles: Contrast enhancement response of intracranial neoplasma. Its validity for the differential diagnosis of tumors in CT. In: Cranial computerized tomography (W. Lanksch, E. Kazner, eds.), pp. 151–161. Springer, Berlin–Heidelberg–New York 1976.
[43] Taylor, S.: High Resolution Computed Tomography of the Sella. Radiologic Clinics of North America, Vol. 20, Nr. 1, 1982.
[44] Vezina, J. L., T. J. Sutton: Prolactin-secreting pituitary microadenomas. AJR **120** (1974) 46–54.
[45] Vezina, J. L.: Prolactin-secreting pituitary adenomas: Radiologic diagnosis, pp. 351–360. North-Holland Biomedical Press Elsevier, Amsterdam 1978.
[46] Wolpert, S. M.: The Radiology of Pituitary Adenomas. Seminars in Roentgenology, Vol. XIX, nr. 1, 1984.

Comparative study of normal subjects and cases with microadenoma on high-resolution computed tomography

Y. Nakagawa, J. Cervós-Navarro, K. Matsumoto, T. Fukami

Introduction

Computed tomography is now well established and universally accepted as a technique for the detection and preoperative evaluation of pituitary adenomas. However, there are sporadic reports of patients with microadenomas less than 10 mm in diameter that have been visualized by computed tomography [1, 2]. It seemed to be important to determine the exact relationship between the normal pituitary stalk and gland for the accurate morphological diagnosis of pituitary microadenomas. In this study, we are reporting the CT findings of the normal pituitary stalk and gland and compare them with those in 6 patients with microadenomas.

Subjects and methods

The pituitary gland and stalk were studied on a GE CT/T 8800 on 189 consecutive patients without evidence of any pituitary abnormality and 6 patients with microadenoma which were diagnosed radiologically and endocrinologically. The 189 patients in the control group were seen because of disorders such as head trauma, facial spasm, trigeminal neuralgia etc.; intracranial mass lesions were clinically ruled out in all (fig. 1). Following the intravenous drip infusion of contrast medium (30% Conray® 100 ml) continuous scans with 1.5 nm slices were performed parallel to the orbitomeatal line (OM-line) from about 10 mm to 35 mm above the OM-line. In selected cases where the study was indicated for the diagnostic evaluation of the caes (29 patients) metrizamide CT was performed. In all patients, continuous horizontal sections were made through the sella turcica and coronal and sagittal projections were reconstructed. The detection-rate of the pituitary stalk and gland in horizontal views and reconstructed coronal and sagittal projections was determined.

The inclination of the stalk was measured on coronal projection. The form of the pituitary glands was examined. These results were compared with those seen in patients with microadenoma.

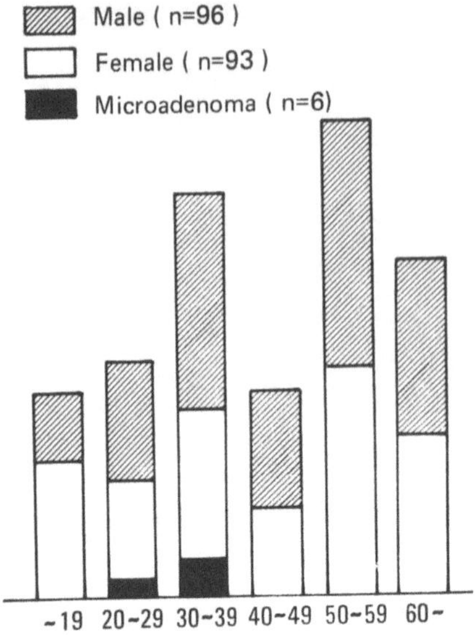

Fig. 1 Distribution of age and sex in 189 normal subjects and 6 cases with microadenoma.

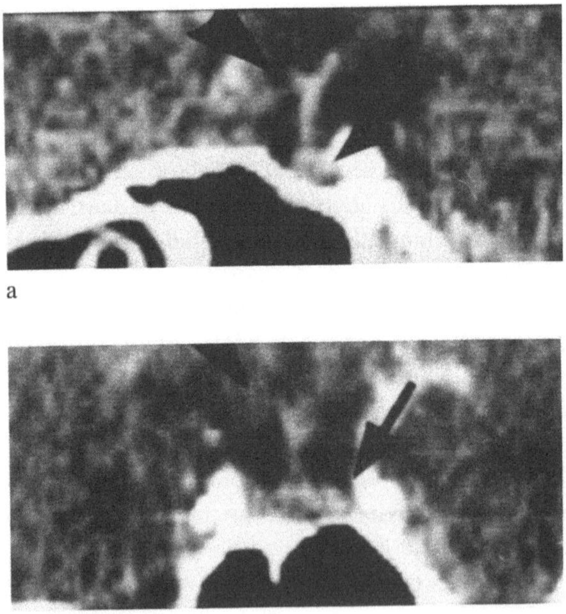

a

b

Fig. 2 Contrast-enhanced CT. Reconstructed sagittal (a) and coronal (b) views. The pituitary stalk (arrow head) and gland (arrow) were demonstrated as a homogeneously enhanced area.

Results

The detection-rate of the pituitary stalk and gland

Following the drip infusion of contrast medium, the pituitary stalk and gland were demonstrated as a homogeneously enhanced area (fig. 2). On metrizamide CT, the silhouette of these structures was shown as a low density area (fig. 3). In may cases, metrizamide was seen within the CSF space in the sella turcica. In the horizontal views, both the pituitary stalk and the gland were demonstrated in 186 out of 189 patients (98.4%). In the reconstructed coronal projections, the pituitary stalks were demonstrated in 179 out of 189 patients (94.2%) and glands in 185 patients (97.9%). In the reconstructed sagittal projections, the stalk was demonstrated in 178 patients (93.6%) and gland in 188 (99.5%). With metrizamide CT, the stalk and gland were demonstrated more clearly than in the contrast-enhanced CT, in all projections and they were visualized in 100% of the cases (tab. 1).

Inclination of the pituitary stalk

The angle of the inclination of the pituitary stalks was measured against a central line that was perpendicular to the cranial line in the reconstructed coronal projections. The mean value of the angle in 189 normal subjects was $1.5 + 1.2°$ (fig. 4). In

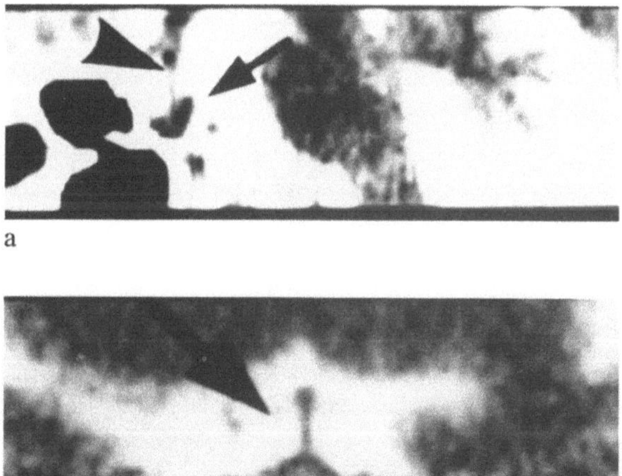

a

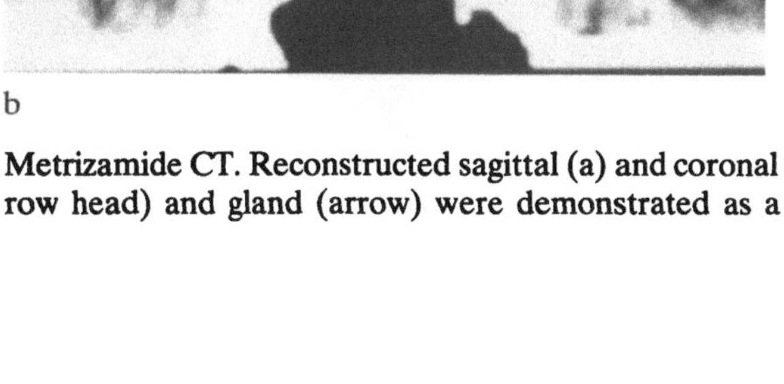

b

Fig. 3 Metrizamide CT. Reconstructed sagittal (a) and coronal (b) views. Pituitary stalk (arrow head) and gland (arrow) were demonstrated as a low density areas.

six patients with microadenoma, the upper surface of the gland on coronal projection was asymmetric and the angle of the inclination of the pituitary stalk increased (fig. 5). Its mean value was $9.3 + 2.4°$. In each case, the stalk was deviated to the side opposite to that on which the microadenoma was found to be located at operation.

Table 1 The detection rate of the pituitary stalk and gland in 189 cases on contrast-enhanced CT and in 28 cases on metrizamide CT

	Horizontal section	Reconstructed Coronal projection	Reconstructed Sagittal projection
CE−CT			
Pituitary Gland	186/189 (98.4%)	185/189 (97.9%)	188/189 (99.5%)
Stalk	186/189 (98.4%)	179/189 (94.2%)	178/189 (93.6%)
Metrizamide CT			
Gland	28/28 (100%)	28/28 (100%)	28/28 (100%)
Stalk	28/28 (100%)	28/28 (100%)	28/28 (100%)

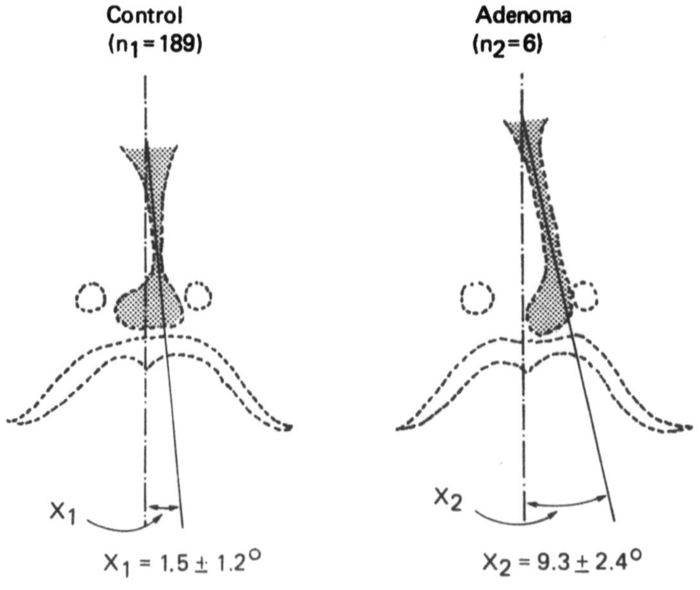

Fig. 4 Inclination of the pituitary stalk.

Correlation between form of pituitary gland and age

The form of the pituitary gland was examined in the reconstructed sagittal projections in the enhanced CT and metrizamide CT and classified into 3 types as follows: type I: an oval gland that filled the whole sella turcica (fig. 6); type II: a gland with an antero-superior intrasellar CSF space (fig. 7); type III: a flattened gland

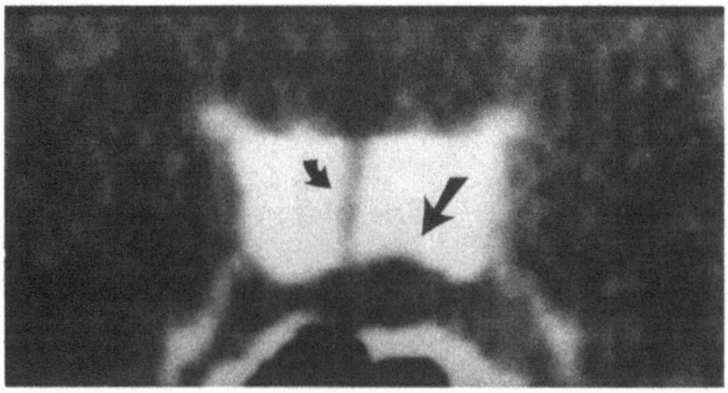

a

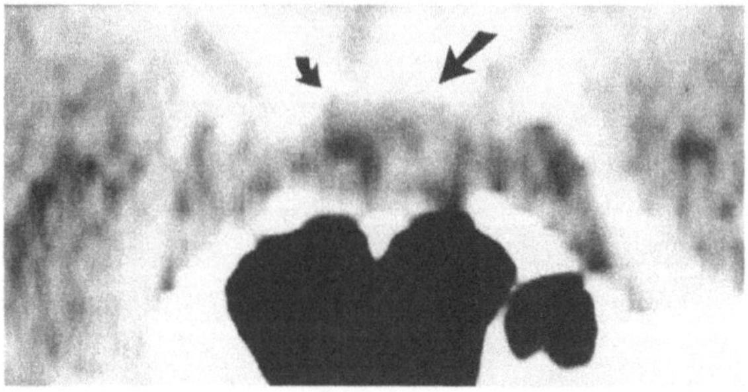

b

Fig. 5 Two cases with prolactinoma on metrizamide CT. A reconstructed coronal view (a) and a high spatial resolution cornal view (b). The upper surface of the gland (large arrow) is asymmetric and the stalk (small arrow) is deviated to the left side.

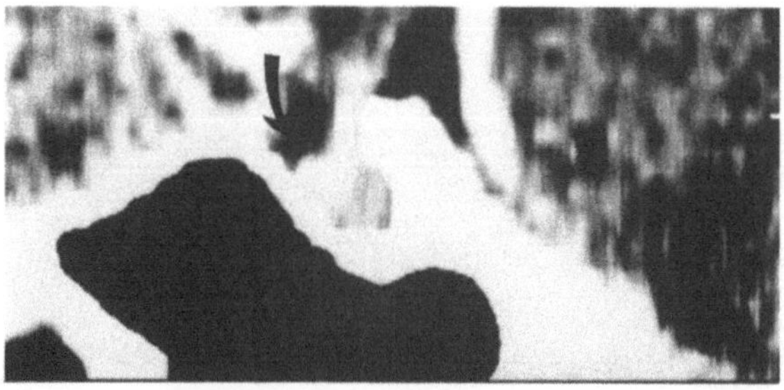

Fig. 6 Sagittal view on contrast-enhanced CT. An oval gland (arrow) filled the whole sella turcica.

localized in the postero-inferior portion of the intrasellar space, with an enlarged CSF space more than half the depth of the sella turcica (fig. 8). Type I was found in 37 out of 189 patients (19.7%). These patients were mainly under the age of 29. Type II was found in 79 patients (42.6%). Type III was seen in 72 patients (38.3%). In 5 out of 6 patients with microadenoma, an oval gland that filled the whole sella turcica was demonstrated. In the remaining patients, type II was shown (fig. 9). It was noteworthy that 29 patients out of 37, who were classified as type I, were under the age of 29 (21 female and 8 male) and that 57 patients out of 72, who were classified as type III, were over the age of 50. The patients who were

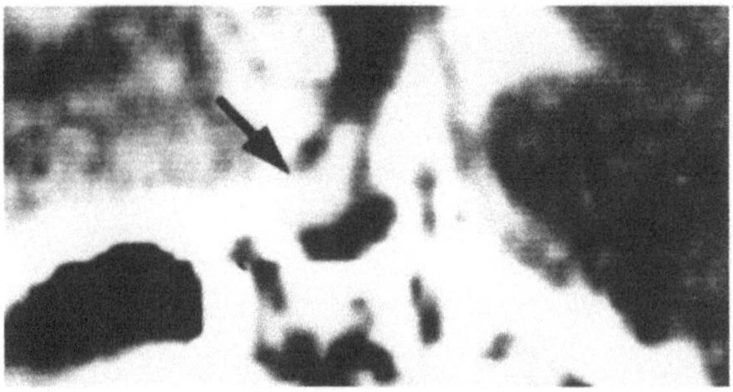

Fig. 7 Metrizamide CT. Metrizamide fills in the antero-superior portion of the intrasellar CSF space.

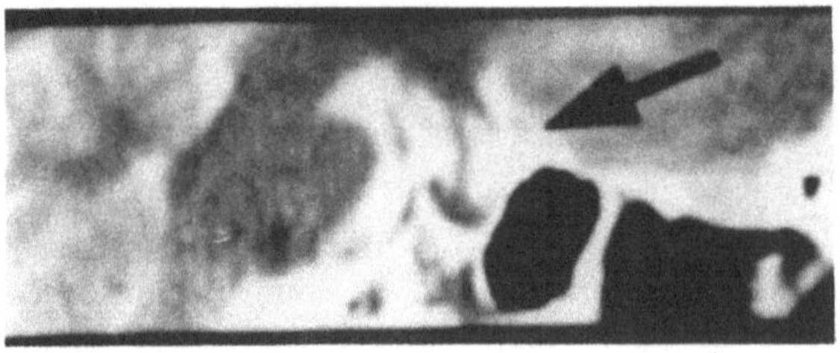

Fig. 8 Metrizamide CT. A flattened gland (arrow) localized in the postero-inferior portion of the intrasellar space.

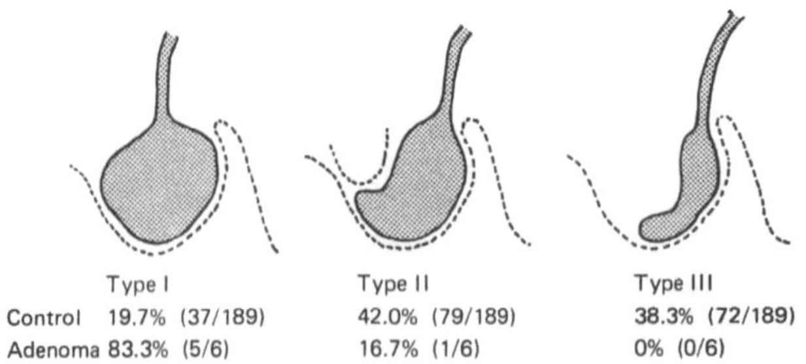

Fig. 9 Classification of the finding on reconstructed sagittal.

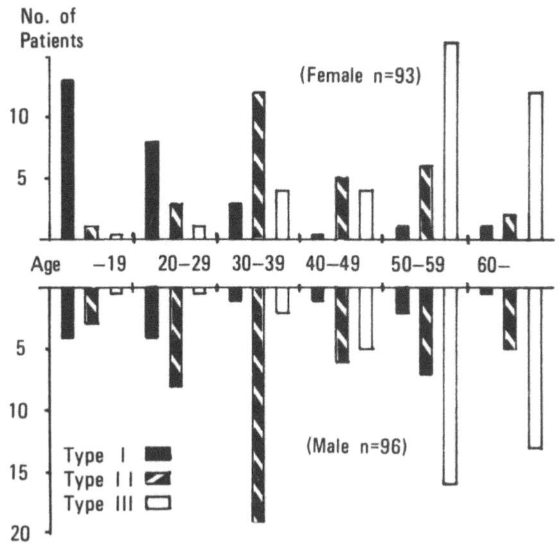

Fig. 10 Correlation between age and form of pituitary gland.

classified as type II were seen at all ages, but especially in the fourth decade (fig. 10).

Discussion

According to the previous reports, pituitary microadenomas in CT studies have frequently been seen as a hyperdense or hyperenhancing mass [3]. Sometimes the microadenoma has been isodense with the pituitary gland or has been hyperdense [4, 5]. The question arises, however, as to whether these enhanced or isodense areas always represent the microadenoma itself. In this study, it was still difficult to distinguish between the normal gland and the area of microadenoma, because most of the normal pituitary glands and stalks in our study were also seen as homogeneously enhanced areas that were very similar to the finding with microadenomas.

The most useful findings which may suppose the existence of microadenoma in the CT were the appearance of the upper surface of the glands and the inclination of the pituitary stalk in the coronal projection [6, 7]. It has been reported that upward displacement of the diaphragma sellae demonstrated in coronal and/or sagittal views in the CT may provide early evidence of an expanding pituitary lesion. In our experience, however, the presence of a convex upper surface of the gland could be seen in normal, especially in younger patients, and did not always indicate that there was a pituitary microadenoma. It was noteworthy that in the patients with *prolactinoma* which were located in the lateral wing of the glands [8], *the upper surface of the gland in the coronal projection had been asymmetric and the angle of inclination of the pituitary stalk had been increased.*

References

[1] Belloni, G., A. Baciocco, P. Borrelli, et. al.: The value of CT for the diagnosis of pituitary microadenoma in children. Neuroradiology **15** (1978) 179–181.
[2] Fukuda, T., Y. Inoue, S. Taniguch: Thin-section CT scan of pituitary gland. Brain Nerve (Tokyo) **34** (1982) 139–144.
[3] Hemminghytt, S., R. K. Kalkhoff, D. L. Daniels, et. al.: Computed tomographic study of hormone-secreting microadenomas. Radiology **146** (1983) 65–69.
[4] Wolpert, S. M., K. D. Post, B. J. Biller, et. al.: The value of computed tomography in evaluating patients with prolactinomas. Radiology **131** (1979) 117–119.
[5] Robertson, H. J., A. Rose, B. Ehmis, et. al.: Trends in the radiological study of pituitary adenoma. Neuroradiology **21** (1981) 75–78.
[6] Svertsen, A., V. M. Haughton, A. L. Williams, et. al.: The computed tomographic appearance of the normal pituitary gland and pituitary microadenomas. Radiology **133** (1979) 385–391.
[7] Sage, M. R., P. C. Blumberg, B. P. Mulligan, et. al.: The diapragma sellae: its relationship to the configuration of the pituitary gland. Radiology **145** (1982) 703–308.
[8] Hardy, J.: Transsphenoidal surgery of hypersecreting pituitary tumors. Excerpta Medeca Int. Congr. Ser. **303** (1973) 179–198.

III Endocrinological and clinical aspects

Actions of dopamine receptor agonists at the pituitary level

E. Flückiger

In 1976 it became firmly established [38] that prolactin secretion from the anterior pituitary of mammals was mainly controlled in an inhibitory mode by dopamine released from the hypothalamus into the portal vessels connecting the median eminence with the anterior lobe of the pituitary. It also became clear that various ergot compounds which inhibit prolactin release do so as agonists at the dopamine receptors of the prolactin cell. These findings agreed with the dopaminomimetic property of certain ergot compounds demonstrated some years earlier at the CNS level [12, 28, 30]. Thus, by 1976 bromocriptine, which had already proven its clinical usefulness to suppress prolactin, to lower GH in some acromegalic patients and to combate symptoms of Parkinsonism, became the standard dopamine receptor agonist [25, 52].

Since then numerous research groups have synthetized and pharmacologically evaluated new chemical structures in order to produce more potent, if possible, more selective dopamine agonists. They contributed many valuable investigational tools for the study of dopamine receptors. As a result today there is a large and still growing choice of dopamine receptor agonists and a bewildering number of dopamine receptor subtypes in the brain and the peripheral tissues. We simplify the issue when in the following we concentrate on the anterior pituitary, especially on the prolactin producing and somatotropin producing cells. A less restricted but short review of ergot compounds and dopaminergic endocrine effects has appeared earlier [24].

Prolactin cells

The prolactin cell responds in vivo and in vitro to nM concentrations of dopamine and dopaminomimetics by attenuation of hormone release and synthesis, accompanied by increased intracellular hormone degradation (see reviews by [13, 20, 25]).

To this general statement there exist a few exceptions: Certain induced and transplantable rat pituitary tumours producing prolactin are not sensitive to dopamine and dopaminomimetics (e.g. [15, 16, 48]).

The dopaminergic effect is mediated by specific binding sites located in the cell membrane fraction of anterior pituitary homogenates [4, 7, 9, 13]. Such binding sites are not found in the dopamine insensitive rat pituitary tumour cell clone 235−1 [17]. The similarly insensitive clone GH_3D_6 lacked high affinity binding sites [15]. On the other hand, cell membranes of the rat pituitary tumour 7315a although dopamine insensitive, had high affinity binding sites [16], indicating that these cells lack an effector. A high degree of correlation between K_i values of various drugs observed with [^{3}H]spiroperidol binding to bovine anterior pituitary membranes and the K_i values similarly obtained using 7315a tumour membranes was found [16], indicating that the physico-chemical nature of the dopaminophilic binding sites on these tumour cells is not different from those of cells of normal pituitaries. Dopaminophilic binding sites on prolactin cells occur in two affinity forms [4, 7, 10]. The K_d values for the high affinity sites of agonists were found to correlate closely with the potencies of the same drugs to inhibit prolactin release in vitro [9, 10]. Human prolactinoma cell membranes did not differ in the K_d values from material of normal human pituitaries [4]. Treating rats chronically with oestrogens did not change the K_d value for the high affinity binding sites, while the K_d value of the low affinity binding sites for [^{3}H]-domperidone was increased together with the number of low affinity binding sites [6].

By anatomic definition the dopamine receptor of the prolactin cell is a post synaptic or post junctional dopamine receptor. Recently a novel dopamine receptor agonist, claimed to be selective for presynaptic dopamine receptors, 3-PPP [2], was unexpectedly found to suppress prolactin serum levels in reserpinized rats dose-dependently, both enantiomers being similarly active [23]. The authors concluded that the dopamine receptor of the prolactin cell is pharmacologically similar to the dopamine autoreceptor of the rat brain. This introduces a novel element to the pharmacological characterization of dopamine receptor subtypes, although the pharmacological characterization of 3-PPP itself is far from clear [42]. An independent piece of evidence that the prolactin cell dopamine receptor may differ from post-synaptic dopamine receptors in the rat brain is the in vitro observation that dihydro-α-ergokryptine is more potent than bromocriptine in inhibiting prolactin release but much less potent in inhibiting [^{3}H]acetylcholine release from rat striatum slices [26]. Very recently another DA autoreceptor selective agonist, DPAI, was also described to lower serum prolactin levels in rats by a direct action [11].

Dopamine binding sites can be made visible by immunocytochemical methods (see [13]). Such studies demonstrated the internalization of binding sites after cluster formation. Possibly this process is responsible for the fact that dopaminophilic binding sites were detected in the cytosol fraction of bovine anterior pituitary homogenates [32, 54], and that dopamine was found in the rat pituitary associated with subcellular particles indistinguishable from prolactin secretory granules. The amount of dopamine in these granules was augmented by pretreating the rats with L-DOPA and reduced after bromocriptine [29].

The biochemical steps which occur between the interaction of a dopaminomimetic with its acceptor in the cell membrane and the final event, i.e. inhibition of hormone secretion, intracellular degradation and attenuated synthesis are still not clear.

As Ca^{2+} is implied in hormone release, a possible way to suppress this could be to attenuate Ca^{2+} influx [20]. But bromocriptine was not found to alter basal or ionophore stimulated Ca^{2+} influx [51], although it inhibited ionophore A 23187 stimulated prolactin release. Thus it must be assumed that the dopamine signal acts through a different mechanism.

After a period of uncertainty it is now agreed that the dopamine signal leads to a reduction in cAMP content of the normal and adenomatous prolactin cell [18, 19, 22, 33, 41]. However, the question whether this reduction in "second messenger" concentration is one of the causes of the inhibition of hormone secretion is not quite settled, although this functional link is much favoured (see [20] for discussion).

Recently, analysis of the link between the dopamine signal and prolactin secretion inhibition was moved one step further by the demonstration [50] that " prolactin secretion may be regulated by a Ca^{2+}-calmodulin dependent process that positively interacts with the cAMP system; the inhibitory action of dopamine seems to be produced by interfering with this system". This also includes phospholipids, such as phosphatidylinositol, phosphorylation of which is reduced by dopamine or bromocriptine [8].

Reduction of cAMP content as the result of dopaminergic stimulation of the prolactin cell may also directly lead to reduced prolactin gene transcription [44, 45].

Rat pituitary cell cultures exposed for 4 days to ergokryptine (between 10^{-11}M and 10^{-8}M), showed dose-dependent and parallel diminution of prolactin synthesis and cAMP concentration [45]. The effect of 10^{-8}M ergokryptine was antagonized dose-dependently by coincubation of cholera toxin or by cAMP analogs. The slowly developing effect on prolactin synthesis was presented by an inhibitory action of ergokryptine on prolactin messenger RNA transcription [44, 46], whose effect was fully established in minutes instead of days, and could also be antagonized by the addition of cAMP. It is probably due to a slow decay of the prolactin messenger RNA that the fast inhibition of its transcription affects prolactin synthesis only with delay. This is in contrast with two other observations which indicate that a faster effect on synthesis may also be possible: dopamine (500 nM) and bromocriptine (2 nM) added to female rat hemipituitaries and incubated for six hours were not only found to reduce prolactin release into the medium but also to diminish the total amount of newly synthetised prolactin [39, 53]. Other dopaminomimetics studied did not show this effect. At present there is no explanation for this fast expression of synthesis inhibition by some but not by other dopanimomimetics.

Prolonged treatment of mice with bromocriptine produced a reduction in pituitary prolactin content and concentration [55, 56]. In male rats continuously treated with oestrogens to stimulate prolactin cells, dopaminomimetics reduced serum prolactin levels, diminished nuclear diameters, DNA synthesis and depressed mitotic activity in the pituitary [21, 31, 37, 53]. This indicates that continued dopaminergic stimulation of prolactin cells may lead to an attenuation of cell metabolism and mitotic processes. Although the link between the acutely observed biochemical changes induced by dopaminergic stimulation of prolactin cells and the longterm sequelae have not yet been elucidated, it is of interest to note that in human prolactinoma cellular changes in the same directions have also been observed. Thus, reduction in cell size, composed of shrinkage of nuclear size and of cytoplasmatic cross area, have been demonstrated [3, 34, 49].

Somatotropin (GH) producing cells

Although normal subjects do not respond to dopaminomimetics with lowering GH serum levels, certain acromegalic patients respond to dopamine, L-DOPA or dopaminomimetic drugs like bromocriptine by a decrease [36]. This effect is in many patients therapeutically relevant [52]. In vitro studies showed this effect to be a direct one at the level of the GH producing adenoma cell [43]. Pure GH secreting adenoma cells had less [^{3}H]-apomorphine binding sites than prolactinoma cells, and did not show specific [^{3}H]-domperidone binding [5]. Lack of [^{3}H]-spiroperidol binding to pure GH adenoma membranes had also been noted earlier [14]. Thus, GH adenoma cells seem to differ from prolactin secreting adenoma cells with respect to the nature of their dopaminophilic binding sites.

Several reports indicate that in vitro the normal human anterior pituitary also responds to dopaminergic agents with reduced GH secretion [1, 35, 40], in contrast to what is observed in vivo. Thus, in vivo this sensitivity to dopaminomimetics is successfully overridden by non-dopaminergic hypothalamic factors. In the rat in vivo bromocriptine did not influence GH [21, 57]. In in vitro experiments with dissociated rat anterior pituitary cells dopamine, apomorphine, bromocriptine and a number of other dopaminomimetics in concentrations up to 10^{-6}M did not lower GH secretion (R. Marbach and R. Haller, unpublished results), indicating a basic difference between normal human and rat GH producing pituitary cells.

Other dopamine sensitive anterior pituitary cells

As some patients with Cushing's disease or with Nelson's syndrome respond to bromocriptine with a lowering of adrenocorticotropin (ACTH) serum levels, it is of interest to note that in one in vitro study of such human adenoma cells inhibition of ACTH secretion by dopaminergic stimulation could be demonstrated [1].

Although of little relevance in a discussion of pituitary adenomas it should be mentioned here that rat thyrotropin (TSH) producing cells may also show dopaminergic inhibition, at least under static conditions [27], while under dynamic conditions (perifused cells) no such effect was found [47]. This discrepancy in the results of the two careful studies is very puzzling.

Summary

The actions of dopamine receptor agonists at the pituitary level are described and discussed using mainly data concerning prolactin and somatotropin producing cells. These two cell types contribute in an important way to the formation of pituitary adenomas in man.

Dopamine receptor subtyping is still in progress. Linking the dopamine signal to biochemical intracellular events has been especially studied with respect to prolactin regulation. Recent progress in the field is presented.

Important clinical phenomena, such as the rapid shrinkage and reexpansion of prolactinoma volume in response to dopaminomimetic treatment or its withdrawal are still not satisfactorily explained.

References

[1] Adams, E. F., I. E. Brajkovich, K. Mashiter: Growth hormone and prolactin secretion by dispersed cell cultures of a normal human pituitary: effects of thyrotropin releasing hormone, theophylline, somatostatin and 2-Br-α-ergokryptine. Acta Endocrinol (Kbh.) **98** (1981) 345–351.

[2] Arnt, J., A. V. Christensen, J. Hytel, et. al.: Effects of putative dopamine receptor agonists in pharmacological models related to dopaminergic and neuroleptic activity. Eur. J. Pharmacol. **86** (1983) 185–198.

[3] Bassetti, M., A. Spada, G. Pezzo, et. al.: Bromocriptine treatment reduces the cell size in human macroprolactinomas: A morphometric study. J. Clin. Endocrinol. Metab. **58** (1984) 2268–2273.

[4] Bression, D., A. M. Brandi, M. P. Martres, et. al.: Dopaminergic receptors in human prolactin secreting adenomas: a quantitative study. J. Clin. Endocrinol. Metab. **51** (1980) 1037–1043.

[5] Bression, D., A. M. Brandi, A. Nousbaum, et. al.: Evidence of dopamine receptors in human growth hormone (GH)-secreting adenomas with concomitant study of dopamine inhibition of GH secretion in a perifused system. J. Clin. Endocrinol. Metab. **55** (1982) 589–593.

[6] Bression, D., A. M. Brandi, M. LeDafniet, et. al.: Modifications of the high and low affinity pituitary domperidone-binding sites in chronic estrogenized rats. Endocrinology **113** (1983) 1799–1805.

[7] Calabro, M. A., R. M. MacLeod: Binding of dopamine to bovine anterior pituitary gland membranes. Neuroendocrinology **25** (1978) 32–46.
[8] Canonico, P. L., R. M. MacLeod: The role of phospholipids in hormonal secretory mechanisms. In: Neuroendocrine Perspectives, Vol. 2 (E. E. Müller, R. M. MacLeod, eds.), p. 123. Elsevier, Amsterdam 1983.
[9] Caron, G. M., M. Beaulieu, V. Raymond, et. al.: Dopaminergic receptors in the anterior pituitary gland. J. Biol. Chem. **253** (1978) 2244–2253.
[10] Caron, M. G., B. F. Kilpatrick, A. DeLean: The dopamine receptor of the anterior pituitary gland. In: Dopamine Receptors (C. Kaiser, J. W. Kebabian, eds.), p. 73. American Chemical Society, Washington, D.C., 1983.
[11] Clemens, J. A., R. W. Fuller, L. A. Phebus, et. al.: Stimulation of presynaptic dopamine autoreceptors by 4-(2-Di-N-Propylaminoethyl) indole (DPAI). Life Sci. **34** (1984) 1015–1022.
[12] Corrodi, H., K. Fuxe, T. Hökfelt, et. al.: Effect of ergot drugs on central catecholamine neurons: Evidence for a stimulation of central dopamine neurons. J. Pharm. Pharmacol. **25** (1973) 409–411.
[13] Cronin, M. J.: The role and direct measurement of the dopamine receptor(s) in the anterior pituitary. In: Neuroendocrine Perspectives, Vol. 1 (E. E. Müller, R. M. MacLeod, eds.), p. 169. Elsevier Biomedical Press, Amsterdam 1982.
[14] Cronin, M. J., C. Y. Cheung, C. B. Wilson, et. al.: [^{3}H]-spiperone binding to human anterior pituitaries and pituitary adenomas secreting prolactin, growth hormone, and adrenocortical hormone. J. Clin. Endocrinol. Metab. **50** (1982a) 387–391.
[15] Cronin, J. M. N. Faure, N., J. A. Martial, et. al.: Absence of high affinity dopamine receptors in GH_3 cells: a prolactin secreting clone resistant to the inhibitory action of dopamine. Endocrinology **106** (1980b) 718–706.
[16] Cronin, M. J., C. A. Valdenegro, S. N. Perkins, et al.: The 715a pituitary tumor is refractory to dopaminergic inhibition of prolactin release but contains dopamine receptors. Endocrinology **109** (1981) 2160–2166.
[17] Cronin, M. J., S. N. Perkins, D. A. Keffer, et. al.: Failure of dopamine and bromocriptine to affect prolactin release and cell growth in the dopamine-receptor deficient 235–1 clone. Mol. Cell. Endocrinol. **28** (1982) 229–246.
[18] Cronon, M. J., M. O. Thorner: Dopamine inhibits adenylate cyclase in human prolactin-secreting pituitary adenomas. Nature **278** (1982) 252–254.
[19] Cronin, M. J., G. A. Myers, R. M. MacLeod, et. al.: Pertussis toxin uncouples dopamine agonist inhibition of prolactin release. Am. J. Physiol. **244** (Endocrinol. Metab. 7) (1983) E499–E504.
[20] Dannies, P. S., S. W. Tam: Mechanism of regulation of prolactin release. In: Cellular Regulation of Secretion and Release (P. M. Conn, ed.), p. 529. Academic Press, New York 1982.
[21] Davies, C., J. M. Jacobi, H. M. Lloyds, et. al.: DNA synthesis and the secretion of prolactin and growth hormone by the pituitary gland of the male rat. J. Endocrinol. **61** (1974) 411–417.
[22] DeCamilli, P., D. Macconi, A. Spada: Dopamine inhibits adenylate cyclase in human prolactin-secreting pituitary adenomas. Nature **278** (1979) 252–254.
[23] Eriksson, E., K. Modigh, A. Carlsson, et. al.: Dopamine receptors involved in prolactin secretion pharmacologically characterized by means of 3-PPP enantiomers. Eur. J. Pharmacol. **96** (1983) 29–36.
[24] Flückiger, E.: Interactions of ergot compounds with dopamine receptors and endocrine functions. J. Neural Transm. Suppl. **18** (1983) 189–204.

[25] Flückiger, E., E. del Pozo, K. von Werder: Prolactin, Physiology, Pharmacology and Clinical Findings. Monographs on Endocrinology, Vol. 23. Springer-Verlag, Berlin–Heidelberg–New York (1982).
[26] Flückiger, E., R. Markstein: Receptor Pharmacology of ergot compounds. In: Prolactin and Prolactinomas (G. Tolis, eds.), p. 105. Raven Press, New York 1983.
[27] Foord, S. M., J. R. Peters, C. Dieguez, et. al.: Dopamine receptors on intact anterior pituitary cells in culture: Functional association with the inhibition of prolactin and thyrotropin, Endocrinology **112** (1983) 1567–1577.
[28] Fuxe, K., T. Hökfelt: Central monoaminergic systems and hypothalamic function. In: The Hypothalamus (L. Martini, M. Motta, F. Fraschini, eds.), p. 123. Academic Press, New York 1970.
[29] Gudelsky, G. A., D. D. Nansel, J. C. Porter: Uptake and processing of dopamine by cells of the anterior pituitary gland. Endocrinology **107** (1980) 30–34.
[30] Hökfelt, T., K. Fuxe: On the morphology and the neuroendocrine role of the hypothalamic catecholamine neurones. In: Brain-Endocrine Interactions. Median Eminence: Structure and Function (K. M. Knigge, E. E. Scott, A. Weindl, eds.), p. 181. Karger, Basel 1972.
[31] Jacobi, J. M., H. M. Lloyd, J. D. Meares: Nuclear diameter in the anterior pituitary gland of the rat: Effects of estrogen, bromocriptine, and haloperidol. J. Histochem. Cytochem. **30** (1982) 677–681.
[32] Kerdelhue, B., A. S. Weisman, R. I. Weiner: A dopaminergic binding site in the high speed supernatant of steer anterior pituitary homogenates. Endocrinology **109** (1981) 307–309.
[33] Labrie, F., P. Borgeat, J. Drouin, et. al.: The role of cyclic nucleotides in the control of anterior pituitary gland activity. In: Cyclic Nucleotides II (J. W. Kebabian, J. A. Nathanson, eds.), p. 525. Springer-Verlag, Berlin–Heidelberg–New York 1982.
[34] Landolt, A. M., H. Minder, V. Osterwalder, et. al.: Bromocriptine reduces the size of cells in prolactin-secreting pituitary adenomas. Experientia **39** (1983) 625–626.
[35] Lawton, N. F., A. J. Evans, R. O. Weller: Dopaminergic inhibition of growth hormone and prolactin release during continuous in vitro perifusion of normal and adenomatous human pituitary. J. Neurol. Sci. **49** (1981) 229–239.
[36] Liuzzi, A., P. G. Chiodini, L. Botalla, et. al.: Decreased plasma growth hormone (9h) levels in acromeglics following CB 154 administration. J. Clin. Endocrinol. Metab. **38** (1974) 910–912.
[37] Lloyd, H. M., J. D. Meares, J. Jacobi: Effects of oestrogen and bromocriptine on in vivo.
[38] MacLeod, R. M.: Regulation of prolactin secretion. In: Frontiers in Neuroendocrinology, Vol. VI (L. Martini, W. F. Ganong, eds.), p. 169. Raven Press, New York 1976.
[39] MacLeod, R. M., I. Nagy, I. S. Login, et. al.: The roles of dopamine, cAMP, and calcium in prolactin secretion. In: Central and Peripheral Regulation of Prolactin (R. M. MacLeod, U. Scapagnini, eds.), p. 27. Raven Press, New York 1980.
[40] Marcovitz, S., C. G. Goodyear, H. Guyda, et. al.: Comparative study of human fetal, normal adult, and somatotropic pituitary function in tissue culture. J. Clin. Endocrinol. Metab. **54** (1982) 6–16.
[41] Markstein, R., P. Herrling, H. Wagner: Bromocriptine mimics dopamine effects on the cyclic-AMP system of the rat pituitary gland. In: Proc. 7th Internat. Congress on Pharmacology (J. R. Boissier, P. Lechat, eds.), p. 848, Abstract No. 26–23. Pergamon Press, Oxford–Paris 1978.
[42] Markstein, R., D. Lahaye: In vitro effect of the racemic mixture and the (−)enantiomer of N-n-propyl-3-(3-hydroxyphenyl)-piperidine (3-PPP) on postsynaptic dopa-

mine receptors and on a presynaptic dopamine autoreceptor. J. Neural Transm. **558** (1983) 43–53.
[43] Mashiter, K., E. Adams, M. Beard, et. al.: Bromocriptine inhibits prolactin and growth hormone release by human pituitary tumours in culture. Lancet **II** (1977) 197–198.
[44] Maurer, R. A.: Transcriptional regulation of the prolactin gene by ergocryptine and cyclic AMP. Nature **294** (1981) 94–97.
[45] Maurer, R. A.: Regulation of prolactin gene expression. In: Cellular Regulation of Secretion and Release (P. M. Conn, ed.), p. 267. Academic Press, New York 1982a.
[46] Maurer, R. A.: Adenosine 3′, 5′-monophosphate derivatives increase prolactin synthesis and prolactin messenger ribonucleic acid levels in ergocryptine-treated pituitary cells. Endocrinology **110** (1982b) 1957–1963.
[47] Price, S. M., J. R. Peters, C. Dieguez, et. al.: Dopamine receptors on intact anterior pituitary cells in culture: Functional associate with the inhibition of prolactin and thyrotropin. Endocrinology **112** (1983) 1567–1577.
[48] Prysor-Jones, R. A., J. S. Jenkins: Effect of bromocriptine, ergotamine and other ergot alkaloids on the hormone secretion and growth of a rat pituitary tumor. J. Endocr. **86** (1980) 147–153.
[49] Rengachary, S. S., T. Tomita, B. F. Jefferies, et. al.: Structural changes in human pituitary tumor after bromocriptine therapy. Neurosurgery **10** (1982) 242–251.
[50] Schettini, G., M. J. Cronin, R. M. MacLeod: Adenosine 3′,5′-monophosphate (cAMP) and calcium-calmodulin interrelation in the control of prolactin secretion: Evidence for dopamine inhibition of cAMP accumulation and prolactin release after calcium mobilization. Endocrinology **112** (1983) 1801–1807).
[51] Tam, S. W., P. S. Dannies: Dopaminergic inhibition of ionophore A23-187-stimulated release of prolactin. Fed. Proc. **39** (1980) 553.
[52] Thorner, M. O., E. Flückiger, D. B. Calne: Bromocriptine, A Clinical and Pharmacological Review. Raven Press, New York 1980.
[53] Thorner, M. O., J. A. Burdman, M. T. Calabrese, et. al.: Dopamine agonists and prolactinomas: clinical and basic considerations of the mechanism of action. In: Lisuride and Other Dopamine Agonists (D. B. Calne, et. al., eds.), p. 213. Raven Press, New York 1983.
[54] Weiner, R. I., J. E. Beach, B. Kerdelhue: Characterization of anterior pituitary membrane and cytosol dopamine receptors. In: Apomorphine and Other Dopaminomimetics, Vol. 2: Clinical Pharmacology (G. H. Corsini, G. I. Gessa, eds.), p. 187. Raven Press, New York 1981.
[55] Yanai, R., H. Nagasawa: Suppression of mammary hyperplastic nodule formation and pituitary prolactin secretion in mice induced by ergocornine and 2-Br-α-ergocryptine. J. Nat. Cancer Inst. **45** (1970a) 1105–1112.
[56] Yanai, R., H. Nagasawa: Effects of ergocornine and 2-Br-α-ergocryptine (CB 154) on the formation of mammary hyperplastic alveolar nodules and the pituitary prolactin levels in mice. Experientia **26** (1970b) 649–650.
[57] Yanai, R., H. Nagasawa (1974): Effect of 2-Br-α-ergokryptine on pituitary synthesis and release of prolactin and growth hormone in rats. Horm. Res. **5** (1974) 1–5.

Dopamine and prolactinomas*

G. Faglia, A. Spada, P. Moriondo, G. Giannattasio, R. Elli, R. C. Scaperrotta, M. Nissim

Introduction

Over the past few years, the possible pathogenetic events promoting the development of prolactinomas have been extensively investigated and debated. As dopamine (DA) is considered the major factor regulating prolactin (PRL) secretion by inhibiting its synthesis and release, particular attention has been payed to possible alterations in the dopaminergic control of PRL secretion in prolactinomas.

On this line, it was proposed that a defective central dopaminergic tone could result in lactotrophic hyperplasia progressing to pituitary tumour [1–3]. This "hypothalamic" hypothesis was opposed to the " pituitary" hypothesis of an autonomous adenohypophyseal hyperfunction.

In this chapter the current concepts and our own contributions regarding the role of DA in the pathogenesis of prolactinomas will be briefly reviewed and discussed.

Evidence for DA defect

In 1978 Fine and Frohman [1] reported that a pharmacological manipulation which selectively enhances the central dopaminergic tone was unable to suppress serum PRL levels in patients affected with prolactinomas. Patients and controls were given L-dopa after pre treatment with carbidopa, the peripheral inhibitor of L-dopa conversion into DA. As L-dopa, but not carbidopa, easily crosses the blood-brain barrier, this manoeuvre results in a selective activation of the central DA followed by a marked decrease in serum PRL levels in normal controls, but not in patients with prolactinomas. This was interpreted to reflect a defective dopaminergic neurotransmission. The same interpretation was given to the lack of PRL suppression after the administration of indirect dopaminergic agents, such as no-

* This work was supported in part by Ministero della Pubblica Istruzione and Consiglio Nazionale della Ricerche (Roma), grant no.: 83.02574.04.115.04912.

mifensine [2, 4], which increases DA release at the presynaptic receptor sites of DA neurons.

In our hands, although a wide variability of responses was observed in individual patients [5], L-dopa administration after carbidopa pretreatment (50 mg carbidopa every 6 hrs for 4 doses followed by 100 mg L-dopa + 35 mg carbidopa) or nomifensine (200 mg) induced a significantly less pronounced decrease in the serum PRL levels in patients with prolactinomas than in normal controls (tab. 1).

Table 1 Effects of different pharmacological manipulations on serum PRL in normal women and in patients with prolactinomas

Treatment	Serum PRL, Δ% ± SE over baseline		
	Controls (n)	Patients (n)	p
Dopamine	−60.8 ± 3.5 (5)	−44.2 ± 41.0 (16)	<0.05
L-dopa + carbidopa	−77.6 ± 4.2 (6)	−35.4 ± 5.3 (12)	<0.005
Nomifensine	−61.3 ± 6.2 (10)	−17.4 ± 6.1 (20)	<0.005
Domperidone	+1220.5 ± 9.5 (8)	+50.0 ± 6.4 (32)	<0.001
Metoclopramide	+1100.5 ± 8.9 (6)	+50.5 ± 5.6 (17)	<0.001
Sulpiride	+715.4 ± 9.2 (10)	+23.6 ± 5.1 (9)[a]	<0.001
Sulpiride during DA infusion	–	+142.3 ± 12.0 (9)[b]	<0.05*

The drugs were administered at the following doses: Dopamine, 0.06 μg/Kg/min for 180 min; Carbidopa, 50 mg every 6 h for 4 doses followed by 35 mg + L-dopa 100 mg; Nomifensine, 200 mg orally; Domperidone, 10 mg i.v.; Metoclopramide, 10 mg i.v.; Sulpiride, 100 mg i.m.; Dopamine, 4 μg/Kg/min for 180 min + Sulpiride, 100 mg i.m. at 120 min.

* a *vs* b.

Also in favour of a central DA defect was the finding that patients with prolactinomas showed an impaired PRL responsiveness to DA receptor blockers, such as sulpiride, metoclopramide or domperidone [6, 7, 8], which was partially restored after DA pre infusion [6, 9] (tab. 1).

Taken together, the above data were consistent with the hypothesis of a defective central dopaminergic activity in prolactinomas.

Evidence against DA defect

The investigation of pituitary hormones under DA inhibitory control other than PRL, such as thyrotropin (TSH) and luteinizing hormone (LH) has recently provided considerable evidence against the hypothesis of a central DA defect.

The administration of DA receptor blockers, such as metoclopramide or domperidone, induced greater serum TSH [10] and LH [11] increases in patients with prolactinomas than in normal controls.

These exaggerated responses are suggestive of an increased hypothalamic DA activity probably reactive to hyperprolactinaemia.

The exaggerated TSH response to dopaminergic disinhibition occurs both in macro- and in microprolactinomas (tab. 2). In fact, the TSH net incremental area under the curve (nAUC) after the administration of the dopaminergic blocker metoclopramide (10 mg i. v.) was significantly greater in 8 microadenomas and in 6 macroadenomas than in normal controls, without any difference between the two groups of patients with prolactinomas. On the contrary, serum PRL increase, though defective in all patients, was more severely impaired in macroprolactinomas (macroprolactinomas, PRL $\Delta\% \pm SE: 15.6 \pm 4.8$, microprolactinomas, PRL$\Delta\% \pm SE: 60.1 \pm 5.8$; $p<0.05$). These data suggest that the residual normal pituitary tissue is still receiving DA from the hypothalamus irrespective of the adenoma size, while the amount of DA reaching the adenomatous lactotrophs is probably smaller in macroadenomas.

Table 2 Effect of L-dopa + carbidopa on TSH response to metoclopramide in normal women, compared with the effect of metoclopramide alone in patients with micro- or macroprolactinomas

Treatment	TSH net AUC μU/ml/60 min		
	Normal women (5)	Micro-prolactinomas (8)	Macro-prolactinomas (6)
Metoclopramide	30.9 ± 3.8[a]	91.2 ± 22.8[c]	79.0 ± 30.7[d]
Metoclopramide after L-dopa + Carbidopa	70.3 ± 16.7[b]	143.0 ± 31.4	–

Metoclopramide (10 mg i.v.) was administered alone, or after oral administration of L-dopa 100 mg in Carbidopa pretreated subjects (50 mg every 6 h for 4 doses + 35 mg with L-dopa).

p values: a *vs* b <0.001 b *vs* c N.S.
a *vs* c <0.001 b *vs* d N.S.
a *vs* d <0.001 c *vs* d N.S.

The hypothesis of an increased central dopaminergic activity is also supported by the finding that the administration of L-dopa + carbidopa to normal women was able to increase the serum TSH response to metoclopramide from 30.9 ± 3.8 to 70.3 ± 16.7 nAUC uU/ml/60 min, a value not statistically different from that observed in women with prolactinomas (tab. 2).

The investigation of LH secretion revealed that the central dopaminergic tone is not diminished in patients with prolactinomas. The administration of L-dopa + carbidopa to 8 women with prolactinomas caused a serum LH decrease similar to that observed in normal controls (tab. 3) suggesting that the enhancement of DA neurotransmission was unaffected in patients with prolactinomas.

Further evidence against the hypothesis of a central catecholaminergic defect has been recently given by Dallabonzana et. al. [12] who observed that nomifensine administration was able to increase serum growth hormone (GH) levels in patients

Table 3 Effects of L-dopa + Carbidopa or Dopamine on serum LH in normal women and in patients with prolactinomas

Treatment	Serum LH, Δ% over baseline		p
	Controls (n)	Prolactinomas (n)	
L-dopa + Carbidopa	−28.0 ± 4.3 (6)	−22.0 ± 6.3 (8)	N.S.
Dopamine	−19.6 ± 9.8 (4)	−18.5 ± 7.4 (8)	N.S.

L-dopa + Carbidopa (see tab. 1), Dopamine, 0.06 μg/Kg/min.

with prolactinomas. As nomifensine activates catecholaminergic neurotransmission at the central level [13], it is likely that the GH increase might reflect the ability of the hypothalamus to release DA.

It is difficult to explain the apparently conflicting data suggesting a DA defect on one hand and normal or even increased central dopaminergic tone on the other hand, unless assuming that either a primary hyposensitivity of tumorous lactotrophs to DA, or a defect in microcirculation preventing DA from reaching the adenomatous cells, do exist [14].

DA-sensitivity of prolactinomas

Although a persistent sensitivity of prolactinomas to DA is suggested by the findings that the administration of dopaminergic agents is able to suppress PRL secretion in most adenomas, it is well known that there is a wide spectrum of sensitivity to such agents irrespectively of basal PRL levels and tumour size. In our experience, chronic administration of relatively high doses of bromocriptine up to 25 mg/day was unable to fully normalize serum PRL in 26 out of 117 prolactinomas, in agreement with previous reports [15, 16].

A more accurate evaluation of the sensitivity of tumorous lactotrophs to DA was carried out studying the *in vivo* and *in vitro* effects of DA, at concentrations in the physiological range, on PRL release. The infusion of 0.06 μg/Kg/min DA was effective in reducing serum PRL in all the patients tested, though the inhibition was less pronounced than in normal controls (tab. 1: Δ% PRL: −44.2% ± 4.1 in 16 prolactinomas *vs* −60.8% ± 3.5 in normal controls; $p < 0.05$).

Moreover, previous studies [17] we performed in 14 patients with PRL secreting pituitary tumours (6 macro- and 8 microadenomas) demonstrated that the infusion of 4 μg/Kg/min DA was able to suppress homogeneously serum PRL by 76.3% (range 60–89%). Decreasing progressively the DA infusion rates a great variability of sensitivity to DA was observed. At the DA infusion rates of 0.5, 0.125, 0.06, and 0.01 μg/Kg/min, a PRL suppression of more than 50% with respect to the basal values was recorded in 12, 6, 3 and 1 patients, respectively.

These data, suggestive of a reduced lactotroph sensitivity to DA in PRL secreting adenomas, are in agreement with those previously reported by Bansal et. al. [18], Spelta et al. [16], and Serri et al. [19]. Bansal et al. [18] observed that the greatest decrement in serum PRL levels occurred at the DA infusion rate of 1 μg/Kg/min in normal controls, while in hyperprolactinaemic patients the maximal decrement was recorded at the DA infusion rate of 4 μg/Kg/min. Spelta et al. [16] and Serri at al. [19] described a significantly smaller PRL inhibition in prolactinomas than in normal controls at the DA infusion rates of 0.04 and 0.02 μg/Kg/min, respectively.

In this respect the interpretation of the results obtained by L-dopa + carbidopa administration according to Fine and Frohman [1] should be reconsidered. In fact in our hands this pharmacological manipulation induced in 12 prolactinomas a PRL suppression of 35.4 ± 5.3% which was significantly smaller than in normal women (77.6 ± 4.2% $p < 0.005$), while the LH inhibition was similar in the two groups (Δ% LH, prolactinomas: −22.0% ± 5.3; controls −28% ± 4.3; p N.S.) (tabs. 1 and 3) and superimposable to that observed during 0.06 μg/Kg/min DA infusion.

These results suggest that patients with prolactinomas are still able to increase DA release following L-dopa + carbidopa in adequate amount, but their PRL suppression is not normal because of a reduced sensitivity to DA.

The *in vitro* secretion studies [20], carried out on cultured tissue fragments from 15 prolactinomas (6 macro- and 9 micro-adenomas) demonstrated a very wide range of PRL suppressibility to DA. The analysis of the data revealed a strict correlation between PRL suppressibility and the tumour size. In fact, at a given DA concentration (5×10^{-7}M) the percent inhibition of PRL release was significantly higher in macro- than in micro-prolactinomas (72.0% ± 4.8 *vs* 20.3% ± 8.8; $p < 0.002$). The dose response curves of DA on PRL release indicated that the different degrees of responsiveness of the two types of tumours can be primarily ascribed to the different ED_{50}s for DA (5×10^{-8}M in macro- and 8×10^{-7}M in microprolactinomas) (tab. 4). These data, indicating a low sensitivity of microprolactinomas to DA might reflect either a defect in DA receptor number and/or affinity, or a post-receptorial disturbance.

Table 4 *In vitro* PRL release from human prolactinomas in basal conditions and after DA

Prolactinomas	PRL release µg/mg protein/30 min	PRL release % inhibition		
	Baseline	DA concentration		
		10^{-8}	10^{-7}	10^{-6} M
Macroadenomas				
Mean ± SE	4.7 ± 1.3	20.3 ± 8.0	60.0 ± 5.1	79.6 ± 7.4
Range	1.6 – 15.0	(10.2 – 26.2)	(55.1 – 64.0)	(78.0 – 85.2)
Microadenomas				
Mean ± SE	1.4 ± 0.4	10.3 ± 2.7	15.0 ± 3.0	57.6 ± 6.0
Range	0.1 ± 4.7	(9.8 – 11.0)	(9.2 – 20.0)	(38.2 – 79.2)

Defect in microcirculation

As it is conceivable that the DA receptor is modulated by the amount of neurohormone reaching the lactotrophs, the different sensitivity to DA in prolactinomas might reflect alterations in the blood supply progressing along with the tumour growth. In this respect, the morphological characteristics of the microvasculature of prolactinomas might be of great interest.

From preliminary observations, the frequency of capillaries in prolactinomas was much higher (about 9-fold) in micro- than in macroprolactinomas (tab. 5). This finding can be explained if one assumes that the growth rate of the capillaries in these adenomas is very low and cannot keep up with the parenchymal cell growing rate. The different frequency of capillaries in micro- and macroadenomas could have important consequences as to the regulation of PRL secretion. In fact, the low frequency of capillaries in macroprolactinomas might explain the existence of a DA defect at the lactotroph level in spite of a normal or even increased central DA

Table 5 Frequency of capillaries in micro- and macroprolactinomas

Prolactinomas	n	Capillaries/0.1 mm² tissue section
Macroadenomas	(3)	
Mean		5.0
Range		(1 – 11)
Microadenomas	(4)	
Mean		45.5
Range		(35 – 59)*

* $p < 0.001$

tone. Moreover, the differences in blood supply might play a role in the modulation of DA receptors in the two types of tumour.

Conclusions

Evidence is accumulating that:

1. In contrast with the "hypothalamic" hypothesis that a central DA defect is the leading event in the pathogenesis of prolactinomas, the central dopaminergic activity is not impaired but even increased in patients with PRL secreting tumours.
2. Tumoral lactotrophs are hyposensitive to DA.
3. Alterations in intra-tumoral microcirculation have been documented. In particular, a significant difference exists in the frequency of capillaries which appear much higher in micro- than in macroprolactinomas.

References

[1] Fine, S. A., L. A. Frohman: Loss of central nervous system component of dopaminergic inhibition of prolactin secretion in patients with prolactin-secreting pituitary tumors, J. Clin. Invest. **61** (1978) 973–980.

[2] Müller, E. E., A. R. Genazzani, S. Murru: Nomifensine: Diagnostic test in hyperprolactinemic states. J. Clin. Endocrinol. Metab. **47** (1978) 1352–1357.

[3] Van Loon, G. R.: A defect in catecholamine neurons in patients with prolactin-secreting pituitary adenoma. Lancet **2** (1978) 868–871.

[4] Camanni, F., A. R. Genazzani, F. Massara, et. al.: Prolactin responsiveness to nomifensine in patients with hyperprolactinemia of tumorous or uncertain etiology. J. Clin. Endocrinol. Metab. **51** (1980) 650–653.

[5] Moriondo, P., P. Travaglini, M. Nissim, et. al.: Evaluation of two inhibitory tests (nomifensine and L-dopa + carbidopa) for the diagnosis of hyperprolactinemic states. Clin. Endocrinol. (Oxf) **13** (1980) 525–533.

[6] Faglia, G., P. Moriondo, P. Beck-Peccoz, et. al.: Use of neuroactive drugs and hypothalamic regulatory hormones in the diagnosis of hyperprolactinemic states. In: Neuroactive Drugs in Endocrinology (E. E. Müller, ed.), pp. 263–278. Elsevier/North-Holland, Amsterdam 1980.

[7] Barbarino, A., L. De Marinis, E. Menini et. al.: Prolactin-secreting pituitary adenomas: Prolactin dynamics before and after transsphenoidal surgery. Acta Endocrinol. (Kbh) **91** (1979) 397–409.

[8] Camanni, F., A. R. Genazzani, F. Massara, et. al.: Prolactin-releasing effect of domperidone in normoprolactinemic and hyperprolactinemic subjects. Neuroendocrinology **30** (1980) 2–6.

[9] Crosignani, P. G., E. Reschini, M. Peracchi, et. al.: Failure of dopamine infusion to suppress the plasma prolactin response to sulpiride in normal and hyperprolactinemic states. J. Clin. Endocrinol. Metab. **45** (1977) 841–844.

[10] Scanlon, M. F., M. D. Rodriguez-Arnao, A. M. McGregor, et. al.: Altered dopaminergic regulation of thyrotropin release in patients with prolactinomas: Comparison with other tests of hypothalamic-pituitary function. Clin. Endocrinol. (Oxf) **14** (1981) 133–143.

[11] Quigley, M. E., S. J. Judd, G. B. Gilliland, et. al.: Functional studies of dopamine control of prolactin secretion in normal women and women with hyperprolactinemic pituitary microadenomas. J. Clin. Endocrinol. Metab. **50** (1980) 994–999.
[12] Dallabonzana, D., B. Spelta, L. Botalla et. al.: Effects of nomifensine on growth hormone and prolactin secretion in normal subjects and in pathological hyperprolactinemia. J. Clin. Endocrinol. Metab. **54** (1982) 1125–1128.
[13] Gerhards, H. G., A. Carenzi, A. Costa: Effects of nomifensine on motor activity dopamine turnover rate and cyclic 3′,5′-adenosine monophosphate concentrations of rat striatum. Naunyn-Schmiedeberg's Arch. Pharmacol. **286** (1974) 49–52.
[14] Yen, S. S. C.: Neuroendocrine regulation of the menstrual cycle. In: Neuroendocrinology (D. T. Krieger, Y. C. Hughes, ed.), pp. 259–272. Sinauer Associates Inc. Publishers, Ma, USA, 1980.
[15] Thorner, M. O., H. F. Schran, W. S. Evans, et. al.: A broad spectrum of prolactin suppression by bromocriptine in hyperprolactinemic women: A study of serum prolactin and bromocriptine levels after acute and chronic administration of bromocriptine. J. Clin. Endocrinol. Metab. **50** (1980) 1026–1033.
[16] Spelta, B., D. Dallabonzana, G. Oppizzi, et. al.: Do patients with tumoral hyperprolactinemia have a hypothalamic dopamine deficiency? J. Endocrinol. Invest. **5** (Suppl. 1) (1982) 46.
[17] Faglia, G., A. Spada, P. Moriondo, et. al.: What is the role of dopamine in the pathogenesis of prolactinomas? In: Pituitary hyperfunction. Physiopathology and Clinical Aspects (G. M. Molinatti, F. Camanni, E. E. Müller, eds.), pp. 279–288. Raven Press, New York 1984.
[18] Bansal, S., L. A. Lee, P. D. Woolf: Abnormal prolactin responsivity to dopaminergic suppression in hyperprolactinemic patients. Am. J. Med. **71** (1981) 961–966.
[19] Serri, O., O. Kuchel, M. T. Buu, et. al.: Differential effects of a low dose of dopamine infusion on prolactin secretion in normal and hyperprolactinemic subjects. J. Clin. Endocrinol. Metab. **56** (1983) 255–259.
[20] Spada, A., S. Nicosia, L. Cortelazzi, et. al.: *In vitro* studies on prolactin release and adenylate cyclase activity in human prolactin secreting pituitary adenomas. Different sensitivity of macro- and microadenomas to dopamine and vasoactive intestinal polypeptide. J. Clin. Endocrinol. Metab. **56** (1983) 1–10.

Rhythmometric study of the circadian profile of plasma prolactin in patients with prolactinoma or empty sella syndrome

E. Ferrari, F. Agrimonti, P. A. Bossolo, R. Frajria, M. M. Daguati, L. Magnani, G. Marelli, A. Cozzi, A. Angeli

Introduction

Hyperprolactinaemia is a very frequent finding in patients with gonadal disorders, and it is often difficult to discriminate cases of prolactinoma from cases of "empty sella" or of "functional" hyperprolactinaemia.

The diagnosis is generally easy in the presence of an evident enlargement of the pituitary fossa, but PRL-secreting adenomas are frequently very small ("microadenomas"), and false positive and false negative results may occur even with the most sensitive neuroradiological procedures [2, 16]. Furthermore, also the diagnostic validity of several pharmacological tests evaluating PRL secretion has been questioned [14].

The aim of this study was to verify the diagnostic and prognostic value of the evaluation of the circadian chrono-organization of PRL secretion in prolactinoma and in the empty sella syndrome.

Data of the literature concerning the circadian rhythmicity of PRL secretion in pituitary tumours and in the empty sella syndrome are poor and often conflicting. Furthermore, all of these studies simply presented hormonal values recorded at different times of the 24 hour cycle, without any statistical validation of the rhythm and any computation of its phase and amplitude. Therefore, from a chronobiological point of view, such studies may be defined as limited to the "macroscopical" approach.

Subjects and methods

The study concerns 34 women aged 19–46 years with proven pituitary PRL-secreting adenomas (PRL-Ad.), and 25 patients (20f. and 5 m.) aged 25–59 years with primary empty sella syndrome (E.S.). A number of these cases were the object of a preliminary report [5].

The diagnosis was made in every case on the basis of clinical, endocrinological and neuroradiological findings (X-ray and tomography of the pituitary fossa, and cranial CT). An extra-sellar expansion of the pituitary tumour was present in 5 patients. In most of the patients with pituitary adenoma diagnosis was confirmed at neurosurgery. Twenty patients with PRL-Ad. were re-examined within 1–2 months after selective transsphenoidal adenomectomy. Clinically healthy subjects, sex- and age-matched, were chosen as controls.

The study included the rhythmometric and dynamic assessment of PRL and cortisol secretion. The circadian pattern of plasma cortisol was chosen as the reference rhythm, due to its very good reproducibility. In every case the study was performed at least 7 days after hospital admission, in order to allow synchronization of subjects to the same life schedule (meals at 08.00, noon and 18.00; sleep in darkness from 21.00 to 06.00 approximately). No patient was given any therapy for at least 7 days before the study.

In order to accustom subjects, the rhythmometric study was preceeded by one night of simulated experimental conditions. Both in patients and in controls blood samples were collected every 4 h. for 24 h., through an indwelling catheter inserted in the antecubital vein before the sleep span. Plasma was stored at −20 °C until assayed. Plasma PRL and cortisol were evaluated by RIA methods, using commercial kits (PRL: Biodata, Milano; Cortisol: Sorin, Saluggia). The sensitivity of the methods was 8 ng/ml and 1 mcg/dl respectively; intra- and inter-assay variations were always less than 10%.

Data were analyzed by conventional statistical methods and by the single and the population mean cosinor procedures [7]. These methods allow the validation of 95% statistical significance of the circadian rhythm of the function studied, and the evaluation of the parameters of the rhythm, namely the mesor M (a rhythm-adjusted mean), the amplitude A (equivalent to one half the total rhythmic variability) and the acrophase Ø (the lag from a defined time point of the crest time of the variable), with the corresponding 95% confidence limits.

As far as the dynamic assessment was concerned, PRL secretion was evaluated by one stimulation test (TRH 200 mcg i.v.) and two suppression tests (bromocriptine 5 mg orally, and nomifensine 200 mg or.); all these tests were carried out in the morning, beginning at 08.30. Cortisol secretion was assessed both by insulin-induced hypoglycaemia (0.1 U./kg i.v. at 08.30) and by pulse stimulation using a small dose of synthetic corticotropin (Synacthen 2,500 ng i.v.) given at 08.30 and at 20.30 on different days. The succession of the tests varied randomly.

In every case the absolute and per cent changes of plasma hormonal levels from basal values were considered for statistical analysis (Student's t test). In order to avoid the possibility of erroneous evaluations due to spontaneous fluctuations in PRL secretion, the responses of plasma PRL to suppression tests were expressed as the mean of the percent changes from basal levels of the values recorded between 120 and 240 min. after the drug administration, according to Camanni et al. [3].

Data obtained in patients were compared with those obtained in age- and sex-matched clinically healthy subjects. The ranges of control responses are listed in tab. 1.

Table 1 Per cent changes from basal values of plasma PRL and plasma cortisol in different tests in control subjects

Function and test	n	$\bar{x} \pm SD$	range	
Prolactin				
– TRH test	30	+480 ± 271	+150.2	+800.5
– bromocriptine test	10	−83.6 ± 8.7	−72.8	−98.7
– nomifensine test	10	−47.3 ± 13.5	−29.6	−70.2
Cortisol				
– I.T.T.	20	+141.0 ± 68.0	+45.5	+515.9
– Synacthen test 08^{30}	34	+108.7 ± 56.1	+31.3	+220.0
– Synacthen test 20^{30}	34	+279.8 ± 129.1	+40.4	+560.4

Results

Figure 1 displays the mean chronograms of plasma PRL and plasma cortisol in PRL-Ad. and in E.S. At any time of the 24 hour cycle plasma PRL levels are much higher in patients with prolactinoma than in controls, with a wide inter-individual variability. The occurrence of higher PRL values during the night could be viewed as being compatible with a rhythmic pattern of plasma PRL throughout the 24 hours, if one looks "macroscopically" at the mean chronogram. In patients with E.S. plasma PRL levels are a little higher than in controls throughout the 24 hours, but the circadian profile is similar to that of the control subjects.

The circadian profile of plasma cortisol is very similar in the two groups of patients and in controls, even if the plasma cortisol levels are at the lower limits of the control range or even noticeably reduced, particularly in the morning.

Table 2 summarizes the results of the population mean cosinor analysis of rhythmometric data. A statistically significant circadian rhythm of plasma PRL is not detectable in the group of patients with PRL-Ad., whereas the same rhythm is highly significant in patients with E.S., with a delay of about 2 hours of the circadian acrophase, with respect to controls.

On the contrary, the circadian rhythm of plasma cortisol reaches statistical significance both in PRL-Ad. and in E.S. In comparison with controls, a slight reduction

Table 2 Results of the population mean cosinor analysis

Variable	n	P	Mesor ± SE	Amplitude A. (95% C.I.)	Acrophase*
pl. Prolactin ng/ml					
PRL-secreting adenomas	34	.583	145.0 ± 32.9	21.7	−51°
Empty sella	25	.001	23.6 ± 4.1	6.5 (3.4 − 9.0)	−52° (−33°/−82°)
Controls	6	.03	19.9 ± 1.5	4.13 (.6 −7.7)	−13° (−314/−88°)
pl. Cortisol mcg/dl					
PRL-secreting adenomas	33	.001	10.9 ± .7	3.40 (2.1 − 4.7)	−141° (−121/−162°)
Empty sella	25	.001	9.5 ± .4	3.04 (2.29 − 3.80)	−131° (−108/−151°)
Controls	14	.001	13.8 ± 1.0	5.98 (5.78 − 6.17)	−127° (−110/−156°)

* phase reference = local midnight 360° = 24 h 15° = 1 h

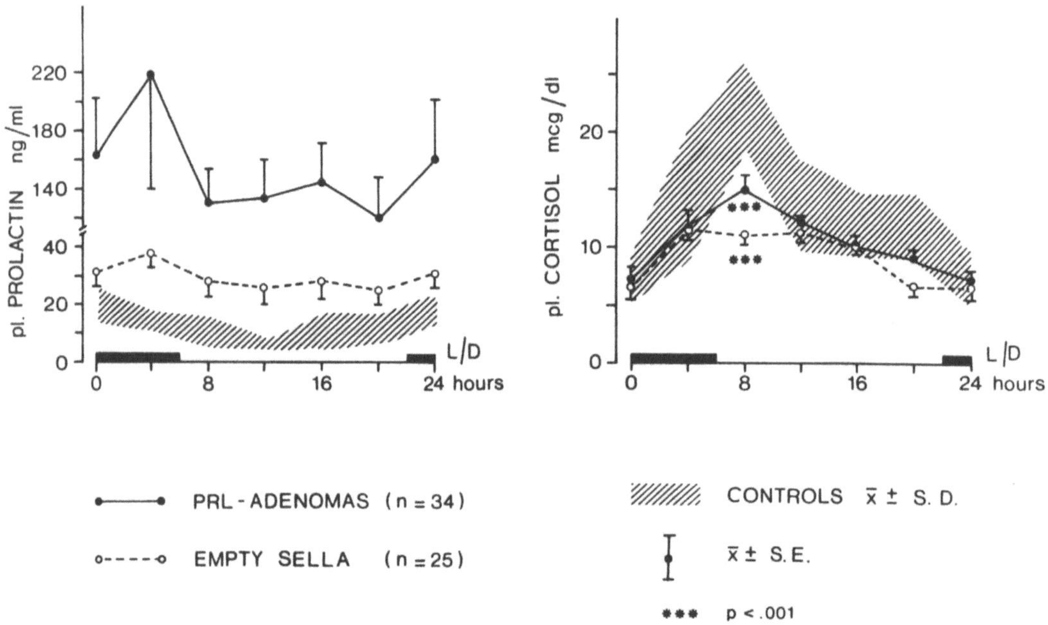

Fig. 1 Circadian profiles of plasma PRL and plasma cortisol in prolactinomas and in the empty sella syndrome.

in the mesor and a significant reduction in the amplitude of cortisol rhythm are evident in the two groups of patients, while the circadian acrophase of this rhythm is coincident in patients and in controls.

Figure 2 and table 3 summarize the results of the rhythmometric study performed in 20 cases of PRL-Ad. before and within 1−2 months after selective transsphenoidal adenomectomy. In 13/20 patients plasma PRL levels were normalized by

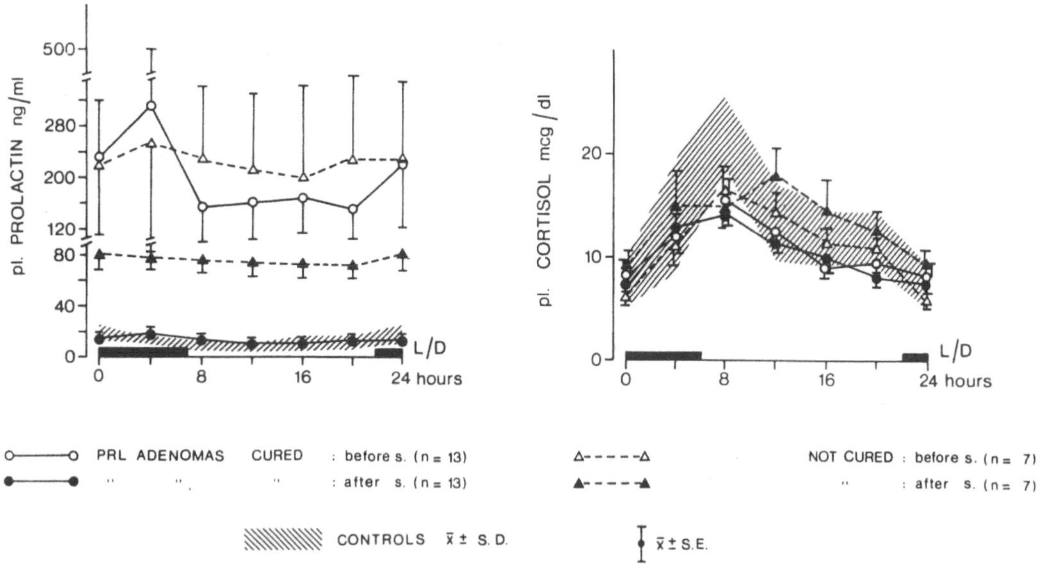

Fig. 2 Circadian profiles of plasma PRL and plasma cortisol in prolactinomas before and after surgery.

Table 3 Results of the population mean cosinor analysis of rhythmometric data of prolactinoma patients before and after surgery [5]

Variable		n	P	Mesor ± SE	Amplitude A	Acrophase*
					(95% C.I.)	
pl. Prolactin ng/ml						
"cured"	before s.	13	.324	127.1 ± 20.1	4.84	−336°
	after s.	13	.013	13.6 ± 2.0	2.70 (.6 − 5.0)	−51° (−358/−100°)
"not cured"	before s.	7	.165	77.8 ± 15.9	7.84	−52°
	after s.	7	.307	75.9 ± 10.1	3.20	−23°
pl. Cortisol mcg/dl						
"cured"	before s.	13	.001	10.5 ± 1.1	3.40 (1.96 − 5.03)	−137° (−101/−164°)
	after s.	13	.001	10.6 ± .8	3.10 (1.76 − 5.04)	−129° (−100/−157°)
"not cured"	before s.	7	.021	10.9 ± 1.0	3.40 (.58 − 9.36)	−168° (−124/−275°)
	after s.	7	.040	13.3 ± 1.5	3.38 (.21 − 7.61)	−166° (−73/−230°)

surgery, whereas in the other 7 cases hyperprolactinaemia still persisted after surgery, although at lower levels. Therefore, according to the results of selective adenomectomy, patients were divided in 2 groups, namely "cured" and "not cured".

In the pre-operative study the circadian profile of plasma PRL is not different in the two groups of patients. After surgery, the circadian profile of plasma, PRL in "cured" patients falls within the normal range. In contrast, the group of "not cured" patients exhibits persistent high levels of plasma PRL, without apparent rhythmic fluctuations.

The analysis of these data by population mean cosinor method shows the recovery after surgery of a statistically significant circadian rhythm of plasma PRL only in the group of "cured" patients.

Plasma cortisol displays a very similar circadian pattern in the two groups of patients, both before and after surgery. By the population mean cosinor analysis a highly significant circadian rhythm of plasma cortisol is always detectable, without significant differences in the rhythm parameters.

Table 4 summarizes the incidence of normal responses of plasma PRL and plasma cortisol to the pharmacological tests in patients with E.S. and with PRL-Ad. Only 1 patient with PRL-Ad. responds normally to the stimulation by TRH, and blunted responses occur in 7/34 cases (20%). In contrast, 62% of the E.S. patients show a normal PRL response to TRH, with blunted responses in the remaining 38% of the cases. Changes in plasma PRL induced by bromocriptine are not different in PRL-Ad. and in E.S. patients.

On the contrary, only 1 patient with PRL-Ad. exhibits a normal decrease in plasma PRL after nomifensine administration, and paradoxical increases in plasma PRL occured in 13/25 cases (52%). 3/8 patients with E.S. (37.5%) respond normally to nomifensine, and blunted responses are observed in 3/8 patients.

The statistical analysis of PRL responses by the Student's t test confirms the validity of TRH and the nomifensine test for the diagnosis of PRL-Ad., and the discriminant value of TRH test in differentiating PRL-Ad. from E.S.

Table 4 Incidence of normal responses of plasma PRL and cortisol to pharmacological tests in empty sella and in pituitary PRL-secreting adenomas [5]

Function and tests	Empty sella		PRL-adenomas whole group		PRL-aden. "cured" before s.		PRL-aden. "cured" after s.		PRL-aden. "not cured" before s.		PRL-aden. "not cured" after s.	
		%		%		%		%		%		%
pl. Prolactin												
– TRH test	13/21	62	1/34	3	1/12	8	5/12	42	0/6	0	0/6	0
– bromocriptine	4/10	40	9/26	35	4/9	44	4/9	44	1/5	20	2/5	40
– nomifensine	3/8	38	1/25	4	0/8	0	2/8	25	0/5	0	1/5	20
pl. Cortisol												
– I.T.T.	19/21	90	20/32	62	6/12	50	8/12	75	4/6	67	5/6	84
– Synacthen 08[30]	11/11	100	24/25	96	9/10	90	9/10	90	5/5	100	5/5	100
– Synacthen 20[30]	11/11	100	21/23	91	8/9	89	8/9	89	4/5	80	4/5	80

The response of plasma cortisol to insulin-induced hypoglycaemia is generally normal in patients with E.S., whereas it is normal only in 20/32 (62.5%) patients with PRL-Ad. The incidence of normal responses of plasma cortisol to pulse stimulation by Synacthen is comparable in E.S. and in PRL-Ad.. Nevertheless, the amplitude of cortisol response to Synacthen is significantly higher in the evening than in the morning only in patients with E.S. ($p < .01$) as well as in normal subjects.

After surgery, the group of "cured" patients shows a significant increase (from 8 to 41%) in the incidence of positive responses of PRL to TRH, in comparison with the pre-operative study. In contrast, in "not cured" patients, no positive responses to TRH occur both before and after adenomectomy.

The decrease in plasma PRL after bromocriptine or nomifensine administration does not seem to be significantly affected by selective adenomectomy in both groups of patients. Nevertheless, a greater incidence of positive responses to nomifensine occurs after surgery in "cured" patients in comparison with the pre-operative study.

Discussion

The results of this study confirm and extend previous observations on the occurrence of consistent abnormalities of the circadian pattern of plasma PRL in PRL-Ad.

Changes of the circadian profile of plasma PRL have been described in tumorous hyperprolactinaemia [1, 4, 9, 11, 13], and the normalization of PRL circadian pattern after adenomectomy was observed only in localized pituitary tumours [10].

The disturbance of the rhythmic variations of plasma PRL throughout the 24 hour cycle does not seem to be related to the enhanced PRL secretion by itself [6]. In fact the circadian pattern of plasma PRL is qualitatively maintained both during pregnancy [1] and in oestrogen-induced hyperprolactinaemia [19]. Moreover, the normality of the circadian profile of plasma PRL in primary empty sella syndrome has been considered as a discriminating feature from PRL-secreting tumours [12].

In the present study, rhythmometric computation yielded a clear-cut differentiation among patients with PRL-Ad. and E.S., respectively. In this regard, our data show a good agreement between the evaluation of the circadian profile of plasma PRL and the assessment of PRL responses to TRH and to nomifensine.

Furthermore, the chronobiological approach seems to be valuable in monitoring the effects of surgery on PRL-Ad. The recovery of the normal circadian periodicity of PRL secretion after surgical removal of the pituitary tumour may represent an index of the re-establishment of the physiological neuro-humoral control of PRL secretion.

As far as plasma cortisol is concerned, the maintainance of its normal circadian rhythm both in PRL-Ad. and in E.S. agrees with previous findings about the normality of the adrenocortical circadian rhythmicity in patients with localized intrasellar lesions [8]. These results may be considered a further argument in favour of the fundamental stability of the circadian chrono-organization of glucocorticoid secretion.

Finally, our study provides the first evidence of a significant reduction in the magnitude of the morning peak, hence of the circadian amplitude of the plasma cortisol rhythm, in patients with hyperprolactinaemia. The mechanisms which may support such a reduction are till now unknown. A possible involvement of dopamine and 5-hydroxy-tryptamine at the adrenal cell level in modulating steroidogenesis has been postulated [15, 17, 18]. Further studies are needed to clarify whether hyperprolactinaemia is associated with peripheral neurotransmitters abnormalities, which in turn could lead to subtle changes of the circadian program of glucocorticoid secretion.

References

[1] Boyar, R. M., J. W. Finkelstein, S. Kape, et al.: 24-hour prolactin secreting pattern during pregnancy. J. Clin. End. Metab. **40** (1975) 1117–1120.

[2] Burrow, G. N., G. Wortzman, N. B. Rewcastle, et al.: Microadenomas of the pituitary and abnormal sella tomograms in an unselected autopsy series. New Engl. J. Med. **304** (1981) 156–158.

[3] Camanni, F., A. R. Genazzani, F. Massara, et al.: Prolactin responsiveness to nomifensine in patients with hyperprolactinemia of tumorous or uncertain etiology. J. Clin. Endocr. Metab. **51** (1980) 650–653.

[4] Cryer, P. E., L. Jacobs, W. H. Daughaday: Regulation of growth hormone and prolactin secretion in patients with acromegaly and/or excessive prolactin secretion. Mt. Sinai J. Med. **40** (1973) 402–413.

[5] Ferrari, E., P. A. Bossolo, F. Baldi et al.: Chronobiological study of pituitary adenomas and of the empty sella syndrome. Chronobiologia **IX** (1982) 241–248.

[6] Frantz, A. G.: Rhythms in prolactin secretion. In: Endocrine Rhythms (D. T. Krieger, ed.), pp. 175–186. Raven Press, New York 1979.

[7] Halberg, F.: Chronobiology. Ann. Rev. Physiol. **31** (1969) 675–725.

[8] Krieger, D. T.: Biorhythms in central nervous system diseases (primarily those of pituitary-adrenal hormones). In: Biorhythms and human reproduction (M. Ferin, F. Halberg, R. M. Richard, L. van de Wielde, eds.), pp. 621–649. John Wiley and Sons, 1974.

[9] Jacobs, L. S., W. H. Daughaday: Physiopathology and control of prolactin secretion in patients with pituitary and hypothalamic diseases. In: Human Prolactin (J. L. Pasteels, C. Robyn, eds.), pp. 189–205. Excerpta Medica Ed., Amsterdam 1973.

[10] Jaquet, P., F. Grisoli, M. Guibout et al.: Prolactin secreting tumors. Endocrine status before and after surgery in 33 women. J. clin. Endocr. Metab. **46** (1978) 459–466.

[11] L'Hermite, M., M. Degueldre, A. Caufriez, et al.: Secrétion de prolactine: intérêt des investigations dynamiques. Path. Biol. **23** (1975) 769–778.

[12] Malarkey, W. B., T. J. Goodenow, R. R. Lanese: Diurnal variation of prolactin secretion differentiates pituitary tumors from the primary empty sella syndrome. Am. J. Med. **69** (1980) 886–890.
[13] Malarkey, W. B., C. Johnson: Pituitary tumors and hyperprolactinemia. Arch. Intern. Med. **136** (1976) 40–44.
[14] Peters, J. R., S. M. Foord, C. Dieguez, et al.: Microprolactinoma and functional hyperprolactinemia: two clinical entities or two phases of the same disease? In: a clinical problem: microprolactinoma (G. M. Molinatti, ed.) pp. 21–34. Excerpta Medica Ed., Amsterdam 1982.
[15] Snider, S. R., O. Kuchel: Dopamine: an important neurohormone of the sympatoadrenal system. Significance of increased peripheral dopamine release for the human stress response and hypertension. Endocr. Review **4** (1983) 291–309.
[16] Swanson, H. A., G. du Boulay: Borderline variants of the normal pituitary fossa. Brit. J. Radiol. **48** (1975) 366–369.
[17] Tait, J. F., S. A. S. Tait, J. B. G. Bell, et al.: Further studies on the stimulation or rat adrenal capsular cells: four types of response. J. of Endocrinol. **47** (1980) 11–27.
[18] Verdesca, A. S., C. D. Westermann, R. S. Crampton, et al.: Direct adrenal cortical stimulatory effect of serotonin. Amer. J. Physiol. **196** (1961) 1065–1072.
[19] Wekemans, M., C. Robyn: The influence of exogenous oestrogen on the circadian periodicity of circulating prolactin in women. J. clin. Endocr. Metab. **40** (1975) 886–891.

Prolactin responses to thyrotropin-releasing hormone, metoclopramide and insulin-induced hypoglycaemia in hyperprolactinaemic and normoprolactinaemic patients

H. M. Heshmati, G. Turpin, N. Gaham, F. Brihmat-Allali, S. Jambart, A. Carayon, J. L. de Gennes

Introduction

The role of hypothalamic dopamine as a major physiological prolactin (PRL)-inhibiting factor is well recognized [1, 2, 3]. Many of the tests of PRL release are based on removing or increasing dopamine-mediated activity with drugs acting at hypothalamic and/or pituitary levels [4–7]. Other agents or conditions such as thyrotropin-releasing hormone (TRH) or insulin-induced hypoglycaemia (IH) are also involved in PRL release [6, 8].

The purpose of this study was to compare the stimulatory effect of TRH, metoclopramide (MC), a dopamine blocking agent, and IH on PRL secretion in various pathological conditions with or without hyperprolactinaemia.

Materials

Two groups of patients were studied. Group 1 included 12 patients (3 males, 9 females), aged 23–50 yrs (mean = 32 yrs) who had a PRL adenoma and hyperprolactinaemia resulting in impotence, gynecomastia, galactorrhoea and amenorrhoea. Group 2 included 12 patients (7 males, 5 females), aged 19–73 yrs (mean = 40 yrs) who had hypothalamic hypopituitarism (4 cases), isolated gonadotropin deficiency (2 cases), acromegaly (1 case), cranio-pharyngioma (1 case), craniostenosis (1 case), primary hypothyroidism (1 case), galactorrhoea (1 case) and primary testicular deficiency (1 case). Three patients in group 1 and 3 in group 2 had previous pituitary surgery and/or radiotherapy. All patients in both groups (except 1 patient with severe untreated primary hypothyroidism, and 1 acromegalic patient with elevated thyroxine levels, in group 2) had normal or sub-normal thyroid and adrenal functions or had replacement therapy by thyroxine and cortisone. No patient was receiving any medication known to interfere with the PRL secretion.

Methods

Dynamic tests were performed on 3 different days, at 08–09 AM, after an overnight rest and fast, with TRH (200 μg, iv) for PRL and thyrotropin (TSH) determination, with MC (2.5 mg, iv) for PRL determination, and with insulin (0.10 U/kg, iv) for glucose, PRL and growth hormone (GH) determination. Blood was sampled before (2 baseline determinations) and during the test (15, 30, 60, 90 and 120 min after the injection) through an indwelling iv needle. PRL was determined by a double antibody homologous radioimmunoassay (RIA) (standard PRL: 42 IU WHO 71/222). Interassay and intraassay coefficients of variation were 9% and 7% respectively. TSH and GH were measured by previously described RIA [9]. Glucose was determined by an enzymatic method (glucose oxydase). Statistical analysis was performed using the nonparametric Mann-Whitney U test. A P value greater than 0.05 was not considered significant. All reported values represent the mean ±SD. In group 2, 1 patient with severe primary hypothyroidism (TSH: 59 ng/ml) and 1 patient with acromegaly (GH: 10.8 ng/ml) were not included for TSH and GH calculations respectively. An increase of more than 50% above basal values for

Table 1 Basal PRL, TSH and GH levels in patients with (group 1) and without (group 2) PRL adenoma

	Group 1 (n = 12)		Group 2 (n = 12)		Group 1 vs Group 2
	Basal	(n)	Basal	(n)	
PRL (ng/ml)	621 ± 988	(12)	18 ± 17	(12)	P < 0.001
TSH (ng/ml)	0.83 ± 0.67	(10)	0.63 ± 0.22	(10)	NS
GH (ng/ml)	1.1 ± 1.1	(12)	1.2 ± 0.5	(10)	NS

Table 2 PRL and TSH responses to 200 μg iv TRH injection in patients with (group 1) and without (group 2) PRL adenoma

		Group 1 (n = 12)		Group 2 (n = 12)	
PRL	Increment (ng/ml)	363 ± 919	(n = 12)	81 ± 166	(n = 12)
	Positive response	4		11	
TSH	Increment (ng/ml)	1.54 ± 1.77	(n = 10)	0.77 ± 0.45	(n = 10)
	Positive response	10		8	

PRL and TSH, a peak of more than 10 ng/ml for GH and a nadir of less than 55 mg/dl for glucose were considered as positive responses of these parameters to TRH, MC and insulin.

Results

In the basal state, the mean PRL level was significantly higher in group 1, while mean TSH and GH levels were similar in both groups (tab. 1). Two patients in group 2 (1 craniopharyngioma, 1 primary hypothyroidism) had hyperprolactinaemia. Under TRH, a positive response was observed in 33% and 92% of cases for PRL and in 100% and 80% of cases for TSH, in groups 1 and 2 respectively (tab. 2). Under MC, a positive response was observed in 8% and 83% of cases for PRL, in groups 1 and 2 respectively (tab. 3). Under insulin, the mean glucose level fell from 77 ± 7 mg/dl to 29 ± 12 mg/dl in group 1 and from 78 ± 10 mg/dl to 38 ± 13 mg/dl in group 2. A positive response was observed in 17% and 17% of cases for PRL and in 58% and 20% of cases for GH, in groups 1 and 2 respectively

Table 3 PRL response to 2.5 mg iv MC injection in patients with (group 1) and without (group 2) PRL adenoma

		Group 1 (n = 12)	Group 2 (n = 12)
PRL	Increment (ng/ml)	194 ± 397	57 ± 67
	Positive response	1	10

Table 4 PRL and GH responses to 0.10 U/kg iv insulin injection in patients with (group 1) and without (group 2) PRL adenoma

		Group 1		Group 2	
		(n = 12)		(n = 12)	
PRL	Increment (ng/ml)	213 ± 461	(n = 12)	4 ± 9	(n = 12)
	Positive response	2		2	
GH	Peak (ng/ml)	14.6 ± 12.5	(n = 12)	5.4 ± 6.7	(n = 10)
	Positive response	7		2	

(tab. 4). Positive responses of PRL to TRH and MC were present in 0% and 75% of cases, in groups 1 and 2 respectively. Positive responses of PRL to TRH, MC and IH were present in 0% and 17% of cases, in groups 1 and 2 respectively.

Discussion

In normal subjects, TRH acts directly on pituitary lactotropes to stimulate PRL release. MC blocks dopamine receptors of the hypothalamus and the pituitary, causing an increase in PRL levels. The stimulatory effect of IH on PRL secretion is mediated within the hypothalamus. A normal response to these tests requires the integrity of the hypothalamic pituitary axis for PRL release [6, 8].

The relative importance of hypothalamic dysfunction and intrinsic pituitary abnormality in the pathogenesis of PRL adenomas has been the subject of many studies. A number of tests of PRL secretion have been proposed to discriminate between tumorous and non-tumorous hyperprolactinaemia [3, 4, 7, 10, 11]. In PRL adenoma, there is a blunted or absent PRL response to TRH in vivo [5, 6] and in vitro [12]. The response returns to normal after complete tumour removal [5, 6]. In post-partum women and in patients with hypothalamic hyperprolactinaemia, the response of PRL to TRH is normal [4]. The response of PRL to MC or other dopaminergic blocking agents is diminished or absent in PRL adenoma and in hypothalamic hyperprolactinaemia [4–7], but normal in hyperprolactinaemic post-partum women [5, 7]. The normal response to MC is found after successful surgery of the PRL tumour [5, 6]. In PRL adenoma, there is an alteration in hypothalamic dopamine secretion due to the short-loop feedback effect of PRL [6, 7, 13, 14]. The release of PRL in patients with PRL adenoma is not refractory to physiological concentrations of dopamine, but there is an abnormality of the peripheral dopamine metabolism [15]. In vitro studies show that the inhibition of PRL release and adenylate cyclase activity caused by dopamine is higher in macroadenomas and lower or absent in microadenomas [16]. In hypothalamic hyperprolactinaemia, there is a dopamine deficiency at the pituitary level [4]. The response of PRL to IH is blunted or absent in PRL adenoma and in hypothalamic disturbances [6, 8].

Our results are in agreement with most of the above findings and we conclude that:

Firstly, in normoprolactinaemic and hyperprolactinaemic patients without PRL adenoma, the responses of PRL to TRH and MC are common. The response of PRL to IH is rather rare.

Secondly, in hyperprolactinaemic patients with PRL adenoma, the responses of PRL to TRH, MC and IH are usually diminished or absent. This supports the presence of altered PRL tumour cell receptors and autonomous secretion of the tumour.

References

[1] Frohman, L. A., M. E. Stachura: Neuropharmacologic control of neuroendocrine function in man. Metabolism **24** (1975) 211–234.

[2] Smythe, G. A.: The role of serotonin and dopamine in hypothalamic-pituitary function. Clin. Endocrinol. **7** (1977) 325–341.

[3] Serri, O., O. Kuchel, N. T. Buu, et al.: Differential effects of a low dose dopamine infusion on prolactin secretion in normal and hyperprolactinemic subjects. J. Clin. Endocrinol. Metab. **56** (1983) 255–259.

[4] Ferrari, C., P. Rampini, R. Benco, et al.: Functional characterization of hypothalamic hyperprolactinemia. J. Clin. Endocrinol. Metab. **55** (1982) 897–901.

[5] Barbarino, A., L. De Marinis, G. Maira, et al.: Serum prolactin response to thyrotropin-releasing hormone and metoclopramide in patients with prolactin-secreting tumors before and after transsphenoidal surgery. J. Clin. Endocrinol. Metab. **47** (1978) 1148–1151.

[6] Tucker, H. St. G., H. V. Lankford, D. F. Gardner, et al.: Persistent defect in regulation of prolactin secretion after successful pituitary tumor removal in women with the galactorrhea-amenorrhea syndrome. J. Clin. Endocrinol. Metab. **51** (1980) 968–971.

[7] Massara, F., F. Camanni, M. Martra, et al.: Reciprocal pattern of the TSH and PRL responses to dopamine receptor blockade in women with physiological or pathological hyperprolactinemia. Clin. Endocrinol. **18** (1983) 103–110.

[8] Woolf, P. D., L. A. Lee, W. F. Leebaw: Hypoglycemia as a provocative test of prolactin release. Metabolism **27** (1978) 869–877.

[9] Turpin, G., H. M. Heshmati, M. Roger, et al.: Le dosage des stimulines hypophysaires dans le liquide céphalorachidien chez le sujet normal et en pathologie hypothalamo-hypophysaire. Adénome hypophysaire sécrétant ou non sécrétant, selle turcique vide, syndromes hypothalamiques. Ann. Endocrinol. (Paris) **41** (1980) 21–30.

[10] Camanni, F., A. R. Genazzani, F. Massara, et al.: Prolactin responsiveness to nomifensine in patients with hyperprolactinemia of tumorous or uncertain etiology. J. Clin. Endocrinol. Metab. **51** (1980) 650–653.

[11] Pineda, G., M. Valdes, M. Castro, et al.: Pituitary microadenoma: diagnostic studies. Clin. Endocrinol. **10** (1979) 583–594.

[12] Chihara, K., J. Iwasaki, N. Minamitani, et al.: Prolactin secretion from human prolactinomas perifused in vitro: effect of TRH, prostaglandin E1, teophylline, dopamine and dopamine receptor blockers. Acta Endocrinol. **105** (1984) 6–13.

[13] Molitch, M. E., R. H. Goodman, K. D. Post, et al.: Surgical cure of prolactinoma reverses abnormal prolactin response to carbidopa/L-dopa. J. Clin. Endocrinol. Metab. **55** (1982) 1118–1123.

[14] De Marinis, L., A. Mancini, G. Maira, et al.: Postoperative evaluation of dopaminergic tone in prolactinoma patients. II. Plasma thyrotropin response to metoclopramide. J. Clin. Endocrinol. Metab. **58** (1984) 405–409.

[15] Ho, K. Y., G. A. Smythe, M. Duncan, et al.: Dopamine infusion studies in patients with pathological hyperprolactinemia: evidence of normal prolactin suppressibility but abnormal dopamine metabolism. J. Clin. Endocrinol. Metab. **58** (1984) 128–133.

[16] Spada, A., S. Nicosia, L. Cortelazzi, et al.: In vitro studies on prolactin release and adenylate cyclase activity in human prolactin-secreting pituitary adenomas. Different sensitivity of macro- and microadenomas to dopamine and vasoactive intestinal polypeptide. J. Clin. Endocrinol. Metab. **56** (1983) 1–10.

Evidence for functional impairment of growth hormone secretion in prolactinoma

E. Jungmann, P.-H. Althoff, G. J. Hermann, K. Schöffling

Introduction

In the adult, prolactinomas are the most common pituitary tumour. In prepubertal children, however, prolactinomas are very rarely found. Recently, our group described a 13-year-old boy with prolactinoma – induced growth failure and hypogonadism [12]. Decreased basal growth hormone (HGH) levels were found which were unresponsive to insulin-induced hypoglycaemia. Since the parents of the patient refused pituitary operation, bromocriptine treatment was started. Together with a prompt decrease in prolaction levels and radiological evidence for pituitary tumour shrinkage the patient showed a rapid catch-up growth and normalization of sexual maturation. It was presumed, therefore, that the growth failure in this patient was caused by a functional impairment of growth hormone secretion comparable to the prolactin-induced decreases in TSH levels in adult prolactinoma patients [11]. To examine our hypothesis the present study was aimed to assess impaired growth hormone secretion in patients with prolactinoma and to find out which mechanism(s) might be involved.

Methods

After giving informed consent, 6 till then untreated patients with prolactinoma (5 women, 1 man, aged 22–66 years) participated at this study. Prolactinoma was suspected by the finding of increased prolactin levels which were unresponsive to TRH stimulation and confirmed by neuroradiology. 4 of the patients harboured a microprolactinoma, in 2 a suprasellar extension was found which necessitated transsphenoidal operation. 6 healthy male volunteers (aged 19–30 years) served as controls. A minimum of 2 days was allowed between each examination. From 10.00 P.M. prior to the day of testing all subjects were fasting, abstained from smoking and avoided strenous physical activity. None of the subjects took any medication known to influence HGH or prolactin levels.

The subjects remained supine throughout the tests. Bromocriptine 2.5 mg p.o. ('Pravidel', Sandoz AG) and, in controls only, 1 tablet of placebo was given at zero time (8.00 A.M.). Metoclopramide 10 mg i.v. ('Paspertin', Kali Chemie) was injected after 120 min. Moreover, metoclopramide was injected i.v. in the controls 120 min. after pretreatment with bromocriptine or furosemide 40 mg i.v. ('Lasix', Hoechst AG). In no experiment were adverse side effects of drugs registered. Commercially available radioimmunoassay kits were used for the determination of prolactin (Serono AG) and HGH (Sorin, Sallugia). Results are given as median ± standard error of median or as individual hormone levels. Statistical evaluation was made by paired Wilcoxon test.

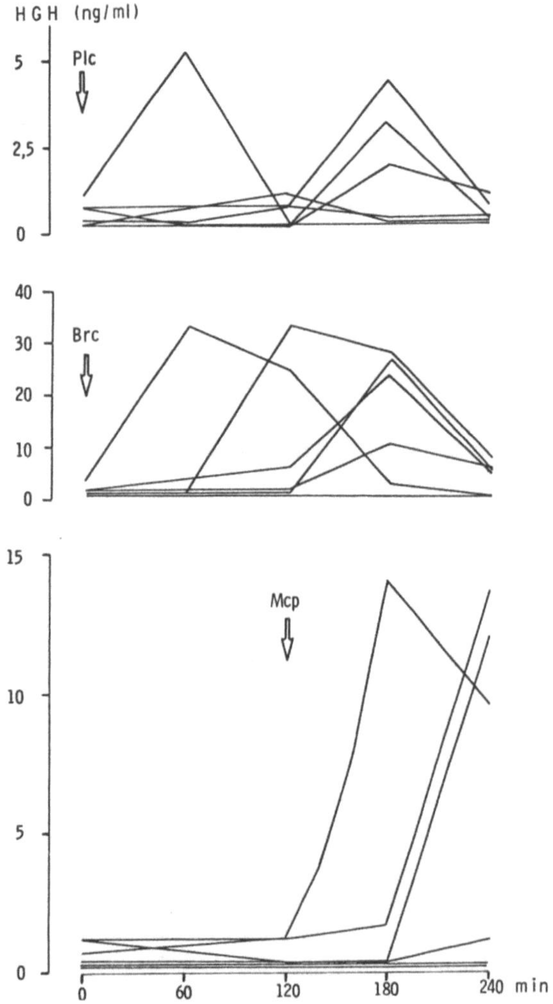

Fig. 1 Human growth hormone (HGH) responses to placebo (Plc), bromocriptine (Brc, 2.5 mg p.o.) or metoclopramide (Mcp, 10 mg i.v.) in 6 young healthy volunteers.

Results

In the placebo experiment, spontaneous HGH spikes never exceeded 5 ng/ml. Therefore, higher HGH levels in the following tests were taken for significant responses to stimulation. Thus, in the controls significant HGH responses to bromocriptine were seen in 5 and to metoclopramide in 3 out of 6 volunteers (fig. 1). In prolactinoma, comparatively smaller HGH responses to bromocriptine were found

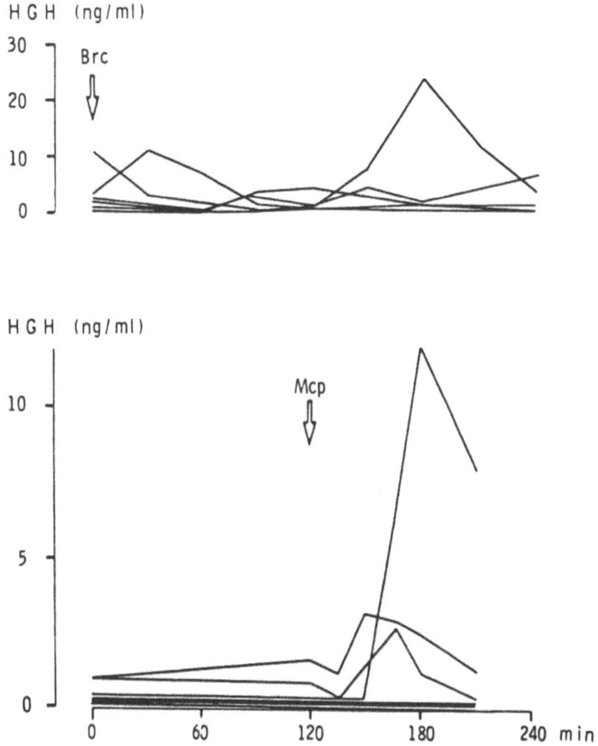

Fig. 2 Human growth hormone (HGH) responses to bromocriptine (Brc, 2.5 mg p.o.) or metoclopramide (10 mg i.v.) in 6 patients with prolactinoma.

in 2 and to metoclopramide in 1 out of 6 patients (fig. 2). Prolactin levels were decreased by bromocriptine both in controls and patients with prolactinoma ($p < 0.05$). As expected, in prolactinoma prolactin responsiveness to metoclopramide was decreased ($p < 0.05$) (fig. 3). After pretreatment with bromocriptine, both the HGH and prolactin responses to metoclopramide were blunted (fig. 4). After furosemide pretreatment, the prolactin response was decreased and the growth hormone response blunted (fig. 5).

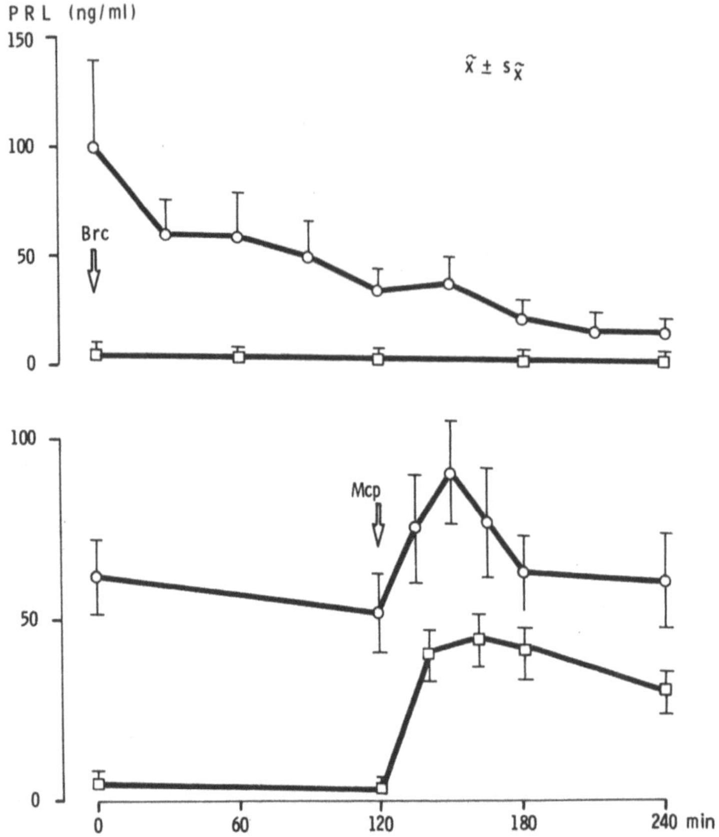

Fig. 3 Prolactin responses to bromocriptine (Brc, 2.5 mg p.o.) or metoclopramide (Mcp, 10 mg i.v.) in 6 patients with prolactinoma (○—○) and in 6 healthy volunteers (□—□). $x \pm S_x$.

Discussion

Like l-dopa, bromocriptine can serve as a stimulation test for HGH secretion [4]. Recently, metoclopramide stimulation of HGH secretion has been introduced as a reliable test for HGH deficiency in prepubertal patients [2]. In none of the common tests for HGH stimulation are all subjects expected to respond in an equal and reproducible manner [6]. Therefore, taking both tests together and taking into consideration that only adult subjects were studied, our conclusion appears justified that HGH secretion is in fact more or less impaired in all prolactinoma patients. The mechanism is still unknown, by which metoclopramide increases HGH levels in responsive subjects. Apparently, muscarinic receptors are involved [7]. The stimulatory action of bromocriptine on HGH secretion in normal subjects is also

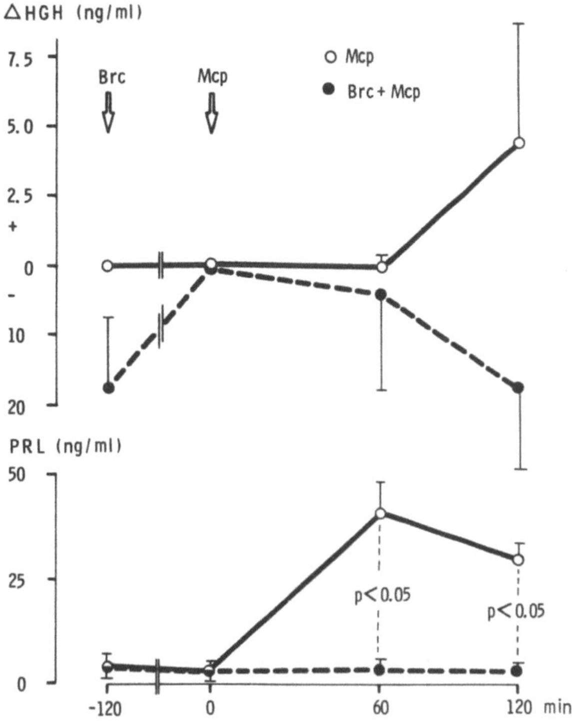

Fig. 4 Effect of bromocriptine pretreatment (Brc, 2.5 mg p.o.) on the responses of growth hormone (HGH) and prolactin (PRL) to metoclopramide (Mcp, 10 mg i.v.) in 6 healthy male volunteers. $\hat{x} \pm S_{\bar{x}}$.

unexplained. Except for 9, 10 – transdihydrolisuride all dopaminergic agents including dopamine itself stimulate HGH in healthy man [5]. Apparently, other than dopaminergic D2 – receptors are involved which are probably situated in the hypothalamus [3, 8]. On the contrary, dopaminergic stimulation is known to decrease HGH release at the pituitary level both in healthy and acromegalic subjects [10]. Thus, bromocriptine has been introduced into the therapy of acromegaly [1, 4, 13]. After pretreatment with dopaminergic stimulation HGH responsiveness to insulin-induced hypoglycaemia or a dopaminergic agonist (l-dopa) was found to be blunted [14]. Similarly, pretreatment with bromocriptine or enhancement of endogenous dopaminergic activity by furosemide [9] abolished the rise in HGH concentration after metoclopramide injection in responsive healthy volunteers. Therefore, we conclude from the analogy with the decrease in TSH levels [11] that the impaired HGH secretion in prolactinoma is due to an increased dopaminergic inhibition of HGH secretion at the pituitary level which is caused by feedback stimulation of inhibitory dopaminergic mechanisms by prolactin excess [13] and is, thus, reversible after successful bromocriptine treatment.

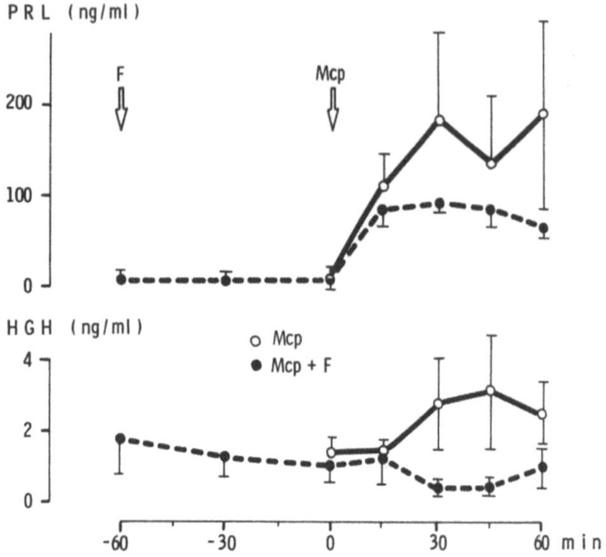

Fig. 5 Effect of furosemide pretreatment (F, 40 mg i. v.) on the responses of human growth hormone (HGH) and prolactin (PRL) to metoclopramide (Mcp, 10 mg i. v.) in healthy male volunteers. $\bar{x} \pm S_{\bar{x}}$.

References

[1] Althoff, P.-H., B. Böttger, C. Rosak, et al.: Bromocriptin – zur Pharmakotherapie endokriner Erkrankungen. Inn. Med. **9** (1982) 189–198.

[2] Cohen, H. N., I. D. Hay, J. A. Thomson, et al.: Metoclopramide Stimulation: A Test of Growth Hormone Reserve in Adolescent Males. Clin. Endocr. **11** (1979) 89–93.

[3] Cronin, M. J., W. S. Evans: Dopamine Receptors in the Normal and Abnormal Anterior Pituitary. Clinics in Endocrinology and Metabolism **12** (1983) 15–30.

[4] Del Pozo, E., O. Lancranjan: Clinical Use of Drugs Modifying the Release of Anterior Pituitary Hormones. Frontiers in Neuroendocrinology **5** (1978) 207–248.

[5] Dorow, R., M. Breitkopf, K.-J. Gräf, et al.: Neuroendocrine Effects of Lisuride and Its 9, 10 – Dihydrogenated Analog in Healthy Volunteers. In: Lisuride and Other Dopamine Agonists (D. B. Calne, R. Horverski, R. J. McDonald, W. Wuttke, eds.). Raven Press, New York 1983.

[6] Frasier, S. D.: A Review of Growth Hormone Stimulation Tests in Children. Pediatrics **53** (1974) 929–937.

[7] Jungmann, E., P.-H. Althoff, G. J. Hermann, et al.: The Effect of Pizotifen, a Serotonin Antagonist, and of Pirenzepine, a Muscarinic Antagonist, on Hormonal Responses to Metoclopramide in Healthy Man. Arzneimittelforschung **34** (1984) 1022–1024.

[8] E. Jungmann, G. J. Hermann, P. Grützmacher, et al.: Die dopaminerge Hemmung der Aldosteron- und Prolactinsekretion: Einfluß von Urämie und Hyperkaliämie. Verh. Dtsch. Ges. Inn. Med. **90** (1984) 1231–1234.

[9] van Loon, G. R., M. J. Sole: Plasma Dopamine: Source, Regulation, and Significance. Metabolism **29** (Suppl. 1) (1980) 1119–1123.

[10] Marcovitz, S., C. G. Goodyer, H. Guyda, et al.: Comparative Study of Human Fetal, Normal Adult, and Somatotropic Adenoma Pituitary Function in Tissue Culture. J. Clin. Endocrinol. Metab. **54** (1982) 6–16.

[11] Scanlon, M. F., M. D. Rodriguez-Arnao, A. M. McGregor, et al.: Altered Dopaminergic Regulation of Thyrotropin Release in Patients with Prolactinomas: Comparison with Other Tests of Hypothalamic-Pituitary Function. Clin. Endocr. **14** (1981) 133–143.

[12] Schumm, P.-M., F. Kollmann, Chr. Leitner, et al.: Involution of an Adolescent's Prolactinoma by Long-Term Treatment with Bromocriptine. Intern. Workshop: Pituitary Hyperfunction. Milan, 9–11 Sept. 1982.

[13] Thorner, M. O., E. Flückiger, D. B. Calne: Bromocriptine. A Clinical and Pharmacological Review. Raven Press, New York 1980.

[14] Woolf, P. D., R. Lantigua, L. A. Lee: Dopamine Inhibition of Stimulated Growth Hormone Secretion: Evidence for Dopaminergic Modulation of Insulin- and L-Dopa-Induced Growth Hormone Secretion in Man. J. Clin. Endocrinol. Metab. **49** (1979) 326–330.

TSH response to dopamine receptor blockade in women with PRL-secreting microadenoma: Long effect of surgical removal

M. Montini, M. Salmoiraghi, M. D. Pagani, D. Parodi, D. Gianola, L. Ferrari, R. Benco, I. Nosari, P. Sala, V. Cassinari, G. Pagani

Introduction

An increased dopaminergic inhibition of TSH release has been demonstrated by several authors [9, 10] in patients with prolactin secreting pituitary tumours. In this pathological state, a short loop positive feed-back action of prolactin has been postulated to be responsible for the increased hypothalamic dopaminergic activity. In contrast, the so called functional hyperprolactinaemia is thougt to be characterized by a primary reduction in central nervous system (CNS) dopamine activity [5, 7]. For these reasons the acute effect of dopamine receptor blockade on TSH release has been utilized for the differential diagnosis of hyperprolactinaemic states [4, 10]. In this report we have tested this hypothesis by comparing the TSH and PRL release following acute dopamine receptor blockade with domperidone (DOM) in 6 women with autonomous hyperprolactinaemia due to a proven PRL-secreting pituitary microadenoma (PMA), before and after its surgical removal and restoration of baseline and post-stimulative PRL levels.

Patients and methods

We studied 6 women, aged 17–44, with a galactorrhoea-amenorrhoea syndrome. A prolactin secreting pituitary microadenoma was diagnosed on the basis of: (a) basal hyperprolactinaemia (mean of 4 samples at 08.00 a.m.); (b) blunted or absent responses of PRL to TRH (200 mcg) and domperidone (10 mg), in comparison with the increases observed in normal subjects [4]; (c) an abnormal radiological picture of the pituitary fossa, confirmed by computerized tomography scanning (CAT-scanner Pfizer 0450). Each patient then underwent transphenoidal removal of the pituitary tumour which was confirmed by histology. Before the surgical event, we studied the TSH and PRL response to domperidone in every patient after an informed, written consent.

The domperidone test was done at 08.00 a.m., with the patient fasting and recumbent, with an indwelling catheter placed in an arm vein and kept open with saline solution. Blood sampling was done every 15 minutes for half an hour before and two hours following DOM (10 mg) intravenous injection. Serum PRL and TSH were measured by the double antibody radioimmunoassay method (CEA-Sorin kit).

Functional investigations of pituitary secretion of GH, ACTH, LH and FSH, were performed separately by the LHRH test (25 mcg iv) and insulin (0.1 U/kg) induced hypoglycaemia. The tests were repeated in every subject 1 month after surgery and only in 5 patients 6 and 12 months after surgery (because one patient conceived and was investigated 18 months after surgery).

Results

In all patients the pituitary reserves of gonadotropins, GH and ACTH were normal either before or after surgery.

The preoperative baseline PRL levels were elevated with a blunted response to TRH in all subjects. Following DOM the PRL secretion areas were reduced in comparison with those observed in women with normal cycles during the early follicular phase [4].

After surgery, PRL secretion areas after DOM, showed significant increases in four patients while in patient 3 and 4 there was considerable variation (tab. 1). In all patients PRL per cent increases induced by DOM ($\Delta\%$ above baseline values) were very small before surgery and became normal in the post operative period (fig. 1).

Preoperative TSH baseline values were normal in our cases, and showed an exaggerated response to DOM with secretion areas greater than 200 μU/ml/120 minutes, which we consider the upper limit of a normal response [4].

Table 1 PRL secretion area in 6 microprolactinoma bearing patients

Patient	Before surgery	After surgery			
		1	6	12	18
Z. M. R.	1872	2288	6858	4654	
R. M.	1967	3720	3039	3717	
S. L.	3215	2258	2649	2932	
L. M.	1285	1324	3987	616	
T. S.	2065	1254	3697	5716	
R. L.	1157	3216	pregnancy		10471

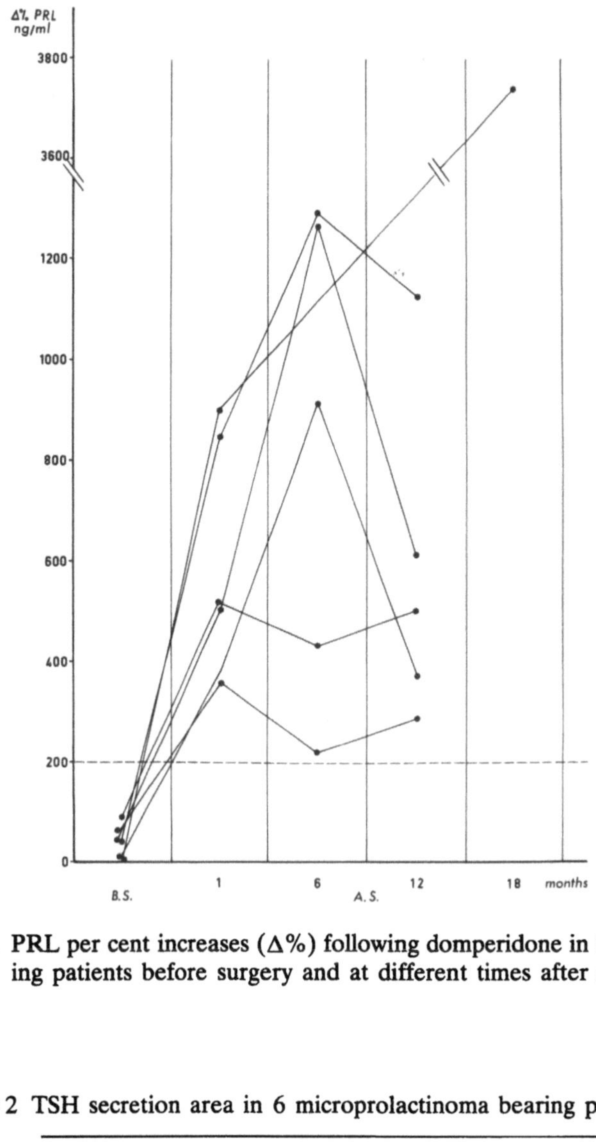

Fig. 1 PRL per cent increases (Δ%) following domperidone in 6 microprolactinoma bearing patients before surgery and at different times after surgery.

Table 2 TSH secretion area in 6 microprolactinoma bearing patients

Patient	Before surgery	After surgery			
		1	6	12	18
Z. M. R.	234.00	9.75	149.00	108.75	
R. M.	286.25	95.75	123.50	14.00	
S. L.	258.00	120.00	195.00	72.50	
L. M.	250.00	36.00	73.00	9.50	
T. S.	245.00	34.75	76.25	31.00	
R. L.	276.00	180.00	pregnancy		178.00

After surgery all patients had perfectly normalized TSH secretion areas, following DOM (tab. 2).

Also the TSH net increases after DOM showed a similar degree of variation; in fact they were higher than normal values in the preoperative period and were normalized by surgery (fig. 2).

Finally, in each patient, regular menstrual cycles were restored and in one case pregnancy occurred three months after surgery.

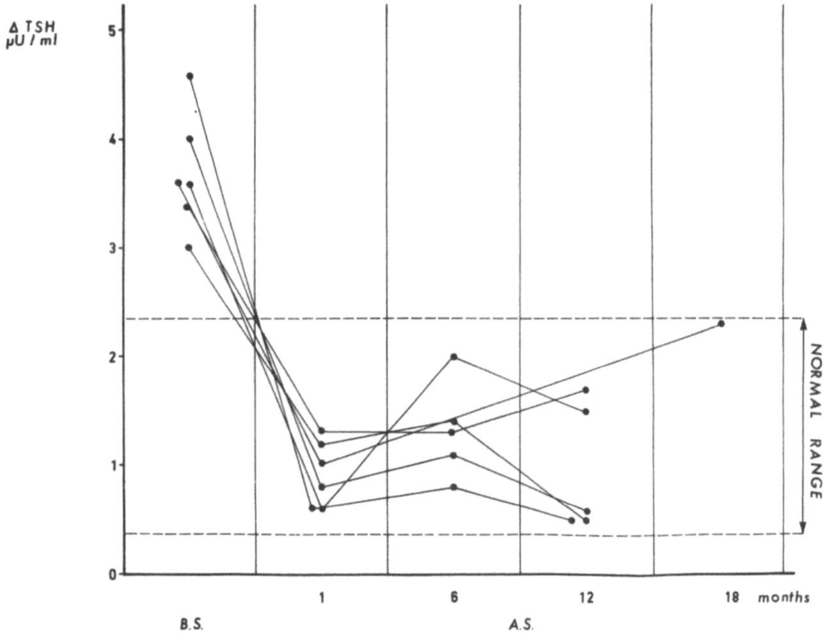

Fig. 2 TSH net increases (Δ) following domperidone in 6 microprolactinoma bearing patients before surgery and at different times after surgery.

Discussion

Our findings confirm the existence of an exaggerated dopaminergic inhibition of TSH secretion in patients with microprolactinoma. This fact may be due to a positive short-loop feed-back of enhanced PRL levels on dopaminergic neurons of the median eminence [10]. In fact, the selective removal of the adenomatous lactotroph, at least in our cases, is able to restore the physiological dopamine control on PRL and TSH secretion.

On the basis of this data we can hypothesize that, in our cases, the development of the microprolactinoma may depend on a primary alteration in lactotrophic cells at the dopamine receptor or post-receptor site [11, 13].

This hypothesis can justify the lack of lactotroph responsiveness to dopaminergic blockade and the consequent rise, in hypothalamic dopamine turnover and activity which are able to exert an exaggerated inhibition on thyrotropic cells [3].

Nevertheless, recent observations from Camanni et. al. [1] have shown the inability of surgical removal to restore a normal PRL secretory pattern after nomifensine in five patients with microprolactinoma. The authors suggest a hypothalamic pathogenesis of pituitary microprolactinoma in accordance with the hypothesis of Fine and Frohman [2]. Van Loon [12] and Ho et. al. [6].

In addition, in an other eight cases of microprolactinoma in women we have observed the existence of an exaggerated hypothalamic opioid activity (Naloxone supressible), which was able to alter reciprocally the dopamine inhibitory action on lactotrophic (diminished) and thyrotropic (enhanced) cells [8].

We can therefore speculate that the development of microprolactinoma may not be homogeneous and may reflect genetic and environmental factors acting either at the pituitary or hypothalamic level. Concerning our operated cases it is very important to follow the secretory patterns of PRL and TSH to confirm the absence of any disturbance in the hypothalamic dopaminergic control of pituitary hormonal secretion.

References

[1] Camanni, F., E. Ghigo, E. Ciccarelli, et. al.: Defective regulation of Prolactin secretion after successful removal od prolactinomas. J. Clin. Endocrinol. Metab. **57** (6) (1983) 1270–1276.

[2) Fine, S. A., L. A. Frohman: Loss of central system component of dopaminergic inhibition of prolactin secretion in patients with prolactin secreting pituitary tumours. J. Clin. Invest. **61** (1978) 973–980.

[3] Foord, S. M., J. R. Peters, C. Dieguez, et. al.: Dopamine receptors on intact anterior pituitary cells in culture: functional association with the inhibition of prolactin and thyrotropin. Endocrinology **112** (5) (1983) 1567–1577.

[4] Gelli, D., G. Pagani, M. Montini, et. al.: Effect of sulpiride on TSH secretion in patients with tumoral and functional hyperprolactinaemia. J. Endocr. Invest. **4** (Suppl. 2) (1981) 25.

[5] Gudelsky, G. A., J. Simpkins, G. P. Muller, et. al.: Selektive action of prolactin on cathecolamine turnover in the hypotalamus and on serum LH and FHS. Neuroendocrinology **22** (1976) 206–209.

[6] Ho, K. Y., G. A. Smythe, M. Duncan: Dopamine infusion studies in patients with pathological hyperprolactinaemia: evidence of normal prolactin suppressibility but abnormal dopamine metabolism. J. Clin. Endocrinol. Metab. **58** (1) (1984) 123–128.

[7] Hokfeldt, T., K. Fuxe: Effect of prolactin and ergot alkaloids in the tubero-infundibular dopamine (DA) neurons. Neuroendocrinology **4** (1972) 100–122.

[8] Pagani, G., M. Montini, R. Benco, et. al.: Reciprocal response of PRL and TSH to sulpiride during opiate receptor blockade in pituitary microprolactinoma, p. 85. First International Meeting of I.S.E., "Recent Progress in Opioid Research", Florence, 3–5 Oct., 1983.

[9] Quigley, M. E., S. S. C. Yen: Evidence for increased dopaminergic inhibition of secretion of thyroid stimulating hormone in hyperprolactinaemic patients with pituitary microadenoma. American J. Obst. Gynecol. **137** (1980) 653–655.
[10] Scanlon, M. F., M. D. Rodriguez Arnao, A. M. Mc Gregor, et. al.: Altered dopaminergic regulation of thyrotropin release in patients with prolactinomas comparison with other dynamic test of prolactin secretion. Clinical Endocrinology **14** (1980) 133–143.
[11] Tallo, D., W. B. Malarkey: Adrenergic and dopaminergic modulation of growth hormone and prolactin secretion in normal and tumour bearing human pituitaries in monolayer culture. Endocr. and Metab. **53** (6) (1981) 1278–1284.
[12] Van Loon, G. R.: A defect in catecholamine neurons in patients with prolactin secreting pituitary adenomas. Lancet **2** (1978) 868–871.
[13] Webb, C. B., J. L. Thominet, H. Barowsky, et. al.: Evidence for lactotrophe dopamine resistence in hydiopathic hyperprolactinaemia. J. Clin. Endocrinol. Metab. **56** (6) (1983) 1089–1093.

Prolactin and TSH responses to TRH and domperidone in delayed puberty

V. Popović, D. Micić, R. Han, S. Radmanović, M. Nešović, S. Pavlica, P. Dordević, D. Manojlović, J. Mićić, D. Durić

Introduction

The distinction between isolated gonadotropin deficiency and delayed puberty is difficult. Spitz et. al. [5] have suggested that an impaired prolactin response to challenge with TRH may facilitate the diagnosis of isolated gonadotropin deficiency and differentiate this condition from delayed puberty. These authors found an impaired response of prolactin to TRH and possibly to metoclopramide also, in patients with isolated gonadotropin deficiency.

The aim of this study was to compare prolactin responses to TRH and domperidone, a peripheral dopaminergic antagonist, in patients with delayed puberty.

Material and methods

Patients

Ten patients (6 male and 4 female) with delayed puberty were studied. They were 14.5 to 18 years old and had delayed sexual development for their age according to Tanner (stage 2). None were obese. Their bone age was between 13 to 16 years (delayed in comparison to their chronological age). All subjects were followed till spontaneous sexual development.

Tests

TRH test was performed with 200 mcg i.v. (Relefact, Hoechst) and samples for prolactin and TSH determinations were taken at 0, 20, and 60 minutes. The next day 10 mg of domperidone were given i.v. and samples for prolactin and TSH were taken at 0, 30, 60, 90 and 120 minutes. The peak hormonal responses in the tests were then compared.

Assays

Testosterone was determined using BIODATA kits with a normal range from 3–9 ng/ml. Prolactin was determined using BIODATA kits with a normal range from 5–25 ng/ml and intraassay CV was 9.7% The TSH was determined using INEP kits with a normal range from 1–8 mU/l and an intraassay CV of 10%.

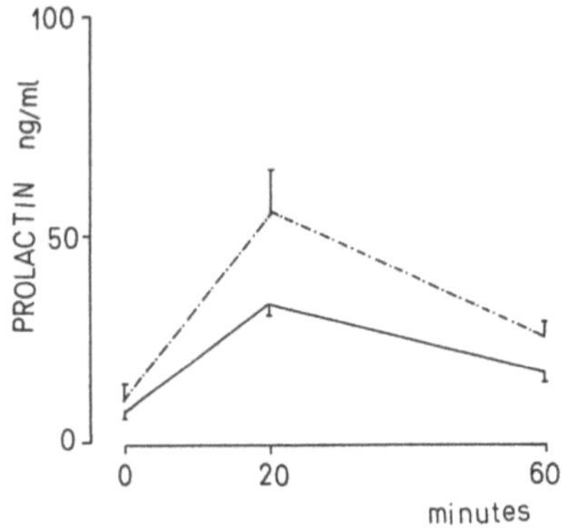

Fig. 1 Prolactin response to TRH in patients with delayed puberty
boys ————; girls –·–·–·–·–

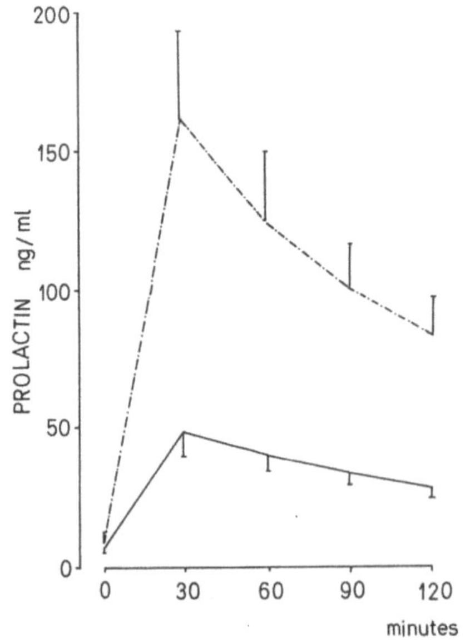

Fig. 2 Prolactin response to domperidone in patients with delayed puberty
boys ————; girls –·–·–·–·–

Results

The mean basal testosterone level in boys with delayed puberty was 1.8 ± 0.2 ng/ml. The prolactin and TSH responses to TRH are shown on figures 1 and 2. The peak elevation of prolactin after the TRH test ranged from 32 to 48 ng/ml for boys and 32 to 60 ng/ml for girls. The response of TSH to TRH was normal. The peak prolactin response to domperidone, a dopaminergic agent which does not cross the BBB, ranged from 34 to 65 ng/ml for boys and 65 to 200 ng/ml for girls. The TSH did not change after domperidone administration.

Discussion

We have shown that the prolactin response after domperidone is as effective as after TRH injection, in our patients with delayed puberty and that this test could be possibly used to differentiate this condition from isolated gonadotropin deficiency.

The precise mechanism underlying this difference in prolactin response to TRH in delayed puberty and in patients with isolated gonadotropin deficiency is not known [6]. Certain levels of oestrogen are required to achieve a prolactin response to TRH and in both conditions oestrogens are low. The difference in response might be due to subtle differences in oestrogen levels, or due to different age groups of patients with delayed puberty compared to patients with an isolated gonadotropin deficiency. There is evidence today, that there is a functional interaction between gonadotrophs and lactotrophs [2]. Experimental studies in vitro suggest that gonadotrophs can activate the secretory activity of the lactotrophs through the release of a paracrine humoral factor. It is not known whether these functional interactions are different in isolated gonadotropin deficiency in comparison to patients with delayed puberty.

Domperidone, a dopamine antagonist which does not cross the BBB is not a very good indicator of central dopaminergic activity when its concentration is low [1]. It is a better indicator of dopamine hyperactivity. Metoclopramide, passes through BBB and indicates central dopaminergic activity much better [3]. The prolactin response to metoclopramide in delayed puberty is normal. We have shown a normal response of prolactin to domperidone also.

We did not find any changes in the TSH levels during the domperidone test in patients with delayed puberty.

In patients with isolated gonadotropin deficiency a low basal prolactin and an impaired response to TRH are said to be due to an abnormal steroid milieu [4]. The mechanism of this phenomenon awaits further clarification.

Abstract

We have studied 10 patients with delayed puberty (6 male and 4 female). They were 14.5 to 18 years old and had delayed sexual development for their age (stage 2 Tanner). None were obese. During a TRH test (200 mcg i.v.) samples for prolactin and TSH determinations were obtained. After domperidone (10 mg i.v.) samples for prolactin and TSH were obtained as well. The basal prolactin level was normal (9.2 ± 2.4 ng/ml). The prolactin reponses to TRH in our patients were normal i.e. the peak elevation of prolactin after TRH injection ranged from 32 to 48 ng/ml for boys and 32 to 85 ng/ml for girls. The TSH response to TRH was normal. The peak prolactin response after domperidone ranged from 34 to 65 ng/ml for boys and 65 to 200 ng/ml for girls. The TSH levels did not change after domperidone administration. We have shown that the prolactin response after domperidone administration is as effective as after TRH injection in our patients with delayed puberty and that this test could be used to differentiate delayed from isolated gonadotropin deficiency.

References

[1] Cocchi, D., A. Penalva, A. Novelli: Hypothalamic neurotransmitter function in experimental hyperprolactinaemia. 3rd European Workshop on Pituitary Adenomas. Abstract Book, 7–10 Sept., Amsterdam 1983.

[2] Denef, C.: Functional interrelationship between pituitary cells. 3rd European Workshop on Pituitary Adenomas. Abstract Book, 7–10 Sept., Amsterdam 1983.

[3] Jungmann, E., P. Althoff, U. Schwedes, et. al.: Responsiveness of aldosterone and pituitary hormone secretion to metoclopramide in prolactinoma. 3rd European Workshop on Pituitary Adenomas. Abstract Book, 7–10 Sept., Amsterdam 1983.

[4] Spitz, I., A. Zylber-Haran, S. Trestian, et. al.: The decrease basal and stimulated prolactin levels in isolated gonadotropin. deficiency: a consequence of the low estrogen state. Clin. Endocrinol. (Oxf.) **16** (1982) 423–432.

[5] Spitz, I., H. Hirsh, S. Trestian: The prolactin response to thyrotropin-releasing hormone differentiates isolated gonadotropin deficiency from delayed puberty. N. Engl. J. Med. **308** (1983) 575–579.

[6] Spitz, I., S. Haas, S. Trestian, et. al.: The interrelationship between prolactin and thyrotropin secretion following dopaminergic blockade in patients with mild hyperprolactinaemia without demonstrable pituitary tumour. Clin. Endocrinol. (Oxf.) **19** (1983) 285–294.

Anterior pituitary function in patients with prolactinomas

A. Luger

Introduction

Prolactin secreting pituitary adenomas are known to be able to compromise anterior pituitary function by two separate mechanisms: 1. mechanically, as is the case in macroprolactinomas by compressing the surrounding nonadenomatous tissue and 2. metabolically by the excess production of prolactin.

It was the aim of this study to investigate the pituitary function of patients with prolactinomas by measuring basal and stimulated hormone levels and correlate them to the prolactin levels.

Patients and methods

32 patients with prolactinomas were investigated (tab. 1). 13 patients had microprolactinomas and 19 macroprolactinomas, 18 females and 14 males, whose mean age was 37, ranging from 13 to 54 yrs.

Serum prolactin levels ranged from 48 to 82000 ng/ml. Basal levels of growth hormone (GH), luteinizing hormone (LH), follicle stimulating hormone (FSH), thyroxine (T4), thyroid stimulating hormone (TSH), testosterone (T) and oestradiol (E2) as well as urinary cortisol excretion were measured.

GH secretion was stimulated by 0.5 g/kg body weight arginine, LH and FSH by 100 μg LHRH, and TSH by 200 μg TRH.

All hormones were determined by using commercially available radioimmunoassays.

CT scans where performed in all patients, from which the patients were then classified as having micro- or macroprolactinomas as previously described [1]. Data are expressed as mean ± SD.

Table 1 Data of 32 patients with prolactinomas

No	Sex	Age yrs	PRL ng/ml	GH ng/ml	LH mU/ml	FSH mU/ml	T4 µg/dl	T ng/dl
1	F	22	72	1.2	5.3	4.7	7.8	–
2	F	34	60	1.3	1.6	5.4	9.0	–
3	F	30	5330	0.8	2.2	3.2	6.5	–
4	F	39	400	0.7	4.7	3.2	6.0	–
5	F	19	1700	0.9	2.4	4.2	6.7	–
6	F	26	3750	0.7	2.8	1.7	8.3	–
7	F	31	230	3.2	1.2	1.3	7.5	–
8	F	40	2500	0.6	9.7	3.8	8.9	–
9	F	31	14000	0.5	6.4	0.3	6.4	–
10	F	39	84	1.3	0	1.9	6.4	–
11	F	47	150	0	4.6	1.8	7.9	–
12	F	45	103	0.9	3.6	19.1	4.4	–
13	F	31	351	1.2	3.7	5.4	5.1	–
14	F	40	162	0.4	1.9	3.2	7.7	–
15	F	29	114	0.9	3.5	4.5	7.0	–
16	F	37	339	0.5	0.3	1.3	4.2	–
17	F	51	1375	0.5	2.5	5.7	6.8	–
18	F	54	720	1.3	1.7	4.8	6.6	–
19	M	45	116	0.5	5.2	4.3	6.0	170
20	M	37	48	0.8	6.0	2.1	5.1	285
21	M	53	870	0.8	1.6	2.7	5.3	0
22	M	33	185	1.4	2.4	3.9	7.1	162
23	M	33	1050	1.0	1.5	2.6	4.2	0
24	M	40	418	0.9	2.3	3.3	8.7	112
25	M	46	2680	0.6	2.7	2.9	6.5	340
26	M	40	2111	0.6	1.3	0.2	3.8	90
27	M	27	1750	0.5	7.4	1.6	5.9	0
28	M	35	1104	0.9	1.8	2.4	3.4	100
29	M	13	513	0.7	1.0	4.5	3.9	30
30	M	51	82000	0.6	5.2	3.9	7.3	137
31	M	50	3850	0.9	3.3	4.5	6.7	0
32	M	36	1250	0.8	2.8	3.9	8.7	290

Results (see figure 1)

Mean basal GH-levels were 0.9 ± 0.4 ng/ml, and stimulation with arginine led to a mean peak level of only 1.6 ± 0.8 ng/ml. The normal reactivity of GH secretion was found in only 22% of the patients, all of them having microadenomas.

Although testosterone levels in men (122 ± 116 ng/dl) and oestradiol levels in women (38 ± 36 pg/ml, n = 7) were generally in the lower normal range or below the normal range, basal LH and FSH concentrations were not elevated (LH 3.2 ±

2.1 mU/ml and FSH 3.7 ± 3.2 mU/ml). Administration of 100 μg LHRH led to a mean peak value of LH 4.6 ± 2.5 mU/ml and FSH 6.6 ± 5.6 mU/ml. Gonadotropin secretion was suppressed in 16 patients (50%).

Mean basal thyroxine (6.4 ± .7 μg/dl) and TSH levels (2.5 ± 1.3 μU/ml) were in the normal range although subnormal thyroxine levels were found in 5 patients (16%).

Urinary cortisol excretion was normal (mean of 37 ± 16 μg/24 h) in all but 4 patients (13%) who had a macroprolactinoma.

None of the measured parameters correlated with the serum prolactin levels.

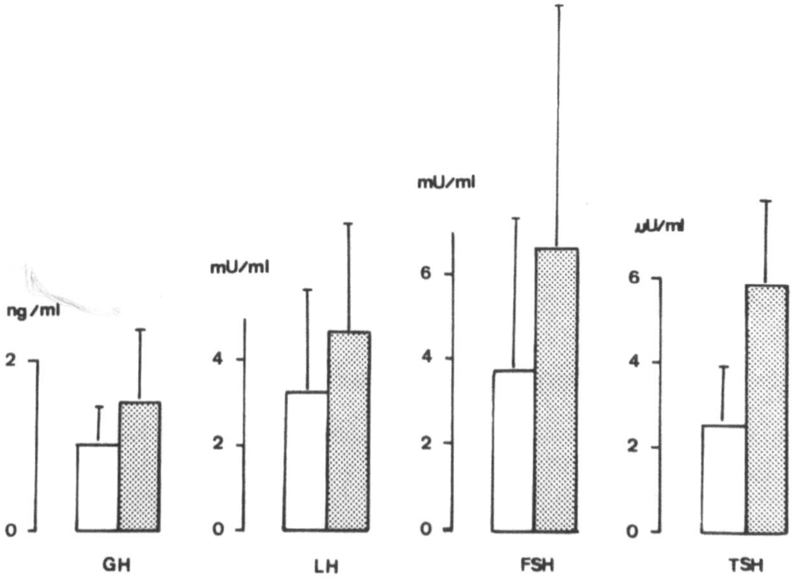

Fig. 1 Basal (open bars) and stimulated (shaded bars) GH, LH, FSH and TSH secretion in 32 patients with prolactinomas.

Conclusions

In this series of 32 patients with prolactinomas a clear order in which pituitary dysfunction occurs could be found. The most sensitive anterior pituitary function in these patients is GH secretion; only 22% were not affected. GH secretion, however, does not have major clinical relevance in adult patients. Disturbances of gonadotropin secretion are often encountered, 50% of our patients had hypogonadotropic hypogonadism.

As previously reported [2, 3], recovery of hypogonadism frequently occurs after normalization of hyperprolactinaemia. It still remains to be established on which level the hypothalamic-pituitary-gonadal axis is affected and to what extent mechanical compression is causally involved. In our patients and in the previously reported series of 22 men with prolactinomas [3] stimulation of the gonadotropins that were in the low normal range was possible. Furthermore, Leydig cell function has been shown to react normally after administration of human choriongonadotropin [3]. Thus diminished LHRH-release by the hypothalamus seems to be the cause of hypogonadism in male patients with prolactinomas. Because exogenous LHRH led to an increase in the gonadotropins, a direct action of prolactin is more likely than the mechanical compression of the monadenomatous tissue. However, in the 14 male patients no correlation between serum prolactin levels on the one side and LH, FSH or testosterone levels on the other side could be found.

Corticotropin and thyrotropin secretion were the two least frequently affected pituitary functions (13 and 16%), all of the patients having macroprolactinomas with impairment of the two other anterior pituitary functions.

In summary, our results show in addition to previous studies [4–6] that impairment of GH-secretion is the most frequently encountered pituitary dysfunction in patients with prolactinomas, followed by hypogonadotropic hypogonadism, thyrotropin and ACTH secretion.

References

[1] Vezina, J. L., T. J. Sutton: Prolactin secreting pituitary microadenomas. AJR **120** (1974) 46–54.
[2] Carter, J. N., J. N. Tyson, G. Tolis, et al.: Prolactin-secreting tumors and hypogonadism in 22 men. N. Engl. J. Med. **299** (1978) 847–852.
[3] Arafah, B. M., A. M. Manni, J. S. Brodkey, et al.: Cure of hypogonadism after removal of prolactin-secreting adenomas in men. J. Clin. Endocrinol. Metab. **52,** (1981) 91–94.
[4] Chang, R. J., W. R. Keye, S. E. Monroe, et al.: Prolactin-secreting pituitary adenomas in women. IV. Pituitary function in amenorrhea associated with normal or abnormal serum prolactin and sellar polytomography. J. Clin. Endocrinol. Metab. **51** (1980) 830–835.
[5] Hagen, C., J. Lindholm, E. Suenson, et al.: Relationship between plasma prolactin concentration and pituitary function in patients with a pituitary adenoma. Clin. Endocrinol. **11** (1979) 671–679.
[6] Flückiger, E., E. del Pozo, K. von Werder: Prolactin – Physiology, Pharmacology and Clinical findings. Springer-Verlag, Berlin–Heidelberg–New York, 1982.

Pituitary adenomas with hyperprolactinaemia in males

C. Muhr, A.-L. Hulting, P. O. Lundberg, S. Werner

Introduction

Studies on hyperprolactinaemic disorders have been focussed on women and considerably less articles deal with men with hyperprolactinaemia. We have thus chosen to investigate a material of male patients with signs of a pituitary tumour and hyperprolactinaemia to further describe this patient group.

Material and methods

Thirty-seven consecutive men with a pituitary tumour and hyperprolactinaemia were studied. Patients with concomitant hypersecretion of GH were excluded. Serum levels of prolactin (PRL), luteinizing hormone (LH), follicle-stimulating hormone (FSH) and plasma levels of testosterone and GH are given as mean values based on 2–4 fasting morning samples. The adrenal function was evaluated by U-cortisol and, in patients with suspected adrenal insufficiency, by the Metyrapone test. The thyroid function was evaluated by serum thyroid stimulating hormone (TSH), T_4 and T_3 and by the thyroid releasing hormone (TRH) test when hypothyroidism was suspected. GH reserve was tested by the L-dopa test (500 mg perorally). TRH, 200 μg, was administered as an intravenous injection and TSH, GH and PRL were analysed.

The roentgenological examination included plain sellar films in anterior-posterior and lateral projections and skeletal tomography in some patients. All patients underwent CT or sella encephalography. The patients were grouped according to the radiographical findings: group I had sellae of normal size with asymmetries indicating microadenomas, group II had enlarged sellae and group III enlarged sellae with local bone erosinons as signs of invasive tumour growth and group IV consisted of patients with enlarged sellae, bone erosions and signs of parasellar invasive tumour growth according to encephalography or CT. Perimetry, as described by Goldmann, and visual acuity were examined in all patients. Patients were ranked 1–37 according to preoperative PRL levels (fig. 7). Pituitary surgery, by transsphenoidal or transfrontal route, was performed in 11 patients. External irradiation was given to 11 patients; in eight patients after previous surgery. All patients were treated with bromocriptine, 1.25–10 mg/day. The follow-up time varied between 6 months and 5 years in all but one patient, who died from pneumonia 3 months after the commencement of bromocriptine treatment.

Results

The age of the patients ranged from 25–73 years (mean 47 years, median 51 years). Basal prolactin levels varied between 50 and 18000 μg/l (mean 2600 μg/l and median 1050 μg/l). Prolactin increments were similar in the different age groups (fig. 1). The results of the roentgenological examinations and the perime-

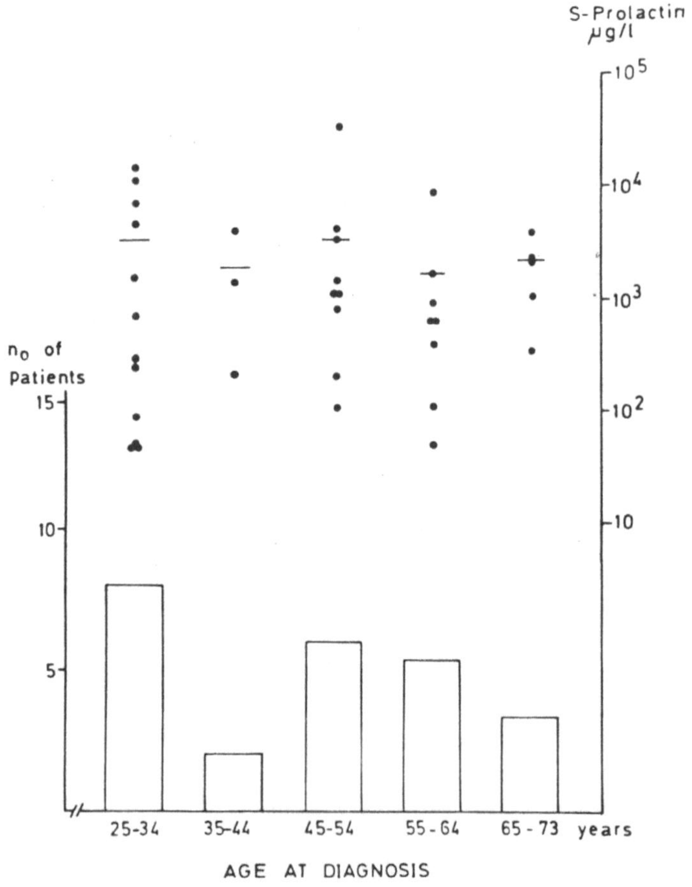

Fig. 1 37 men with prolactinomas grouped according to their age at diagnosis. Their respective S-PRL levels at diagnosis are given at the top of the columns.

Table 1 Roentgenological findings and results of perimetry in 37 men

Sella turcica	no. of patients	no. with suprasellar extension	no. with visual field defects
Group I normal size, asymmetry	5	0	0
Group II enlarged	13	6	5
Group III enlarged, locally eroded (invasive adenomas)	6	5	3
Group IV enlarged, eroded, parasellar tumour growth (invasive adenomas)	13	12	7
	37	23	15

tries are presented in table 1. Five patients showed asymmetric sellae of normal size with no suprasellar tumour extension or visual field defects (group I). Thirteen patients had enlarged sellae with suprasellar tumour extension in 6 and visual field defects in 5 patients (group II). Six patients showed enlarged sellae with bone erosions as signs of invasive tumour growth. Five patients in this group had tumours with suprasellar extension causing visual field defects in 3 patients (group III). Eroded and enlarged sellae with parasellar invasive tumour growth were seen in 13 patients, 12 of whom had tumours with suprasellar extension, in seven cases causing visual field defects (group IV). In groups III and IV with invasively growing tumours the serum prolactin levels were significantly higher than in the rest of the patients (fig. 2). Four patients in group I and 2 patients in group II had prolactin levels ≤ 100 μg/l. These patients had no signs of suprasellar disorders or medical treatment that could have caused their moderate increase in prolactin levels. However, it should be pointed out that moderately elevated prolactin levels per se do not indicate that the pituitary adenoma is prolactin producing but could also be caused by a hypothalamic disturbance with loss of inhibition [5].

Table 2 lists the clinical symptoms according to frequency; no patient was asymptomatic at the time of diagnosis. The most common symptom was decreased libido-potency. Visual field defects, ocular nerve palsies and headache were also frequent. Thirteen patients noticed increased weight (> 4 kg) during the first year with other subjective symptoms of the disease. Secondary hypothyroidism was found in 11 patients and secondary cortisol insufficiency in 7 patients. Galactorrhoea was infrequent.

Table 3 lists the symptom first noted by the patient and the symptom which led to clinical examination. Decreased libido potency was the first subjective symptom in

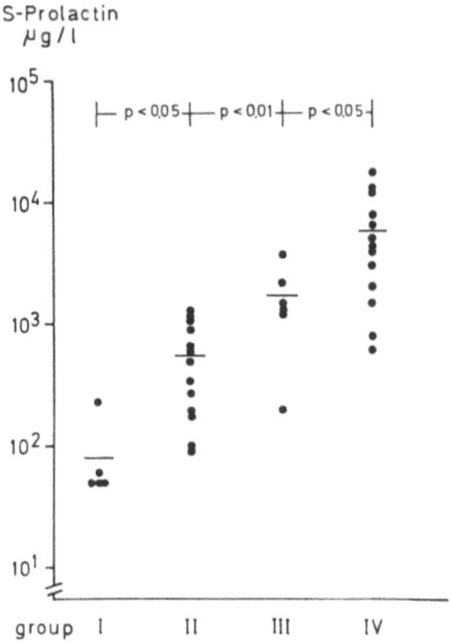

Fig. 2 37 men grouped according to their radiological sella changes and S-PRL levels. Group I: 5 patients with asymmetric sellae of normal size. Group II: 13 patients with enlarged sellae without bone erosions. Group III: 6 patients with enlarged, eroded sellae and Group IV: 13 patients with enlarged sellae, bone erosions and parasellar tumour growth.

Table 2 Clinical symptoms or signs according to frequency in 37 men

Decreased libido/impotence	29
Eye symptoms (visual field defect, ocular nerve palsy)	16
Headache	16
Weight gain, >4 kg	13
Hypothyroidism	11
Cortisol deficiency	7
Gynecomastia	6
Depression	6
Impaired memory, disability to concentrate	5
Epilepsy	3
Galactorrhoea	2

18 patients, but made only 5 patients seek a physician. Visual field defects or ocular nerve palsies usually made the patients contact a physician.

The duration of symptoms varied from 5 months to 35 years. Fifty per cent of the patients had a subjective history of disease for four years or less (fig. 3).

Ten out of the 12 patients with symptom duration of more than 9 years had decreased libido-potency as their first symptom. Out of the 21 patients with symptom

Table 3 The first subjective symptom and the symptom which made the patients seek a physician

	First symptom no. of patients	Symptom leading to clinical examination no. of patients
decreased libido / potency	18	5
headache	8	8
eye symptoms	6	12
hypothyroidism dry skin, cold intolerance	2	5
epilepsy	2	2
galactorrhoea	1	–
cortisol deficiency	–	2
diminished growth of facial hair	–	2
depression	–	1
	37	37

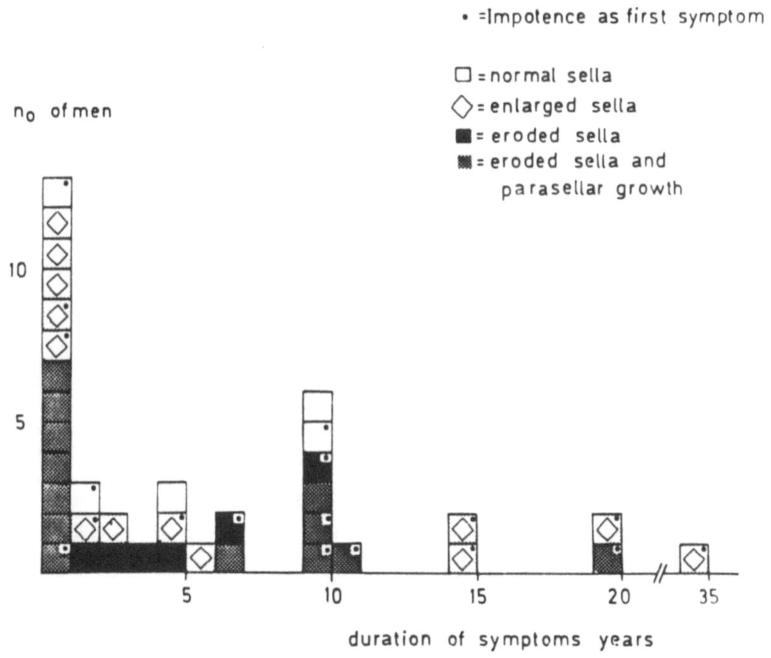

Fig. 3 37 men with prolactinomas arranged according to the subjective duration of symptoms before diagnosis and according to radiographical findings in the sella region. Dots indicate patients with decreased libido and impotence as the first subjective symptom of the disease.

duration less than 5 years 6/10 patients without invasive tumour growth had decreased libido-potency as their first symptom in contrast to 1/11 patients with invasive tumours, indicating that these latter tumours give rise to other symptomatology.

Testosterone and prolactin levels are shown in figure 4; there was no correlation between prolactin and testosterone levels. Twenty-two men had testosterone levels below the lower normal range, 11 nmol/l, only 2 of these patients had normal libido-potency. Ten patients showed testosterone levels between 11 and 16 nmol/l. Altogether 8 patients (aged 25–64 years) indicated by circles in figure 4, had normal libido-potency. The 5 patients with the highest testosterone levels presented a history of disease shorter than 2 years.

In figure 5 prolactin levels are given in relation to LH and FSH; five patients showed LH levels above the upper normal limit, 12 nmol/l. In figure 6 plasma tes-

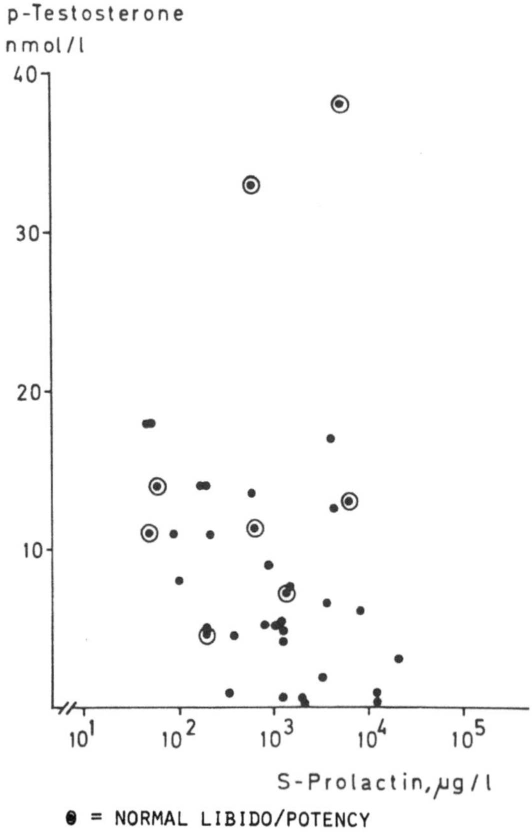

Fig. 4 P-testosterone levels in 37 men with prolactinomas are given in relation to their S-PRL levels. Lower normal range (-2 SD) for P-testosterone is 11 nmol/l. Patients with normal libido and potency are indicated by circles.

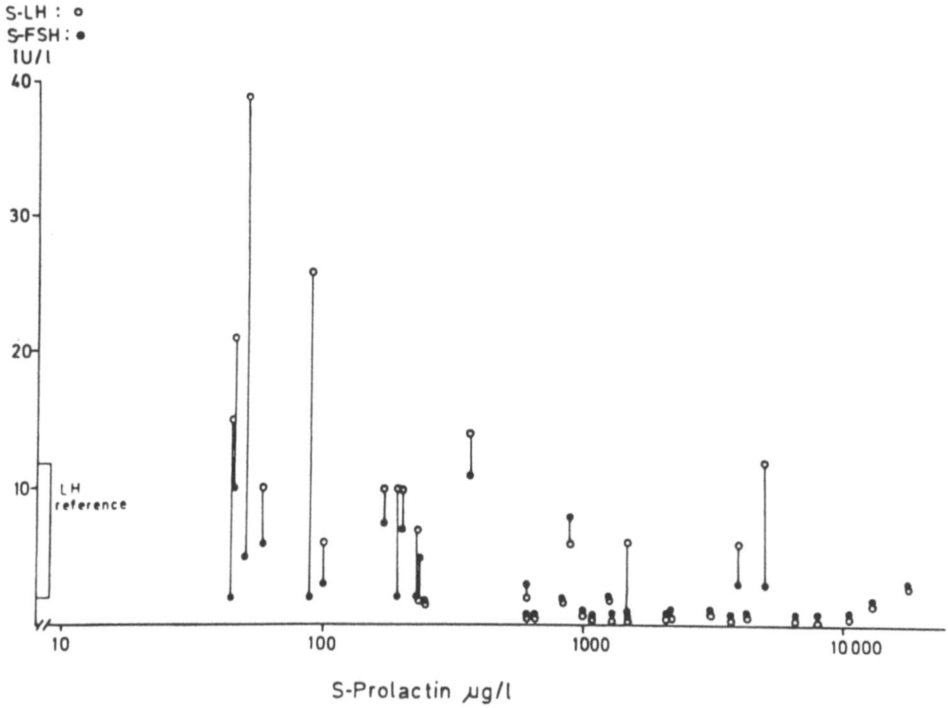

Fig. 5 S-LH (O) and S-FSH (●) in relation to S-PRL levels in 37 men with prolactinomas.

tosterone is related to LH and FSH. Three patients with elevated LH had testosterone levels within the normal range.

Prolactin levels before and during treatment with bromocriptine are shown in figure 7. Patients were ranked 1–37 according to their prolactin concentrations before treatment. Surgery, irradiation or a combination of both did not normalize prolactin levels. Bromocriptine normalized prolactin levels in all but 3 patients; patient no 12 died 3 months after the onset of therapy, the other two showed declining prolactin levels during therapy.

Bromocriptine treatment normalized prolactin levels in 20 patients with testosterone levels below the normal range. Concomitant normalization of testosterone levels were only noted in the 6 patients with initially no signs of LH and FSH insufficiency (fig. 7).

Visual field defects, noted in 15 patients, disappeared during bromocriptine treatment except in 2 patients with parasellar tumour growth and paresis of the oculomotor nerve. Ten large tumours which had not been subjected to surgery or irradiation were studied by CT scan before as well as during bromocriptine therapy. Diminution of tumour size was noted in 8 cases (nos. 4, 9, 10, 11, 14, 15, 18 and 23).

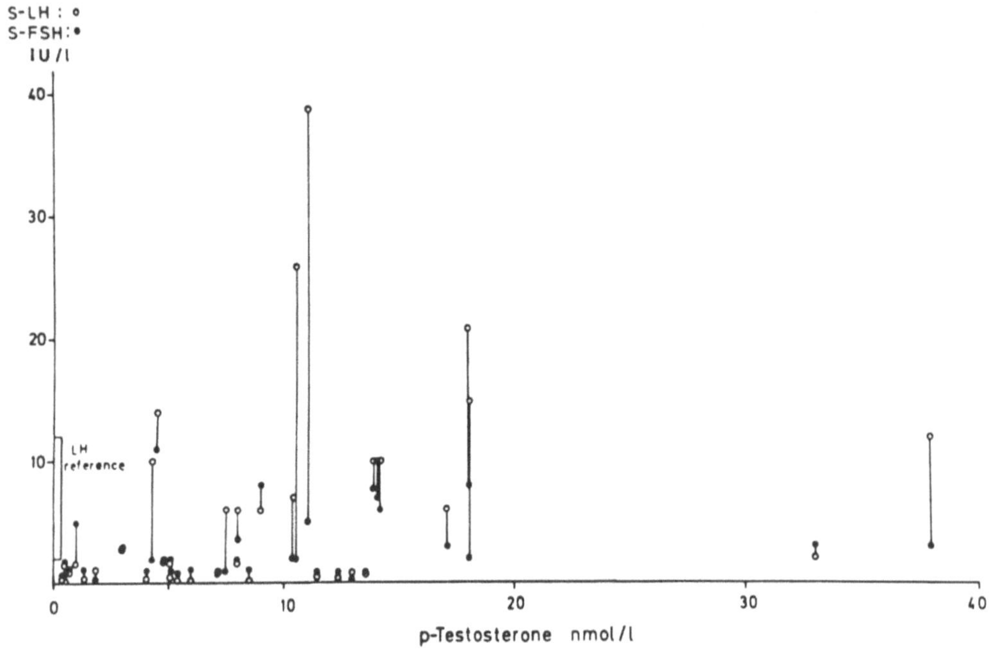

Fig. 6 S-LH (○) and S-FSH (●) in relation to S-testosterone in 37 men with prolactinomas.

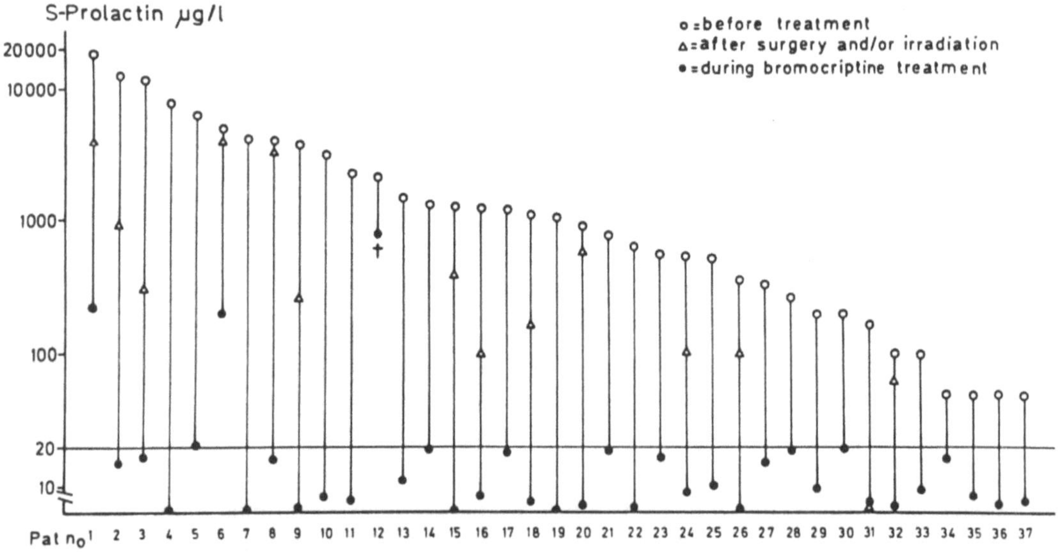

Fig. 7 37 men with prolactinomas listed according to S-PRL levels at diagnosis (○). S-PRL levels 3–6 months after surgery (△; patient nos. 1, 26, 31). S-PRL levels after surgery and external irradiation 50 Gy (△; patient nos. 2, 3, 6, 8, 16, 20, 24, 32). S-PRL after irradiation (△; patient nos. 9, 15, 18), S-PRL during bromocriptine treatment (●).

Discussion

The present study confirms previous reports on male prolactinomas:

a) The most frequent symptom of the disease is decreased libido-potency [1, 2, 3, 8].

b) Pituitary surgery and irradiation are less favourable than bromocriptine treatment with regard to normalization of prolactin levels [1, 3, 4, 7, 8, 9, 10].

c) Pituitary adenomas with an invasive growth pattern have higher serum prolactin levels than adenomas that are not invasive [10].

d) In male patients the diagnosis is often made when local signs of tumour growth result in the development most often of visual field defects [1, 11].

It is evident from this study as well as from a previous one [12] that lack of libido and potency is not considered by many patients a sufficient reason to seek a physician; 9 men lived with these symptoms of hypogonadism for more than 9 years (fig. 3). 7/13 patients with symptoms for less than a year had large tumours with parasellar growth and bone erosions (group IV, fig. 3). Only one of the 7 patients had subjective signs of hypogonadism. Furthermore, 3 of these 7 patients with large tumours had normal testosterone levels.

Fourteen per cent of our patients – 4 with microadenomas (group I) and one patient with a macroadenoma (group II) – showed signs of hypergonadotropic hypogonadism with elevated LH levels and normal or subnormal plasma testosterone (figs. 5 and 6). This has not been reported previously in men with prolactin secreting pituitary adenomas. The finding can be interpreted in different ways. Either gonadotropin secreting tumours with concomitant hyperprolactinaemia are not as rare as reported up to now [13, 14], or in some patients with prolactin producing pituitary adenomas prolactin exerts an inhibitory effect preferentially on the gonad with a secondary increase in LH secretion. Bromocriptine therapy was effective also in these 5 patients. Prolactin as well as LH normalized and testosterone increased.

Surgery or irradiation, performed in 14 patients, did not normalize prolactin levels. During bromocriptine treatment clinical symptoms improved and prolactin levels were normalized in 34/37 patients. Furthermore, medical treatment normalized or improved visual field defects in all affected patients and markedly diminished tumour size in 8/10 patients studied with CT scans before and during bromocriptine treatment.

References

[1] Eversmann, T., R. Echinger, R. Fahlbusch, et al.: Die Hyperprolaktinämie beim Mann: Klinik und Therapie. Schweiz. med. Wschr. **111** (1981) 1782–1789.

[2] Goodman, R. H., M. E. Molitch, K. D. Post, et al.: Prolactin-secreting adenomas in the male. In: The Pituitary Adenoma, pp. 91–108. Plenum, New York 1980.
[3] Carter, J. N., J. E. Tyson, G. Tolis, et al.: Prolactin-secreting tumors and hypogonadism in 22 men. New Engl. J. Med. **299** (1978) 847–852.
[4] Somma, M., H. Beauregard, E. Rasio: Le prolactinome chez l'homme. Résultat thérapeutique chez 40 hommes. Neurochirurgie **27**, Suppl. 1 (1981) 91–94.
[5] Lundberg, P. O., P. O. Osterman, L. Wide: Serum prolactin in patients with hypothalamus and pituitary disorders. J. Neurosurg. **55** (1981) 194–199.
[6] Franks, S., H. S. Jacobs, N. Martin, et al.: Hyperprolactinaemia and impotence. Clin. Endocrinol. **8** (1978) 277–287.
[7] Thorner, M. O., G. M. Besser: Bromocriptine treatment of hyperprolactinaemic hypogonadism. Acta Endocrinol. (Copenh) **88**, Suppl. 216 (1978) 131–146.
[8] Thorner, M. O., W. H. Martin, A. D. Rogol, et al.: Rapid regression of pituitary prolactinomas during bromocriptine treatment. J. Clin. Endocrinol. Metab. **51** (1980) 438–445.
[9] Prescott, R. W. G., P. Kendall-Taylor, K. Hall, et al.: Hyperprolactinaemia in men – response to bromocriptine therapy. Lancet **I** (1982) 245–249.
[10] Muhr, C., P. O. Lundberg, K. Bergström: Prolactin-producing invasive pituitary adenomas. In: Suppl. 256 acc Vol. 103 Advance Abstracts of papers XIV Acta Endocrinologica Congress Stockholm, Sweden, Burson-Marsteller AB, Sweden, p 84, 1983.
[11] Nagulesparen, M., V. Ang, J. S. Jenkins: Bromocriptine treatment of males with pituitary tumours. Hyperprolactinaemia, and hypogonadism. Clin. Endocrinol **9** (1978) 73–79.
[12] Lundberg, P. O., L. Wide: Sexual function in males with pituitary tumors. Fertil. Steril. **29** (1978) 175–179.
[13] Sassolas, G., J. Trouillas, H. Lejeune, et al.: A clinical and biological study of 10 gonadotropic pituitary adenomas revealed by immunocytochemistry and intratumorous assay. 3rd Eur Workshop on Pituitary Adenomas. Amsterdam 1983.
[14] Mashiter, K.: Gonadotrophin-secreting adenomas: *In vitro* studies, clinical aspects and treatment. 3rd Eur Workshop on Pituitary Adenomas. Amsterdam 1983.

Prolactinoma in multiple endocrine neoplasia type I

J. M. Gottswinter, G. Feurle, G. Holz, R. Ziegler

The multiple endocrine neoplasia type I = MEN I is a well known syndrome. However, the same syndrome, including all the facets one could ever expect in it, especially with affection of the anterior pituitary gland by a macro- or microprolactinoma is rather rare.

In 1903 Erdheim, the German pathologist, gave the first description of the combined occurrence of tumours of the parathyroid glands and of the pituitary gland, which caused an acromegaly. 1927 Davidoff and Cushing reported a case in which pituitary, parathyroid and pancreatic adenomas occurred simultaneously. In 1953 Underdahl gave a complete description of MEN I, but he failed to recognize the familial component. In 1954 Wermer noticed the genetic aspect of this syndrome, which explained an increased familiar occurrence. In his honour this entity was called the "Wermer syndrome" or multiple endocrine neoplasia I = MEN I, or formerly, multiple endocrine adenomatosis I = MEA I. The term was changed to MEN I because of the increased number of malignant tumours developing in patients bearing these adenomas. Another syndrome is MEN II, consistent of C-cell carcinoma of the thyroid and pheochromocytoma.

Whereas the combination of tumours of the parathyroids, the pituitary (acidophilic adenomas) and the pancreas is a well known entity, the combination of a Zollinger Ellison syndrome, with tumours of the parathyroid glands and prolactinoma is not so common. We observed among our patients only one with these features (fig. 1). This woman was referred to us at the age of 60 years because of recurring hypercalcaemia. Her family history was unremarkable. Her past history revealed secondary amenorrhoea since the 26th year of life, explained by genital tuberculosis at that time.

An operation for renal calculi was done in 1970. Two years later hypercalcaemia was found and cured by removal of a parathyroid adenoma, but primary hyperparathyroidism recurred only one year after the surgical intervention. In 1981 the patient went to the hospital because of an urinary tract infection; hypercalcaemia as well as a tumour of the upper mediastinum were found and she was referred to us for further investigations.

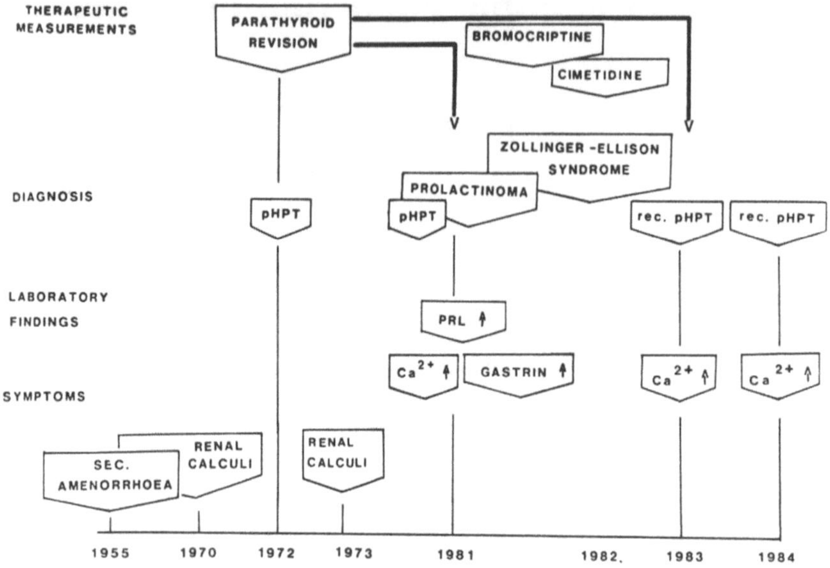

Fig. 1 Clinical course of a patient with MEN I.

Hormone measurements confirmed the suspected pHPT; the parathyroid adenoma was localized in the upper mediastinum as shown by selective venous catheterization and proven at operation. Further endocrine investigations revealed an enlarged sella turcica with markedly elevated prolactin levels of 120 ng/ml, which are thought to be the cause of the longstanding amenorrhoea, instead of the never proven "genital tuberculosis". Neurosurgical treatment of the macroprolactinoma was refused by the patient; we therefore treated with bromocriptine (daily dose 22.5 mg Pravidel). The efficacy of this treatment as shown by the prolactin levels, was abandoned by a reduced compliance of the patient. Gastrointestinal complaints led to further diagnostic procedures and markedly elevated gastrin levels of

Table 1 Clinical signs of MEN I in 85 patients of Ballard et al. [1]

74 patients =	84%	Parathyroid adenoma
55 patients =	65%	Pituitary lesion (15 patients with acromegaly)
69 patients =	81%	Pancreatic tumours (β-cell and NON-β cell tumours)
31 patients =	38%	Adrenal gland affections (adenoma, hyperplasia)
15 patients =	19%	Thyroid disease (goitre, thyroiditis)
49 patients =	58%	Peptic ulcers (often multifocal)
11 patients =	13%	Diarrhoea
11 patients =	13%	Bronchial carcinoids
4 patients =	4%	Multicentric lipomas

1700 pg/ml were found. The diagnosis of a Zollinger-Ellison syndrome was made. All efforts to localize the gastrinoma, including a percutaneous transhepatic pancratic phlebography failed; we then began to treat with H2-receptor antagonists as operation risk for the gastrinoma was considered too high, because the patient suffered from an apoplexy in the meantime.

Unfortunately hypercalcaemia returned in 1982; PTH overproduction was confirmed. Selective venous catheterization again revealed the PTH-source in the mediastinum and at operation the parathyroid adenoma was found attached to the pericardium.

Our patient presents the complete spectrum of MEN I, including parathyroid adenoma, Zollinger-Ellison-Syndrome and prolactinoma. The latter corresponds to some of the so-called "non functioning pituitary adenomas" of earlier reports [2]. The prognosis of patients with MEN I depends on complications such as peptic ulcers, hypoglycaemic coma and metabolic disorders like hypercalcaemia. Snyder et coworkers [5] recommended the following therapeutic procedure: the priority is to abandon the hypercalcaemia, and this means surgical exploration of the parathyroid glands. Secondly it should be tried, to treat the hypergastrinaemia. Because these tumours are often very small or multiple, it is usual to do total gastrectomy or continuously to use H2 receptor antagonists. Snyder [5] reports that satisfying results were even obtainable, when metastatic tumours were evident. We think that in the near future more syndromes of MEN I with hyperprolactinaemia will be detected, if one is aware that hyperprolactinaemia may occur in patients with MEN I. Combinations of MEN I with symptoms of MEN IIb also exist, as reported by Manning et al. [3]. A recently published report from Rieth and Brody [4] showed, that the CT-scan demonstrated pituitary abnormalities in 15 of 21 patients with MEN I; 19 had proved hyperprolactinaemia. Therefore, pituitary evaluation in patients with MEN I has to include prolactin determinations. The clinical presentation of these tumours may vary considerably, as depicted in table 2. Most common is the parathyroid adenoma in this syndrome; pituitary lesions occurred in 65% of the reported patients.

Endocrinopathies may occur one after another, as seen here, so that in the case of one of these endocrine disturbances one should consider the possible coexistance or even later appearance of the others. In cases of proven coexistent MEN investigations of the family history should be done.

References

[1] Ballard, H. S., B. Frame, R. J. Hartsock: Familial multiple endocrine adenoma-peptic ulcer complex. Medicine **43** (1964) 481.

[2] Hoff, F.: Polyadenomatose. Wiener Medizinische Wochenschrift **40** (1965) 813–818.

[3] Manning, G. S., K. A. Stevens, J. L. Stock: Multiple endocrine neoplasia type I. Association with marfanoid habitus, optic atrophy and other abnormalities. Arch. Intern. Med. **143** (12) (1983) 2315–2316.
[4] Rieth, K. G., S. A. Brody: CT of the pituitary gland in multiple endocrine neoplasia type I syndrome. AJNR **4** (3) (1983) 813–815.
[5] Snyder, N., M. Scurry, W. Hughes: Hypergastrinemia in familial endocrine adenomatosis. Ann. Int. Med. **80** (1974) 321.

Recurrence of hyperprolactinaemia detected in long-term follow-up of surgically normalized microprolactinomas

M. Buchfelder, A. Lierheimer, U. Schrell, K. v. Werder, R. Fahlbusch

Introduction

In all hypersecreting adenomas of the pituitary gland the aim of surgical intervention is a normalization of the hormone-excess. In microprolactinomas this objective seemed to be attainable. High normalization rates between 72 and 93% have been reported by specialized surgeons [3, 6–9]. Some years ago we [4] and others [12] had expected that in cases with acute normalization of prolactin-levels hours up to days after the adenomectomy of a microprolactinoma no recurrence of hyperprolactinaemia could be anticipated. However long-term follow-up data were not available at that time.

Materials and methods

In order to assess the longterm prognosis for women with microprolactinoma after selective transsphenoidal adenomectomy we have followed-up 50 women of our Munich and Erlangen series, who had been operated between 1973 and 1983. All of these patients had an acute normalization of serum prolactin levels within one week after the operation. Serial basal measurements of plasma prolactin were made at various intervals after the operation. The normal range of plasma prolactin was up to 500 μU/ml or 25 ng/ml. A relapse was defined as a persistent increase of prolactin above this limit. The follow-up ranged from 1.5 to 10 years with an average of 3.1 years. 18 patients were followed-up for more than 5 years.

Results

In all of the patients serum prolactin-levels normalized acutely hours after the operation and remained within the normal range for up to seven days.

In 8 of the patients, the early postoperative normalization of serum-prolactin for hours up to days after the operation was followed by a slight increase in the follow-up period. As demonstrated in figure 1, the earliest relapse was observed after two months. The longest latency between operation and prolactin re-increase was found to be four years. Not enough data are available to pinpoint the relapse of hyperprolactinaemia in one patient (B.M.), but it must have been between 2 months and 3.5 years after surgery. The patient had been pregnant within this time interval.

The re-increase in prolactin-levels was always slight and exceeded 1360 μU/ml in none of the patients. Recurrent hyperprolactinaemia was always found to be lower

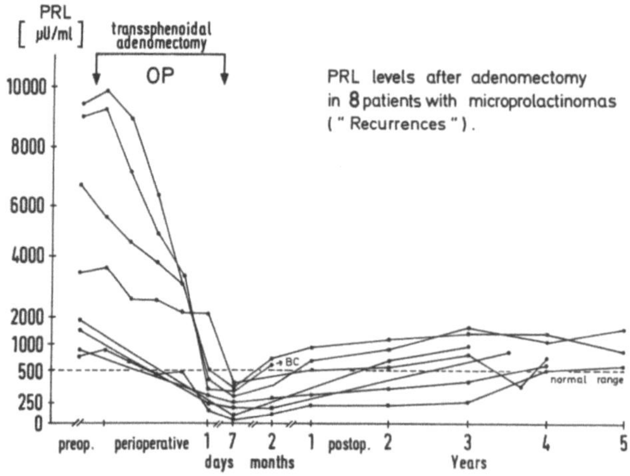

Fig. 1 Prolactin-levels in 8 female patients with an acute normalization of the prolactin-excess after transsphenoidal adenomectomy for microprolactinomas and "recurrences" of hyperprolactinaemia. The acute prolactin-increase during pregnancy in three patients is not documented in this figure. In one patient additional bromocriptine therapy was instituted (BC).

than the initial values before therapy. Only in one patient an additional bromocriptine therapy had to be instituted, because the patient urgently desired to become pregnant.

There was no radiological evidence for tumour recurrence. Three of the eight patients had been pregnant before hyperprolactinaemia was found to recur. The clinical symptoms of the 8 patients with recurrent hyperprolactinaemia before therapy and after prolactin re-increase are summarized in table 1. The patient who was treated with dopamine-agonists became pregnant after the relapse was noted and medically treated. All of the pregnant patients had a resumption of menses after the partus despite slightly elevated prolactin-levels (tab. 1), but in three of them galactorrhoea persisted. However only two of the recurrent hyperprolactinaemic

Table 1 Clinical symptoms before therapy and after recurrence of hyperprolactinaemia in the 8 patients. Each value of serum-prolactin given represents the highest prolactin-level measured after the re-increase

preoperative symptoms	patient	postoperative pregnancy	symptoms (re-appearances)	prolactin μU/ml
secondary amenorrhoea + galactorrhoea	H. M. 30 y.	+	galactorrhoea	750
secondary amenorrhoea	I. H. 42 y.		(anovulatory cycle)	840
secondary amenorrhoea + galactorrhoea	G. L. 39 y.		galactorrhoea	800
secondary amenorrhoea	B. M. 31 y.	+		1020
primary amenorrhoea	D. G. 25 y.			1360
secondary amenorrhoea + galactorrhoea	B. S. 27 y.		(anovulatory cycle)	555
secondary amenorrhoea + galactorrhoea	U. K. 27 y.			630
secondary amenorrhoea + galactorrhoea	B. E. 32 y.	+	galactorrhoea	783

patients had menstrual abnormalisties, 6 had regular menses. Preoperatively all of these patients had been amenorrhoic. Thus the relief of symptoms provided by transsphenoidal microsurgery persisted despite the mild prolactin re-increase. Clinical and biological features before surgery could not predict the long-term outcome. Age, duration of symptoms, prior exposure to oestrogens or dopamine-agonists, as well as the occurrence of pregnancies, do not seem to be significantly different in the groups of recurrent hyperprolactinaemic and long-term normoprolactinaemic patients. Despite post-operative serum-prolactin levels being found to be lower in the long-term normoprolactinaemic group (mean values 215 μU/ml versus 266 μU/ml) there was no significant difference.

Discussion

There are now some published reports about recurrences of hyperprolactinaemia after successful transsphenoidal micro-surgery for prolactinomas and table 2 summarizes them. So far we have found recurrences in 16% of 50 acutely normalized microprolactinomas. We have observed the recurrence of a macroadenoma only once [3]. Four relapses were seen in the 18 patients followed-up for more than 5 years, this represents 22.5%. These data correlate well with the 15% relapse-rate after a similar follow-up period reported by Faglia and Giovanelli et al. [2] from Milan in 1983. Betrand et al. [1] observed three recurrences in 54 female patients followed-up for a shorter interval (mean 20.3 months), one to three years after normalization of prolactin levels by transsphenoidal microsurgery. Even higher recurrence rates were observed by Serri et al. [10] who have followed-up the patients with microprolactinomas operated successfully by Jules Hardy in Montreal between 1970 and 1976. Five to ten years after surgery, 6.2 years in the average,

Table 2 Reported recurrences after successful transsphenoidal microsurgery for prolactinomas. A survey of the literature

author		recurrences	patients with normal PRL	follow-up period
Tindall et al. [11]	(1978)	4	17 (23.0%)	not stated
Laws et al. [8]	(1980)	3	58 (5.1%)	not stated
Derome et al. [3]	(1980)	2	37 (5.4%) microadenoma	not stated
Hardy [6]	(1981)	~12	177 (6.7%)	not stated
Serri, Hardy et al. [10]	(1983)	12	24 (50.0%) microadenoma long-term	6.2 years
Bertrand, Tolis et al. [1]	(1983)	3	55 (5.5%) microadenoma long-term	1.7 years
Faglia, Giovanelli et al. [3]	(1980)	5	37 (14.0%)	not stated
[2]	(1983)	6	39 (15.0%) microadenoma long-term	not stated
Buchfelder, Fahlbusch et al.	(1984)	9	65 (14.0%)	
		8	50 (16.0%) microadenoma long-term	3.1 years

Serri et al. found relapses in 12 out of 24 acutely normalized microprolactinomas, this is 50%! Even in view of the high normalization rate of up to 97% reported by Hardy [6] it looks like the risk of a hyperprolactinaemia relapse increases with time. As in Frantz's et al. series [5] the basal prolactin-levels after adenomectomy were mostly lower than those measured after 4 weeks in our patients.

The recurrence of hyperprolactinaemia after obviously successful transsphenoidal operations for microprolactinomas documented by an acute normalization of the prolactin-excess may be due to the regrowth of residual tumour cells missed by the surgeon during operation. On the other hand, a primary hypothalamic defect might be the cause of the restitution of a microprolactinoma or for the hypersecretion of normal prolactin-secreting cells.

Conclusion

1. Our findings suggest that there is some tendency of microprolactinomas to recur, even after the operation was obviously successful in normalizing the prolactin-excess.

2. The re-increase of acutely normalized prolactin-levels may be delayed for years.

3. Clinical symptoms do not reappear corresponding to the reincreased prolactin-levels.

4. Therefore, a consequent follow-up with yearly determinations of the basal prolactin-levels should be performed in all patients after surgery for prolactinomas.

Acknowledgements

The authors acknowledge with gratitude the collaborative efforts of Drs. H. Junkermann (Universitäts-Frauenklinik Heidelberg), J. Pichl (Medizinische Klinik der Universität Erlangen), H. K. Rjosk (1. Frauenklinik der Universität München) and A. Wolf (Universitäts-Frauenklinik Ulm). They have contributed to the clinical and endocrinological studies of the cases reported and provided us with the follow-up data of patients under their care.

References

[1] Bertrand, G., G. Tolis, J. Montes: Immediate and long-term results of transsphenoidal microsurgical resection of prolactinomas in 92 patients. In: Prolactin and Prolactinomas (G. Tolis, C. Stefanis, T. Mountokalakis, F. Labrie, eds.), p. 441. Raven Press, New York 1983.

[2] Faglia, G., P. Moriondo, P. Travaglini, et al.: Influence of previous bromocriptine therapy on surgery for microprolactinomas. Lancet **I** (1983) 133.

[3] Fahlbusch, R.: Surgical failures in prolactinomas. In: Secorn European Workshop in Pituitary Adenomas (P. J. Derome, C. P. Jedynac, F. Peillon, eds.), p. 273. Asclepios France, Paris 1980.

[4] Fahlbusch, R., M. A. Giovanelli, P. G. Crosignani, et al.: Differentiated therapy of microprolactinomas; Significance of transsphenoidal adenomectomy. In: Pituitary Microadenomas (G. Faglia, M. A. Giovanelli, R. McLeod, eds.), p. 443. Academic Press, London 1980.

[5] Frantz, A. G., P. H. Cogen, C. H. Chang, et al.: Long-term evaluation of the results of transsphenoidal surgery and radiotherapy in patients with prolactinomas. In: Endocrinology of human infertility: New aspects (P. Crosignana, B. L. Rubin, eds.), p. 161. Academic Press, London 1981.

[6] Hardy, J.: Le prolactinome: aspects chirurgicaux. Neurochirurgie **27**, Suppl. 1 (1981) 41.

[7] Jaquet, P., F. Grisoli, M. Guibout, et al.: Prolactin secreting tumours: endocrine status before and after surgery in 33 women. J. Clin. Endocrinol. Metabol. **46** (1978) 459.

[8] Laws, E. R., E. B. Kern: Pituitary tumours treated by transnasal microsurgery. In: Functioning pituitary adenomas (K. Sano, K. Takahawe, T. Fukushima, eds.), p. 25. Proceedings of the first workshop on pituitary adenomas, Tokyo 1980.

[9] Randall, R. V., E. R. Laws, C. F. Abboud, et al.: Transsphenoidal Microsurgical Treatment of Prolactin-Producing Pituitary Adenomas. Mayo Clin. Proc. **58** (1983) 108.

[10] Serri, O., E. Rasio, H. Beauregard, et al.: Recurrence of hyperprolactinaemia after selective transsphenoidal adenomectomy in women with prolactinomas. N. Engl. J. Med. **309** (1983) 280.

[11] Tindall, G. T., C. S. McLanahan, J. H. Christy: Transsphenoidal microsurgery for pituitary tumours associated with hyperprolactinaemia. J. Neurosurg. **48** (1978) 849.

[12] Tucker, H. S. G., S. R. Grubb, J. P. Wigand, et al.: Galactorrhea-amenorrhea syndrome: follow-up of fourty-five patients after pituitary tumour removal. Ann. Int. Med. **94** (1981) 302.

Impairment of pituitary hormone secretion in patients with prolactinoma

G. Leb, H. Warnkross, L. M. Auer, G. Clarici, G. Tscherne, W. Urdl, G. F. Walter, H. Höfler

Introduction

Hormone secreting pituitary adenomas may lead to disturbances of pituitary function in different ways. In patients with pronounced hyperprolactinaemia and enlarged sella or bone destruction of the sella as seen in skull X-rays, prolactin secreting adenomas are the most frequent cause of these changes [1, 2]. On the other hand, the same radiological findings appear together with hyperprolactinaemia usually of a milder degree due to suprasellar extension of a tumour not producing prolactin itself. In this case the tumour impaires transmission of the prolactin inhibiting factor (PIF) by compressing the pituitary stalk, thus leading to an increased prolactin-secretion by the normal pituitary tissue. The same condition may also be found in primary suprasellar lesions, as for instance craniopharyngeomas, owing to destruction of hypothalamic areas responsible for the release of PIF. Hyperprolactenaemia with a normal sella shown in plain skull X-rays may be caused by microprolactinomas or functional hyperprolactinaemia in which a primary disturbance of hypothalamic function is assumed. Frequently hyperprolactinaemia is induced by medication with substances such as neuroleptics, phenothiazine, sulpiride, metoclopramide, and certain antihypertensive drugs. In rare cases primary hypothyroidism leads to hyperprolactinaemia by increased TRH-stimulation which exceeds dopaminergic inhibition.

In macroprolactinomas intrasellar tumour growth may also cause secretory impairment of other pituitary hormones. Usually low basal levels and/or a blunted response to adequate stimulation is present. On the other hand, in functional hyperprolactinaemia and in patients with microadenomas also excessive LH and FSH responses to LHRH stimulation were reported [3].

The aim of our study was to determine preoperatively any impairment of prolactin-secretion and of other pituitary hormones by means of stimulation tests and to assess to what extent these disturbances might be improved or influenced by transsphenoidal surgery. Furthermore, follow-up investigations were performed to establish the need for postoperative replacement therapy.

Material and methods

Pituitary stimulation tests were carried out in 32 patients, 21 females and 11 males, having been operated on for prolactinoma between 1978 and 1983. The mean age of the female patients was 31 years and ranged from 19 to 57 years, the male patients were markedly older on average (49 a) and ranged from 28 to 66 years. Microprolactinomas were observed in 16 female and 1 male patient, whereas a higher incidence of macroprolactinomas was found in males – 10 compared with 5 females (tab. 1). All these female patients had amenorrhoea and galactorrhoea was present in 14, visual field defects in 2, reduction of libido was reported by 5 women. The most frequent symptom in male patients was disturbance of libido and potency in 7 cases, headache and visual field defects were observed in 5 patients. Plain skull X-rays, tomography of the sella and computerized tomography (CT) were done in all patients. Postoperative CT scans were carried out in all macroadenoma patients and in cases where it was necessary due to clinical signs and hormonal findings. A tumour was classified as being a macroadenoma with a diameter of more than 7 millimeters.

Specimens of excised tumorous material and from borderzone areas were examined histologically using routine staining methods for light- and electronmicroscopy. 7 adenomas were found to be eosinophilic or partially eosinophilic, the rest being chromophobe. Imunocytochemical investigations were carried out in tissue specimens from 21 patients, and prolactin (PRL) was detected in 17 of these. In 4 cases of chromophobe adenomas no tissue-prolactin could be detected although preoperative serum-prolactin levels of 760 to 4000 ng/ml were recorded in these patients. All 32 patients were operated on via the sublabial-transseptal-transsphenoidal approach because of recently detected adenomas, except one female patient suffering from recurrent macroadenoma, who had undergone surgery previously in 1975 by subfrontal craniotomy.

Endocrinological investigations included measurement of basal and stimulated serum -PRL, HGH, TSH, LH, FSH and cortisol levels with radioimmunoassay. Pituitary stimulation tests were performed using stimulation by TRH (200 μg/i. v.) LHRH (100 μg i. v.) and insulin-induced hypoglycaemia (0.15 U/kg body weight). Basal and stimulated serum ACTH concentrations were measured in 12 patients. Postoperative follow-up examinations using stimulation tests were done in 13 patients after 2–5 weeks, and in 8 patients 6 months to 2 years following surgery.

The following criteria were applied for the evaluation of pituitary stimulation tests: TRH-test was considered normal when TSH values rose by more than 2.5 U/L and PRL by more than 100% above basal level. Increments following insulin hypoglycaemia were accepted as normal when growth hormone increased above 7 μg/L or more than 100%, ACTH more than 80 ng/L or 100%, and the cortisol rise was more than 100 μg/L or the stimulated values exceeded 240 μg/L. Disturbances of

LH and FSH secretion were presumed when basal levels were below normal or the response to LHRH was smaller than 200% for LH or 100% for FSH. However, a distrurbed secretion was also assumed when high basal LH and FSH levels were present, as well as in cases with excessive stimulation response i. e. more than eight fold for LH and three fold for FSH.

Results and Discussion

Thyrotropin releasing hormone (TRH) stimulates prolactin secretion in normal men whereas in patients with proven prolactinomas TRH leads to varying PRL responses [4, 5]. In most cases with macroprolactinomas the increase in PRL is reduced or lacking but in patients with mild hyperprolactinaemia and microadenomas the PRL response to TRH is also blunted in most instances [6]. The TRH unresponsiveness of PRL secretion in hyperprolactinaemic states may be explained by an ultrashort feedback operating between circulating PRL and lactotroph cells of the pituitary [7, 8]. This is supported by the fact that TRH stimulates PRL release from prolactinoma-tissue in vitro as circulating PRL is not present in the in-vitro experiment. Since an elevated level of circulating PRL inhibits pituitary prolactin secretion from the normal as well as from the adenomatous lactotroph cell [9], evaluation of TRH stimulated PRL levels does not add additional diagnostic information to the basal PRL findings, in the differentiation between functional and adenomatous hyperprolactinaemia. On the other hand, patients with elevated basal PRL levels, in the presence of an enlarged sella, do not necessarily suffer from a prolactinoma [10, 11]. PRL levels above 250 ng/ml are generally indicative of a PRL secreting adenoma, although in some cases such adenomas may also occur when levels are below this limit [12, 13]. The clinical experience that microadenomas are more frequent in females while macroadenomas with higher basal PRL levels are usually found in male patients [11, 14] is supported by our findings. In our patients basal prolactin levels ranged from 160 to 1812 ng/ml in microprolactinomas (16 females, 1 male patient) while in macroprolactinoma-patients (10 male, 5 female) prolactin levels were far higher, particularly in male patients, ranging from 420 to 4000 ng/ml (tab. 1). In 20 subjects, comprising 9 macro- and 11 microadenomas, a prolactin response to TRH of varying degrees was observed, while no stimulation could be seen in the remaining 12 patients. However, in only 2 patients there was a normal increase of more then 100% above basal values. Hyperprolactinaemic patients with a radiologically normal sella also have normal HGH responses to insulin induced hypoglycaemia. Also in patients where proven microprolactinomas do not compress or destroy anterior pituitary tissue, normal HGH secretion has been found [15, 16]. This indicates that PRL itself has no effect on HGH secretion [17]. With enlarged sella suggesting the presence of a macroprolactinoma, impairment of growth hormone secretion or complete somatotroph-

Table 1 Age and sex distribution in 32 prolactinoma patients. Preoperative basal and TRH-stimulated PRL serum levels: mean (range)

	n		age	PRL (ng/ml) basal	PRL (ng/ml) stim.
female	21	100%	30.8		
micro	16	76%	28.6	540 (160–1812)	668 (231–1820)
macro	5	24%	37.8	1505 (520–3300)	1981 (665–3936)
male	11	100%	48.7		
micro	1	9%	48	671	679
macro	10	91%	48.8	1570 (420–4000)	2134 (715–5350)

ic insufficiency is frequently observed [15, 16, 18]. An impaired secretion of LH and FSH in patients with hyperprolactinaemia does not necessarily indicate gonadotrophic cell destruction since this may also be due to a dysfunction of gonadotropin secretion because of elevated circulating PRL levels [13, 18, 19]. The responses of LH and FSH to LHRH in hyperprolactinaemic subjects may therefore vary considerably. Normal responses, excessive but also blunted or absent responses have been reported in prolactinoma patients [13, 15, 19, 20]. Those patients with large prolactinomas and destructions of the gonadotroph show absent or blunted responses to LHRH. However blunted responses of LH and FSH to LHRH-stimulation were also observed in longstanding hyperprolactinaemia; these becoming normal after the lowering of PRL levels [19]. Such findings indicate a lack of endogenous LHRH leading to a secondary atrophy of the gonadotrophs in long-standing hyperprolactinaemia [20]. Pituitary TSH- and ACTH-secretion are rarely disturbed in prolactinoma patients and seem to be rather resistant even in advanced cases [6]. Therefore, most patients with even large macroprolactinomas retain a normal basal and/or TRH-stimulated TSH secretion with normal thyroid function. Likewise hyperprolactinaemia does not seem to have any specific influence on ACTH secretion. Thus in hyperprolactinaemic subjects, normal basal lev-

Table 2 Preoperative examinations in 32 prolactinoma patients

		total	HGH	ACTH	TSH	LH	FSH	Cortisol
Micro-	n	17	1	0	0	12	14	1
prolactinomas	%	100	6	0	0	70	82	6
Macro-	n	15	13	4	3	12	13	6
prolactinomas	%	100	87	27	20	80	87	40

n = number of patients with negative or abnormal stimulation test results for different hormones.

% = percentage of total number of patients examined.

els and a normal rise in both ACTH and cortisol during insulin hypoglycaemia tests were observed [6, 15].

Preoperative stimulation tests were performed in all 32 patients in our study (tab. 2). Growth hormone secretion was impaired in 14 cases, 13 of whom showed macroadenomas. Impairment of ACTH and Cortisol secretion was rare and occurred only in macroadenoma patients. One female patient with a microadenoma of 5 mm in diameter detected by CT showed an insufficient rise in cortisol levels despite a normal ACTH response. High incidence and various patterns of both LH – (24 patients) and FSH – secretion (27 patients) were detected in this series. Blunted or absent responses to LHRH stimulation (FSH 16 and LH 17 patients) as well as low basal levels (LH 5 patients) were observed mainly in macroadenoma patients. However, basal levels above normal (FSH 4, LH 3 patients) along with negative or normal stimulation tests were equally frequent in the macro- and microadenoma groups, whereas excessive stimulation responses (FSH 7, LH 4) were found only in patients with microadenomas.

Table 3 Results of stimulation tests in postoperative follow-up examinations

	preoperative		postop. I		postop. II	
	n	%	n	%	n	%
HGH	14	44%	5	16%	3	9%
ACTH	4	33%	0	0%	0	0%
TSH	3	9%	2	6%	1	3%
LH	24	75%	4	12%	2	6%
FSH	27	84%	4	12%	2	6%
Cortisol	7	21%	3	9%	2	6%

postop. I: 2 to 5 weeks and
postop. II: 6 months to 2 years following surgery.
n = number of patients with negative or abnormal stimulation test results for different hormones.
% = percentage of total number of patients (n = 32).

Postoperative follow-ups with stimulation tests were performed in 13 patients 2–5 weeks (first postoperative control) and in 8 patients a second control was done 6 months to 2 years after surgery (tab. 3). This was done, when persisting impairment of pituitary function was suspected on the basis of clinical symptoms. LH and FSH secretion was restored to normal in all but two males concomittant with a decrease in prolactin levels. Only one female subject with a microadenoma showed a preoperative negative stimulation test for HGH which became normal within one month after surgery (fig. 1). In 6 macroadenoma patients followed-up only one showed a normal HGH secretion postoperatively both after 1 month and 6 months,

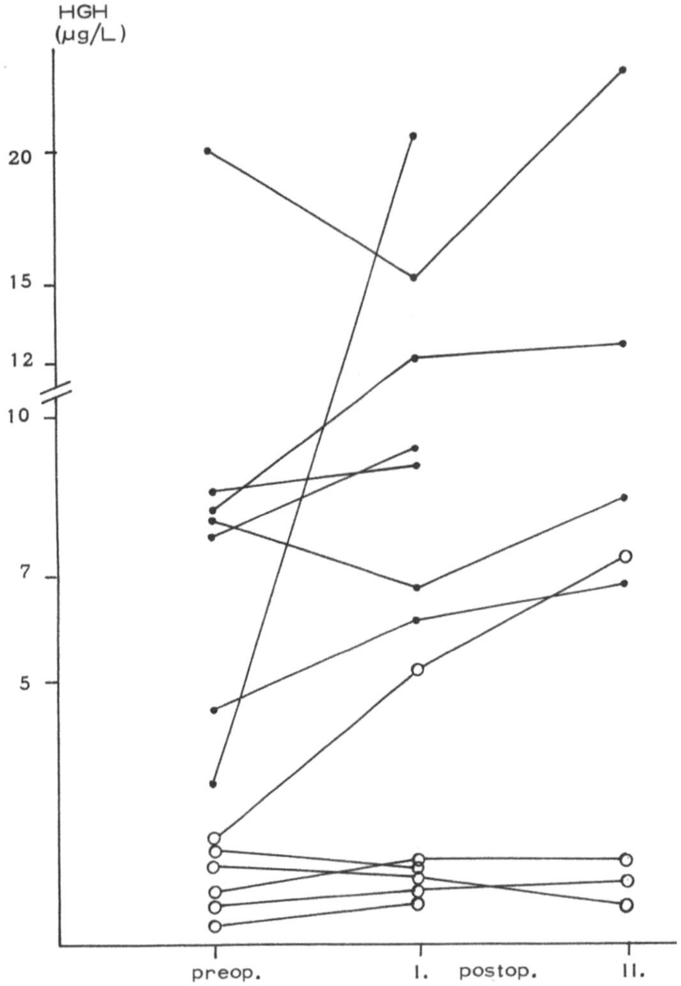

Fig. 1 Stimulated (insulin hypoglycaemia) serum-values of HGH in 7 microprolactinoma (●) and 6 macroprolactinoma (O) patients examined 2 to 5 weeks (postop. I) and in 8 patients examined 6 months to 2 years (postop. II) following surgery.

while 5 patients had negative tests in the first postoperative control examination. Impairment of HGH secretion persisted in 3 patients up to 2 years following surgery. Disturbance of TSH secretion was still present in one female patient and of cortisol secretion in 2 males, out of 8 patients followed up after 2 years, all of them belonging to the macroadenoma group.

Amenorrhoea-galactorrhoea improved in 17 out of 19 females under 40 years of age. During follow-up of 17 microadenoma patients only 3 women showed normal serum prolactin levels in the early postoperative period without a later increase. In a fourth female patient serum-PRL normalized spontaneously after 2 months. In 12 cases PRL levels normalized during postoperative bromocriptine treatment. In one female patient of the microadenoma group PRL levels remained elevated without bromocriptine treatment. Seven female microadenomas and one with a macroadenoma recorded 12 pregnancies and delivered healthy infants. Visual field defects preoperatively observed in 7 macroadenoma patients normalized in 2 cases within one week and in 4 cases within 2 years following surgery. In 1 male patient visiual-field findings improved but no complete normalizition could be achieved. Three patients with macroadenomas required substitution treatment. In two males cortisol replacement was necessary, one of them being additionally treated with testosterone. One female patient who had been operated on twice developed secondary hypothyroidism which required thyroxine replacement.

Our results indicate that on the one hand the preoperative disturbance of LH- and FSH-secretion occurs frequently in prolactinoma patients. Normalization is to be expected in the majority of cases, particularly in microprolactinomas where this secretion-impairment is of a functional nature. In macroadenoma patients, on the other hand, disturbances of HGH, cortisol and TSH secretion have a tendency to persist after surgery and replacement therapy may be required in such patients.

References

[1] Flückiger, F., E. del Pozo, K. von Werder: Prolactin physiology, pharmacology and clinical findings. In: Monographs on Endocrinology, Vol. 23. Springer, Berlin 1982.

[2] Werder, K. von, E. Eversmann, R. Fahlbusch, et al.: Treatment of hyperprolactinemia. In: Frontiers in Neuroendocrinology (W. F. Ganong, L. Martini, eds.). Raven Press, New York 1982.

[3] L'Hermite M., A. Caufriez, M. Badawi, et. al.: Selected aspects of hyperprolactinemia and its management. In: Progress in Prolactin Physiology and Pathology (C. Robyn, M. Harter, eds.). Elsevier North Holland, Amsterdam 1978.

[4] Jacobs, L. S., W. H. Daughaday: Pathophysiology and control of prolactin secretion in patients with pituitary and hypothalamic disease. In: Human prolactin (J. L. Pasteels, C. Robyn, eds.), pp. 189–205. Excerpta Medica, Amsterdam 1973.

[5] Lamberts, S. W. J., J. C. Birkenhäger, H. G. Kwa: Basal and TRH-stimulated prolactin in patients with pituitary tumors. Clin. Endocrinol. (Oxf) **5** (1976) 709–711.

[6] Werder, K. von: Wachstumshormon und Prolaktinsekretion des Menschen. Urban & Schwarzenberg, München–Berlin–Vienna 1975.

[7] Jacobs, H. S., S. Franks, M. A. F. Murphy et. al.: Clinical and endocrine feature of hyperprolactinemic amenorrhea. Clin. Endocrinol. (Oxf) **5** (1976) 439–454.

[8] Lamberts, S. W. J., R. M. MacLeod: The inability of bromocriptine to inhibit prolactin secretion by transplantable rat pituitary tumors. Observations on the mechanism and dynamics of the autofeedback regulation of prolactin secretion. Endocrinology **104** (1979) 65–70.

[9] Knazek, R. A., J. S. Skyler: Secretion of human prolactin in vitro. Proc. Soc. Exp. Biol. Med. **151** (1976) 561–564.

[10] Säger, W.: Hypophysenadenome bei Galactorrhoe. Virchows Arch. Pathol. Anat. **368** (1975) 123–139.

[11] Werder, K. von, R. Fahlbusch, H. K. Rjosk: Hyperprolaktinaemie. Internist **18** (1977) 520–528.
[12] Friesen, H., G. Tolis, R. Shiu, et al.: Studies on human prolactin: Chemistry, radioreceptor assay and clinical significance. In: Human prolactin (J. L. Pasteels, C. Robyn, eds.), pp. 11–23. Excerpta Medica, Amsterdam 1973.
[13] Pozo, E. del, L. Varga, H. Wyss, et. al.: Clinical and hormonal response to bromocriptine (CB 154) in the galactorrhea syndromes. J. Clin. Endocrinol. **39** (1974) 18–25.
[14] Landolt, A. M.: Progress in pituitary adenoma biology. Adv. tech. Standards Neurosurg. **5** (1978) 3–49.
[15] L'Hermite, M., A. Caufriez, E. Virasoro et. al.: Endocrinology of prolactin producing tumors. In: Treatment of pituitary adenomas (R. Fahlbusch, K. von Werder, eds.), pp. 60–77. Thieme, Stuttgart 1978.
[16] Werder, K. von, R. Fahlbusch, R. Landgraf, et. al.: Treatment of patients with prolactinomas. J. Endocrinol. Invest. **1** (1978a) 47–58.
[17] Werder, K. von, O. A. Müller, P. C. Scriba, et. al.: Function and ultrastructure of the pituitary in Forbes-Albright syndrome. In: Human prolactin (J. L. Pasteels, C. Robyn, eds.), pp. 226–230. Excerpta Medica, Amsterdam 1973.
[18] Besser, G. M., L. Parke, C. R. W. Edwards, et. al.: Galactorrhea: Successful treatment with reduction of plasma prolactin levels by Brom-ergocryptine. Br. Med. J. **3** (1972) 669–672.
[19] Rjosk, H. K., K. von Werder, R. Fahlbusch: Hyperprolaktinämische Amenorrhoe. Geburtshilfe Frauenheilkd. **36** (1976) 575–587.
[20] Lachelin, G. C. L., S. Abu Fadil, S. S. C. Yen: Functional delineation of hyperprolactinemic amenorrhea. J. Clin. Endocrinol. **44** (1977) 1163–1174.

IV Surgical treatment

The recurrence of pituitary adenoma – a management challenge

L. Symon

We live in changing times. Up until 10–15 years ago the majority of operations carried out for pituitary tumour were occasioned by visual failure, and the tumours removed were almost always of the type which at that time we described as chromophobe adenoma, that is adenomas without characteristic staining features. In certain specialised centres associated with endocrinologists, a small number of patients with Cushing's syndrome and a rather larger number of patients with acromegaly would proceed to surgery, but in the majority of standard neurosurgical units, operations for acromegaly would occasion less than 10% of the pituitary work and for Cushing's syndrome very much less than that. The secretion of prolactin by somewhere around 70% of so-called inactive adenomas and the realisation that the syndrome of galactorrhoea and amenorrhoea usually had a central cause at the pituitary, has changed the spectrum of pituitary surgery, so that this Symposium may appear appropriately constructed to review surgery of pituitary tumours which many years ago would have passed unrecognised or been untreated.

The challenge to surgical management however is the delineation of whether pituitary tumours have really changed their spots. Are we now dealing with lesions which having been conservatively removed will not recur, or are we dealing with lesions which have the uncertain growth characteristics of pituitary tumours as we have known over many years? Certain of the papers reported in this volume (Roosen and Bock, Aleshire et al.) would suggest that this is not the case.

It seems not unlikely that our new endocrinological expertise has resulted in the more rapid diagnosis of pituitary tumours which in earlier days would have remained silent for many years, or perhaps never reached the stage in which they broke out of the sella and declared their presence by chiasmal compression. The small proportion of endocrine-active tumours in Cushing's disease or acromegaly which proceeded to chiasmal compression was evident to many of us years ago. The explanation was simple, these patients declared themselves by endocrinopathy long before their tumours broke out of the confines of the sella at any rate in an upward direction. This may to some extent raise the question of the proportion of cases with amenorrhoea-galactorrhoea who have gone on to produce large pituitary tumours, a statistic which as yet we simply do not know. Reviewing our own series of almost 300 pitutitary tumours however roughly split equally between males and females, a history of amenorrhoea-galactorrhoea has been far from invariable, even in female patients of child bearing age, perhaps surprising if one considers the large number of patients investigated for this condition at the present time.

We must also acknowledge the differing aims of surgery which we express today, as opposed to those views which were held, in the era of classical surgery for pituitary tumour when the primary indication was visual failure. At the present time as Becker reports in this volume, conservative surgery on the pituitary gland is possible with the preservation of functioning anterior pituitary gland and the avoidance of necessity for hormonal replacement. If this can be achieved without the risk of subsequent recurrence of the tumour then we have indeed reached an ideal world. Even if it cannot be achieved without the complete assurance of absence of further recurrence, the lot of a patients over the years before recurrence takes place may be a great deal more satisfactory, they may for example, if female, go on to have children and the pioneering work of Jules Hardy has indicated the feasibility of this in many instances. It is however clearly incumbent upon us to analyse with care the late results of surgery of any description on the pituitary gland and I make no excuse therefore for drawing to your attention data which tells a largely similar story in the analysis of large pituitary series from Cushing's day to the present time. The pituitary tumour has not changed its spots, and we are likely therefore in pituitary surgery to meet over the years an increasing proportion of recurrences.

A pioneering study of the late surgical results of pituitary surgery was carried out by the late W. R. Henderson, a neurosurgeon who practised in Leeds, England, analysing the 338 cases of pituitary tumours operated on by Harvey Cushing at the Peter Bent Brigham Hospital. This paper was published in the British Journal of Surgery in 1939 [1] as part of a seventieth birthday tribute to Harvey Cushing and it was updated more recently in 1962 by German and Flanigan [2] in a Congress publication from the United States. Table 1 shows statistics which were thought commendable in Cushing's day which, while we would hardly regard them as com-

Table 1 Five year recurrence of pituitary tumours (from [1])

Treatment	Total cases	Recurrence	
		Number	%
Trans sphenoidal	67	45	67
Frontal	40	17	43
Trans sphenoidal and X-ray	49	17	35
Frontal and X-ray	31	4	13
Total cases	187	83	44

mendable today, are considerably better than the results reported in this volume by Aleshire in the management of macro-adenomas, tumours more than 10 mm in size followed up for a mean of 62 months, in which the recurrence rate was over 80%. It may be unfair of me to point out the disparity in recurrence rate between trans-sphenoidal operations even with supplemental x-ray therapy, and what Cushing regarded as the more radical frontal surgery, but it does emphasise the point that where we are dealing with a macro-adenoma, that form of surgery which is most radical is the most likely to achieve a permanent cure and the lowest rate of recurrence.

The definition of recurrence

A further difficulty in relation to defining recurrence of pituitary tumour has arisen as a result of our advancing technology. Our capacity to assess by hormonal marking has resulted in our endocrinological colleagues pointing out that high prolactin level persisting after pituitary surgery may very well indicate that all the tumour has not been removed although a modest elevation in hormonal level below four or five hundred micrograms may not necessarily so indicate. Our radiological colleagues too have, with the advent of the modern fourth generation scanners, an embarrassing capacity to point out residual or recurrent enhancing tissue within the pituitary fossa itself or in the cavernous sinus, pointing in all probability to residual or recurrent tumour. In defining recurrence therefore it is essential that we take the time course of the condition into consideration. Where a presenting symptom complex, hormonal disturbance or visual failure has been suppressed or abolished by primary surgery and has then reappeared we may talk of symptomatic recurrence. I doubt that persistently elevated hormonal levels by themselves, especially if relatively low, need alarm us too greatly, but where as Karagiousov in this volume has pointed out, the symptoms are not suppressed, then clearly we have not effectively treated the tumour even at primary surgery. Only where the primary symptom complex has clearly been influenced and has subsequently relapsed should we consider a verified tumour recurrence.

This to some extent begs the question of radiological appearances. If post-operative Ct scan shows the appearance of the tumour apparently unchanged there are two explanations, either it has not been removed, or its capsule remains and the cavity has filled with material of radio-density indistinguishable from tumour. Recurrent Ct scanning after some months will usually establish this point, the appearances will gradually settle and it will be clear that the pituitary tumour has been substantially influenced by the primary surgery.

In those terms I will present to you data from the series of 289 patients with pituitary tumour treated between 1948 and 1979 by my colleague Valentine Logue and myself in the academic department of Neurological Surgery in the National Hospital, Queen Square and Maida Vale Hospital [3].

The method of surgery in each case was the same and the presenting feature in over 90% of cases was that of chiasmal compression, progressive visual failure. A standard right frontal craniotomy was employed, the best approach for a right-handed surgeon, and we felt it important to achieve access to the mid-line so the medial portion of the flap was always in the midline. We also felt it important to achieve a low approach to the chiasm so that the lateral burrhole was invariably on the floor of the frontal fossa minimising frontal retraction and diminishing both the hazards of post-operative epilepsy and of damage to the frontal lobe. In the early part of this series, of course, the advantages of operating microscopes were not available. Operative mortality fell from 10% in the first decade to less than 1% in the last hundred cases, undoubtedly associated with improved techniques of support and with the use of the operating microscope. We have follow-up on 270 of these cases, a follow-up of at least 20 years being available on 34 cases operated on between 1948 and '59. Between 1960 and '69 we operated on 80 cases of which 70 have complete follow-up of at least 10 years. Between 1970 and '79 175 cases were operated upon of which 120 have follow-up for at least 5 years. Of 9 cases in which we have incomplete follow-up due to loss of contact in a foreign country we have follow-up for approaching 5 years in all, the period of time in which maximal recurrence is known to be likely (tab. 2).

Table 2 Length of post operative follow-up (from [3])

Years	No of cases	Follow up available		No of recurrences
		Complete	Incomplete (op death)	
1948–59	34	30	4	7
1960–69	80	70	10	6
1970–79	175	170	5	0
Total	289	270	19 (10)	

Even before the advent of the operating microscope, a radical removal of the tumour was carried out as far as possible. The usual method of incising the diaphragma sellae evacuating the centre of the tumour, was followed by an extra capsular dissection starting on the left side, identifying the stalk – not so easy in the pre-microscope days but very straight forward now – isolating it on a portion of the sellar diaphragm and then excising the stretched diaphragma and the tumour completely from the suprasellar region. The most difficult aspect of this dissection is undoubtedly the portion of the tumour lying obliquely upwards and to the right behind the angle of the chiasm on the right, especially if it extends into the cavernous sinus region. A method that I have used in large tumours has been to incise the capsule of the tumour separately between the lateral aspect of the optic nerve and the internal carotid artery – a triangular space which is usually free of significant vessels and provides a further lateral entry point – which in combination with the more mid-line access, enables the postero-lateral portion of the capsule to be undercut and the extension into the cavernous sinus liberally removed with dissectors and curved suction. With the microscope it is often now possible to identify and preserve normal pituitary tissue, often visible to one side of the lower end of the stalk, the stalk itself being frequently eccentric, and by its yellow colour easily separable from the greyish tumour. With the microscope also and with, if necessary, the use of angled mirrors, the cavity of the sella can be liberally cleared to its dural lining but there is no doubt that extensive extension into the cavernous sinus is difficult to clear by any method, and here one must rely on post-operative radiotherapy.

Histological characteristics

We found 13 symptomatic recurrences in 30 cases of delayed visual failure in the follow up of our 270 cases (tab. 3). Associated with diminished visual acuity half the cases showed an increase in headache and 2 cases presented with some ophthalmoplegia.

Table 3 Causes of delayed visual failure following transcranial operations and radiotherapy for pituitary adenoma (from [3])

Total number of verified pituitary adenoma	289
Number of post operative deaths	10
Number of cases with delayed visual failure	30
Recurrence of adenoma	
Histologically verified	13
On air study or CT scan	7
Recurrence as a blood cyst	1
Empty sella syndrome	3
Radiation effect	3
Hydrocephalus	3

Nine of the 13 recurrences were below the age of 40 years and there were 7 females and 6 males with a mean age of 37.7 years. Looking at the average age of our pituitary series as a whole, it is clear that this represents the lower age group. We must however conclude therefore that the younger a patient is operated upon the more likely it is that he will survive to present a recurrence, or that younger cases are more aggressive tumours. This is clearly of significance in relation to the possible occurrence of prolactinoma where we are dealing with a young female population with an average age much below the fifth and sixth decade where chiasmal compression maximally presents. Seventy-seven percent of our recurrences were within the first 10 years following surgery and 3 further cases representing 23% of the recurrences occurred after 10 years, the latest being at 15 years. It is clear therefore that prolonged follow-up of pituitary tumours is required before we can be certain that they will not recur. Reviewing the series as a whole, 2 of the cases recurred twice, one at intervals of 8 years, and another at 4 years, leading to a terminal illness. Including these second recurrences therefore, we may speak of 15 episodes and 10 of them subsequently showed recurrence on review could have been considered in present day terms to have had a complete initial radical removal. Ten of the 13 recurrences had had partial removal of varying degrees. Six of them including the 3 radical cases had not had radio-therapy and that represents 46% of the recurrence series, while the absence of radio-therapy was reported in only 10% of our whole series.

Assessment of recurrence of course requires investigation. Not all late visual failures are due to actual regrowth of the tumour. Thus in our analysis in 1982 one sella mass was verified as a blood cyst, 3 cases showed deterioration of vision secondary to late hydrocephalus, 3 were presumed to be due to radiation in the absence of verifiable evidence of a mass lesion, and 3 showed the empty sella syndrome. Figure 1 shows the CT scans of a 70 year old gentlemen, 10 years after a radical transcranial excision of a giant pituitary tumour who had unquestionably

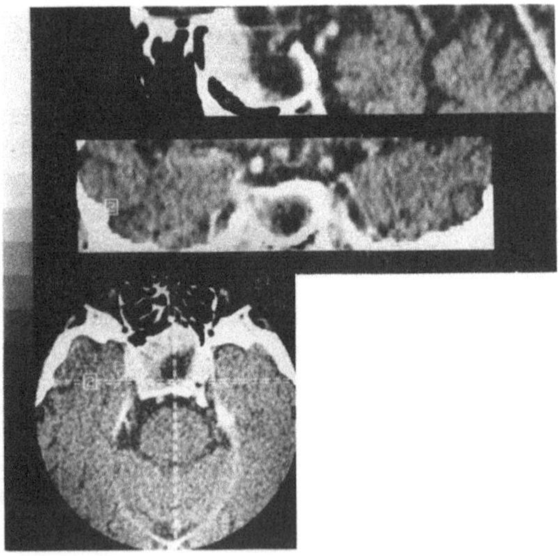

Fig. 1 CT scan, sagittal, choronal and axial, to show a substantially empty sella with the optic chiasm in the upper part of the sella on the sagittal view. Residual pituitary tissue is present.

mildly deteriorating vision over about a year subsequent to his most recent review. The CT scans which are shown in sagittal, coronal and axial planes demonstrate some residual tissue within the sella which enhances, but the sella is clearly mainly empty and the chiasm can be seen to have prolapsed down into it. His general age and the relative mildness of his deterioration contra-indicated further intervention. There has been considerable debate about the significance of histological characteristics in terms of tumour recurrence. This and the susceptibility of tumours to specific chemical suppression with bromocriptine or other suitable agents, has been very considerably amplified by the techniques of selective staining which of course were not available to us at the time of the collection of the greater part of our series. All the cases which were recurred were classified as chromophobe adenomas at the original biopsy but 2 of them showed malignant change at the time of the first recurrence although none went on to the disseminated metastasis which has been occasionally reported. One case showed chromophobe adenoma cells in the CSF. We found it impossible with the exception of frank malignant change in 2 of the recurrences, to attribute clear histological specificity to the likelihood of recurrence. Details of the pertinent operative and histological findings are given in table 4. In a total of 28 operations for recurrent tumour macroscopic degenerative

Table 4 Operative and histological findings (from [3])

Total number of verified recurrent adenomas	13
Radiation not given after first operation	6
Total number of operations performed	28
Partial excision	25
Macroscopic degenerative changes (cystic, necrotic haemorrhagice)	14
Invasive	7
Vascular	8
Capsular invasion	6
Pleomorphism	7
Haemorrhage	4
Malignant change	2

change, cystic formation, necrosis or haemorrhage was visible in 14, that is half of the cases, there was clear invidence of evasion either frankly into extrasellar structures or within the capsule in 13 of the cases, pleomorphism was noted in 7 and malignant change as we have mentioned in 2.

Discussion

We may conclude from neurosurgical experience over 60 years now that our view of pituitary adenomas as usually benign, slowly growing tumours in which malignant change is extremely rare [4] is confirmed. However they undoubtedly spread beyond the sella and although this has been called local malignancy [5] or has been designated an invasive type of tumour [6, 7] there is no certain histological characteristic which identifies such non-carcinomatous lesions. The term carcinoma is properly reserved for cases which either metastasise distantly, that is, not simply by implantation in the neighbourhood but by blood-borne metastasis. It may be possible to recognise these carcinomas or to suspect their histological characteristics by the extensive destruction of the sellar base which they usually show. The occurrence of pleomorphism in capsular invasion [8] is so common in pituitary tumour as a whole and is seen so frequently in series where extensive capsular excision is carried out that these characteristics alone can hardly be regarded as typical. Histologically only 2 of our recurrences showed anything suggestive of malignant change at a second biopsy, none had distant metastases but one did show chromophobe cells in the CSF.

From our own series and that of others [1, 9, 10, 11] most of the recurrences clearly occur within 5 years and only rarely later. The Henderson review of Cushing's series showed the latest known recurrence at 8 years, and in another series of 24 recurrences [11] only 8 of them occurred after 5 years, at 6, 8, 10, 11, 12 and 13 years. Three of our cases recurred after 10 years the latest one being 15 years after operation and we know of a further case since reporting this series, in which a very elderly lady has a prolactin level of over 22,000 and evidence of destruction in the base 20 years after an initial sub-radical chromophobe excision. There is no recurrent evidence of intra-cranial extension or visual failure and the advanced age of the lady precludes further investigation.

If we leave portions of tumour behind, if the tumour is invaded beyond the sellar boundaries, if it has aggressive growth potential [2], or is frankly carcinomatous then we may expect that the tumour will recur. Whether the growth pattern of these tumours is invariably regular or whether they undergo hyperplastic phases or aggressive growth spurts is difficult to say although the presence of tumour necroses, cystic degeneration and haemorrhage [12, 13] would suggest that the recurrent adenoma may well have episodically unusual rapidity of growth.

Our own material has been insufficient to consider the particular growth characteristics of tumours in Nelson's syndrome, but the experience of 4 or 5 cases over the past 10 years indicates that the complete eradication of these almost invariably invasive lesions is extremely difficult and clinical and endocrinological cure is unlikely.

The experiences of Bronson-Ray [10], of Martins [6] and of Guiot [8], of considerable diminution of recurrence rate by radiation is entirely in agreement with our own views. We have never used alpha-particles or the proton beam [4] though these have been suggested as inhibitory to further tumour growth and perhaps capable of eliminating invasive portions of the lesion.

There is no doubt that the current availability of biochemical markers for the functioning adenomas extended as recently by prolactin determinations, is of very great value and complete clinical and biochemical remission of a growth hormone-producing tumour which was locally invasive, and of several prolactin-secreting adenomas, [14] has been reported with bromocriptine.

In our own experience, despite previous suggestions that operation for recurrent adenoma carries a high risk [10, 11] we have found no deaths in the recurrent operations in a total of 28 operations in our own group of 13 recurrent cases. In over half the cases we had further good to excellent visual recovery and mean survival period of 11.5 years after the operation and a good quality of life.

I have avoided entering into the discussion of the correct approach to the pituitary adenoma. While transcranial surgery held almost uniform sway until the late '60's, there is no doubt that it has been extensively replaced by trans-sphenoidal operations in recent years but I am quite certain that whether the trans-sphenoidal or transcranial approach is used total excision of a extensive adenoma may be very difficult. Recurrence has been reported [8, 15] in a very much shorter follow-up period than I have presented to you following the trans-sphenoidal operation and my view remains that with an appreciable suprasellar extension the radical transcranial operation with the use of the operating microscope is most likely when combined with post-operative radio-therapy, to yield the lowest proportion of recurrent lesions.

References

[1] Henderson, W. R.: The Pituitary Adenomata: A follow up study of the surgical results in 338 cases (Dr. Harvey Cushing's series). Brit. J. Surg. **26** (1939) 811–921.

[2] German, W. J., S. Flanigan: Pituitary adenomas, a follow up study of the Cushing Series. Clin. Neurosurg. **10**, Chap. 4, pp. 72–81. Williams and Wilkins, Baltimore 1964.

[3] Symon, L., V. E. Logue, S. Mohanty: Recurrence of pituitary adenomas after transcranial operation. J. Neurol. Neurosurg. and Psych. **45** (1982) 780–785.

[4] Clark, K.: Surgery for the recurrent pituitary adenoma. Clin. Neurosurg. **27** (1980) 309–314.

[5] Jefferson, G.: Extrasellar extension of pituitary adenomas. President's Address, Proc. Roy. Soc. Med. **33** (1970) 433–458.

[6] Martins, A. M., G. J. Hayes, L. G. Kempe: Invasive pituitary adenomas. J. Neurosurg. **21** (1964) 268–276.

[7] Epstein, J. A., B. S. Epstein, L. Motho, et al.: Carcinoma of the pituitary gland with metastasis to the spinal cord and roots of the cauda equina. J. Neurosurg. **21** (1964) 846–853.

[8] Guiot, G.: Consideration on the surgical treatment of pituitary adenomas. In: Treatment of Pituitary (R. Fahlbusch, K. Werger, eds.). Thieme, Stuttgart 1978.

[9] Bakay, L.: The results of 300 pituitary adenoma operations (Professor Herbert Olivecron's series). J. Neurosurg. **7** (1950) 240–255.

[10] Ray, B. S., R. H. Patterson: Surgical experience with chromophobe adenomas of the pituitary. J. Neurosurg. **34** (1971) 726–729.

[11] Wirth, F. P., H. C. Schwartz, P. R. Schwetschenanm: Pituitary adenoma: Factors in treatment. Clin. Neurosurg. **21** (1974) 8–25.
[12] Landolt, A. M.: Ultrastructure of human sellar tumours. Correlation of clinical findings and morphology. Acta Neurochir. (Wein) Suppl. 22 (1975).
[13] Symon, L., J. Jakubowski, B. E. Kendall: Surgical treatment of giant pituitary adenomas. J. Neurol. Neurosurg. Psych. **42** (1979) 973–982.
[14] Spark, R. F., C. Dickstein, J. Pallota: Complete remission of acromegaly with medical treatment. JAMA **241** (1979) 573–579.
[15] Nicola, G.: Transphenoidal surgery for pituitary adenomas with extrasellar extension. Prog. Neurol. Surg. **6** (1975) 142–199.

Transsphenoidal operations for prolactinomas

R. Fahlbusch, M. Buchfelder

Introduction

The treatment of prolactinomas remains determined by the interdisciplinary management by endocrinologists, gynaecologists and neurosurgeons. But the accents of medical and surgical therapy have changed in the last few years since it became known that prolactinomas have to be regarded as heterogenious biological groups.

Patients and methods

Our management of 283 patients with hyperprolactinaemia and pituitary adenomas in Munich up to 1981 is reflected by figure 1. Our normal range for serum prolactin (PRL) is below 500 μU/ml or 25 ng/ml. Seventy-five patients with radiologically detected microadenomas, estimated to be less than 5–7 mm in diameter were not operated. About 10% of these patients underwent observation, 90% were treated medically. 208 patients were operated.

We have performed 174 operations by the transsphenoidal approach, 16 by the transcranial route and 18 using both approaches. Two patients had shunt operations in addition to transsphenoidal surgery. All together we have performed 20% (n = 34) transcranial operations. This percentage could be reduced, mainly by pretreatment with dopamine-agonists in macroadenomas, to less than 2% in the last two years. Between 1981 and March 1984 only one patient (fig. 2) was operated on by the transcranial route.

In this personal series there was neither mortality nor any serious morbidity. The over-all meningitis rate of the transsphenoidal operation is about 1%. In all operated patients with pituitary adenomas, there was a mortality rate of about 1% since 1975, corresponding to the results in other large series [16, 19].

Normalization rate of serum prolactin-levels

The following series (tabs. 1 and 2) is restricted to real prolactinomas. We have eliminated the hormonally inactive tumours with non-tumorous hyperprolactinaemia. Our selection is based on the immunohistochemical examinations and cell-

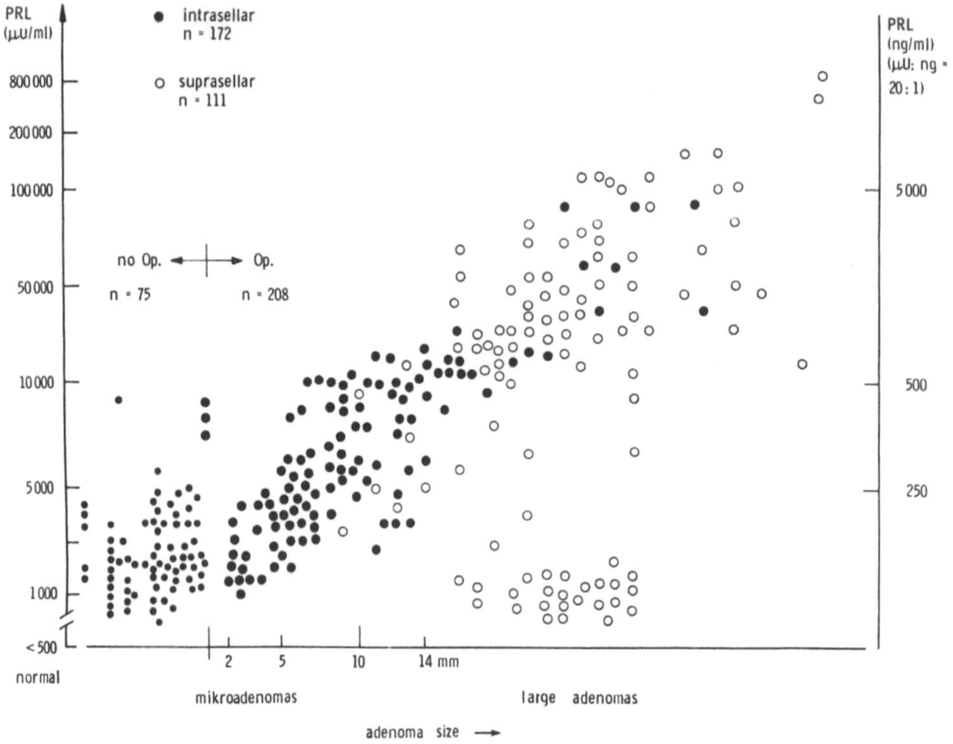

Fig. 1 Relation of radiologically or intraoperatively confirmed localization and tumour size and basal prolactin-levels in 283 patients with pituitary adenomas and hyperprolactinaemia (from R. Fahlbusch, F. Marguth, in: H. Dietz, W. Umbach, R. Wüllenweber: Klinische Neurochirurgie, Bd. II, Klinik und Therapie. Thieme, Stuttgart 1984).

culture studies, performed by K. Mashiter (Endocrine Unit, Hammersmith Hospital, London) in the last 5 years. There are hardly any new aspects, if we compare our present results with our cooperate study reported four years ago [11].

Up to March 1984 the prolactin excess could be eliminated by transsphenoidal and transcranial operations in only 33% of all male and female patients (tab. 1). The best results were obtained in women with microadenomas, in whom prolactin-levels were found to be normal postoperatively in 62%. Table 2 summarizes our results in the last two years by transsphenoidal operations. We were able to improve the normalization rate in microprolactinomas up to 72%.

PRL-levels below 4000 µU/ml or 200 ng/ml could be normalized in 78%, in the last two years in 80%. Even when only patients with a radiologically normal sella (that means with the smallest microadenomas), were operated on by other authors, this normalization rate could not be improved further [27]. The endocrinological

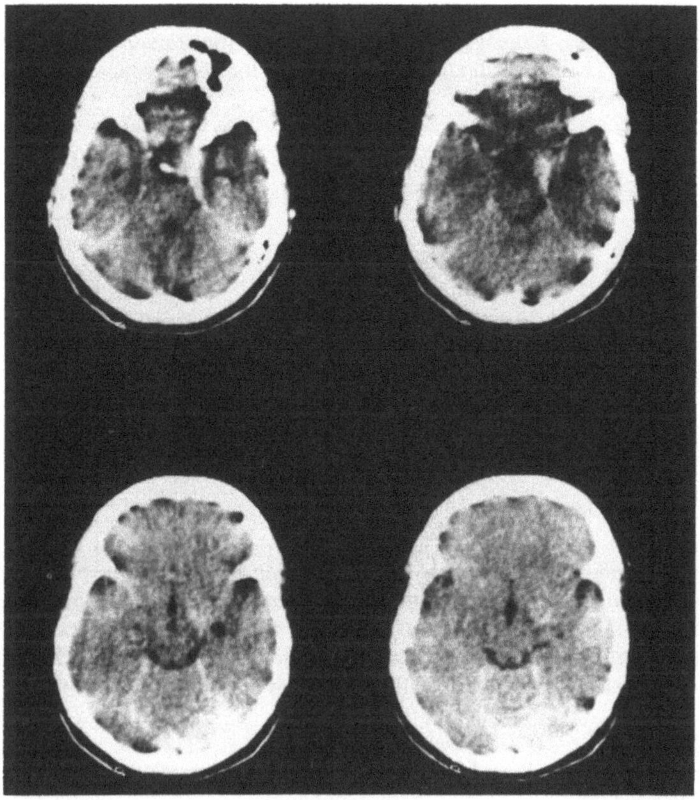

Fig. 2 CT-findings in a 30-year-old female patient (E. K.) with a right para-, supra- and retrosellar macroprolactinoma after pre-treatment with bromocriptine for about 1 year. In this patient the transcranial approach to the tumour had to be used. (It is the only case which could not be operated by the transsphenoidal approach within the last two years.)

results deteriorated, when PRL-levels were above 4000 μU/ml preoperatively, which was in general associated with larger prolactinomas. Particularly in the tumours with parasellar extension, frequently of invasive character, and in tumour stages II with chiasm syndrome and III with compression of the foramen, normalization of the prolactin-levels occured rarely.

In this survey (tabs 1 and 2) we did not distinguish between well-circumscribed and diffuse and invasive adenomas. Invasive tumours are estimated to be 25% to 30% [5] of pituitary adenomas in other series. Thus, prolactin-levels could be normalized in only 2 out of 56 male patients. These patients were young men, aged 16 and 18 who had presented with clinical symptoms of delayed puberty and galactorrhoea and postoperatively had a normal endocrinological development, including

Table 1 Normalization rate in 191 female and 56 male patients with hyperprolactinaemia and various adenoma sizes. Patients were operated on by the transsphenoidal or transcranial approach. The microadenomas were divided into two groups: patients with prolactin-levels below and above 4000 µU/ml

Localisation/ Sex distr.	Microadenoma <4000 µU/ml	>4000	intras.	paras./ sphen.	supras. I	II	III	Total
♀	39/50 (78%)	25/53 (47%)	4/26	2/21	6/16	3/24	0/1	79/191 (41%)
	64/103 (62%)		15%	10%	38%	13%		
♂	1/2	1/3	0/5	0/7	0/6	0/30	0/3	2/56 (4%)
								81/247 (33%)

Sex distr. = sex distribution; intras. = intrasellar adenoma; paras./sphen. = adenoma with extension into the parasellar space or sphenoid sinus; supras. I = adenoma with suprasellar extension without chiasm syndrome; supras. II = suprasellar adenoma with chiasm syndrome; supras. III = suprasellar adenoma with compression of the interventricular foramen.

Table 2 Normalization rate in 49 female and 9 male patients with hyperprolactinaemia and various adenoma sizes operated on by the transsphenoidal approach between 1. 1. 1982 and 30. 3. 1984. The microadenomas were divided into two groups: patients with prolactin-levels below and above 4000 µU/ml

Localisation/ Sex distr.	Microadenoma <4000 µU/ml	>4000	intras.	paras./ sphen.	supras. I	II	III	Total
♀	16/20 (80%)	2/5 (40%)	2/6	1/9	2/6	0/3		23/49
	18/25 (72%)		33%	11%	33%			
♂			0/1		0/3	0/4	0/1	0/9
								23/58 (40%)

Sex distr. = sex distribution; intras. = intrasellar adenoma; paras./sphen. = adenoma with extension into the parasellar space or sphenoid sinus; supras. I = suprasellar adenoma without chiasm syndrome; supras. II = suprasellar adenoma with chiasm syndrome; supras. III = suprasellar adenoma with compression of the interventricular foramen.

normal spermiograms. The mild improvement in our results in microadenomas is not due to the fact that we now are able to identify microadenomas in thin collimation CT-scans [1] which are visualized as hypodense intrasellar lesions (fig. 3). But

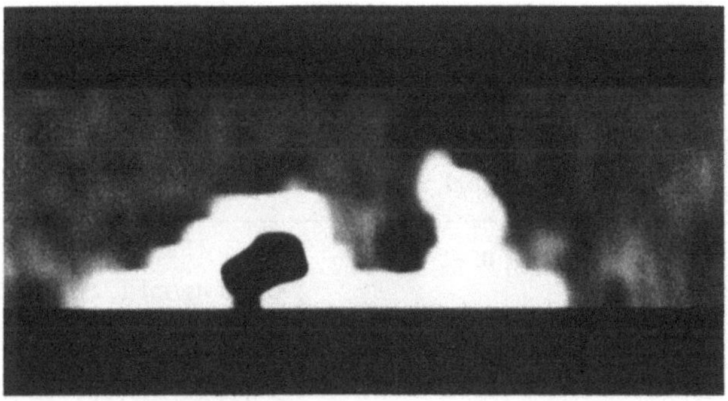

Fig. 3 Typical appearance of a microprolactinoma in thincut CT-scan reconstructions. In the sagittal reconstruction the microadenoma is represented by the hypodense region located dorsobasally. The normal pituitary appears isodense or slightly hyperdense in respect to normal brain tissue.

because we still miss information about the whole extension of tumours, for example with two nodules [2], a systematic surgical exploration of the whole intrasellar space remains necessary.

So far immunohistochemical and especially cell-culture studies of the adenomas and the adjacent structures were performed in 37 patients by Dr. Mashiter. The results led us to operate a little more aggressively. For example we resected the PRL-secreting capsule in 4 cases. As discussed elsewhere more extensively [25] the comparison of adenoma and periadenomatous tissue had not demonstrated new aspects. From histological examinations we know already from the literature [20] that hyperplasia found in the periadenomatous tissue occurs both in patients with normalized and not normalized prolactin-levels.

Influence of preoperative medical treatment on surgery for microprolactinomas

Landolt et al. [18] investigated whether pre-treatment with bromocriptine jeopardizes the results of surgery in microprolactinomas. He found the better normalization rate in 81% of the patients without bromocriptine-treatment, whereas only 33% of the pretreated patients had normal PRL-levels after adenomectomy.

Faglia and Giovanelli et al. [9] did not agree with this interpretation, although a few more patients, who had not had bromocriptine treatment had normal prolactin-levels after adenomectomy. At a first glance it seemed that our series of 75 patients reviewed retrospectively with respect to dopamine-agonist exposure prior to surgery (tab. 3) is comparable to Faglia's results. To point out the discrepancy in

Table 3 Comparison of PRL-normalization rates after surgery for microprolactinomas in relation to previous treatment with bromocriptine (according to Landolt et al. [18] and Faglia et al. [9])

	Landolt (1982) et al.	Faglia (1983) et al.	Fahlbusch (1985) et al.		
	n = 40	n = 49	n = 75		
No Bromocriptine	13/16 (81%)	20/29 (69%)	19/27 (70%)	<200 ng/ml	12/15 (80%)
				>200 ng/ml	7/12 (58%)
Bromocriptine	8/24 (33%) 0/6 <1 year	13/20 (65%)	30/48 (62%)	<200 ng/ml	23/27 (85%)
				>200 ng/ml	7/21 (33%)

Landolt's results, we have divided our patient material into two groups: Patients with prolactin-levels above 4000 μU/ml (200 ng/ml) and patients with PRL-levels below 4000 μU/ml. In the group of larger microadenomas with prolactin-levels above 4000 μU/ml we found normalizations in 33% after pre-treatment with bromocriptine. This is comparable to Landolt's series. In the group without bromocriptine pre-treatment 58% of the patients had normal prolactin-levels after surgery. This discrepancy may also be explained by the fact, that we as well as Faglia et al. [9] always stopped the pre-treatment with bromocriptine weeks or even months before the operation, whereas Landolt continued this therapy in the majority of cases.

These results seem to underline our management for patients who wish to become pregnant:

1. Microadenomas larger than 7 mm in diameter and with PRL-levels above 4000 μU/ml (200 ng/ml) should be operated as the first step of therapy (tab. 4).
2. If these patients had pre-treatment with bromocriptine, this should be interrupted before the operation.

Fertility after transsphenoidal microsurgery

Complications during bromocriptine-induced pregnancies occur only in those patients with larger tumours and most likely in those with suprasellar extension before pregnancy. The incidence is 5,6% [22] or even higher [14]. No complications were observed in 101 pregnancies in 72 hyperprolactinaemic patients in cooperation with H. K. Rjosk and K. v. Werder [24]. In about 25% of our female patients

Table 4 Indications for surgery in prolactinomas

A.	Macroadenomas
	1. Rapidly progressive loss of vision
	2. Desire for pregnancy
	3. Further growth on dopamine-agonists
B.	Microadenomas
	1. Desire for pregnancy: adenoma >7 mm in diameter
	2. No desire for pregnancy: patient's spontaneous decision
A + B	Dopamine-agonists not tolerated or ineffective

surgery was performed in order to enable the patient to become pregnant. In all instances a selective adenomectomy was attempted. Up to the end of 1981, 44 of 47 patients, who desired urgently to become pregnant and were married, had conceived and delivered. Out of these 27 after surgery alone and 17 after additional bromocriptine therapy. This delivery rate corresponds to other authors [15, 28]. These results document the selectivity of our surgical procedure. In the microprolactinomas, operated on in Milan and Munich [11] no additional partial insufficiency of the anterior pituitary had to be substituted by hydrocortisone or thyroid hormones. This is our experience with larger adenomas as well, if they were not operated radically or unless the transcranial approach was used. Diabetes insipidus occurred in the early postoperative phase till the third day in 17% and lasted longer than 3 months in 3%, but was in no case permanent.

The case of a 31-year-old female patient who did not become pregnant after therapy is demonstrated in figure 4. Preoperatively a complete insufficiency of the anterior lobe is rarely observed in patients with microprolactinomas. In this patient intraoperatively an old haemorrhage with calcification as well as blood from a recent haemorrhage was found. After the resection of this space-occupying lesion, there was a slight improvement of pituitary function but no regular periods despite a recovery of gonadotropine secretion.

Long-term results in microprolactinomas

Some years ago we had assumed, that in cases with acute normalization of prolactin-levels hours after the adenomectomy no recurrence of hyperprolactinaemia could be expected. Up to now 50 patients had consequent follow-up with determinations of PRL-levels over a period of 1.5 to 10 years. In 8 of these patients an early normalisation of prolactin-levels occurred after 7 days, in 5 within hours, and was followed by a slight but persistent increase in the PRL-levels up to 1360 μU/ml (fig. 5).

SELECTIVE ADENOMECTOMY OF A MICROPROLACTINOMA AFTER INTRASELLAR HAEMORRHAGE

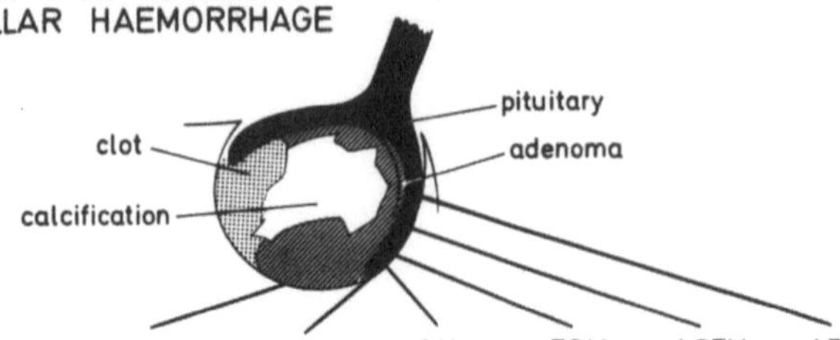

H.K. 31y.	PRL	LH	GH	TSH	ACTH	ADH
PREOPERATIVE	1237 - 1839	4,1 - 6,8	1,4 - 2,0	2,0 - 3,0	4,8 - 5,0	n
POSTOPERATIVE 3 months	363 - 774	3,7 - 6,3	0,4 - 2,4	1,4 - 2,4	14,1 - 16,0	n
POSTOPERATIVE 3 years	471 - 308	2,3 - 8,8	0,7 - 1,0	1,5 - 3,3	10,9 - 14,0	
TEST	TRH	LRH	IHT	TRH	IHT	17 - hours thirst per.
NORMAL VALUES	< 500µU/ml	Δ_{30} > 2ng/ml	Δ_{30} >7 ng/ml	Δ_{30} >2,7µU/ml	plas. cortisol 4-19 µg % Δ_{60} >12 µg %	urine concentr. >750 mOsm/kg

Fig. 4 Selective adenomectomy of a microprolactinoma in a 31-year-old women after intrasellar haemorrhage. After resection of the space-occupying intrasellar lesion, there was only a slight improvement of anterior pituitary insufficiency.

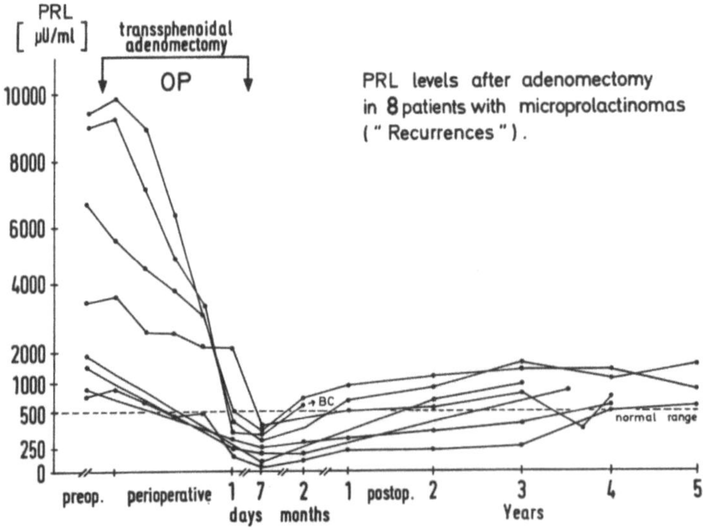

Fig. 5 Prolactin levels in 8 female patients who had an acute normalization of basal prolactin-levels after adenomectomy for a microprolactinoma and "recurrences" of hyperprolactinaemia.

The earliest time span of prolactin re-increase was two months; the latest 4 years. Three patients from our series had a partus before hyperprolactinaemia relapsed. The acute prolactin-increase during pregnancy is not documented in figure 5. After delivery normal menses resumed in spite of slightly increased basal prolactin-levels. Only 2 of the 8 patients had menstrual abnormalities, in three others galactorrhoea persisted or reappeared. It is open whether this reappearance of hyperprolactinaemia is to be regarded as a "recurrence" or a "relapse". The biological significance and a possible hypothalamic influence are under discussion. So far we have found recurrences in 16% of our microprolactinoma patients, which correlates well with the 15% in Faglia's series [9], but Serri et al. [26] report about 50% (12 out of 24) relapses in Hardy's series. So far we have only once observed the recurrence of a macroadenoma. In a 28-year-old female patient (fig. 6) with a su-

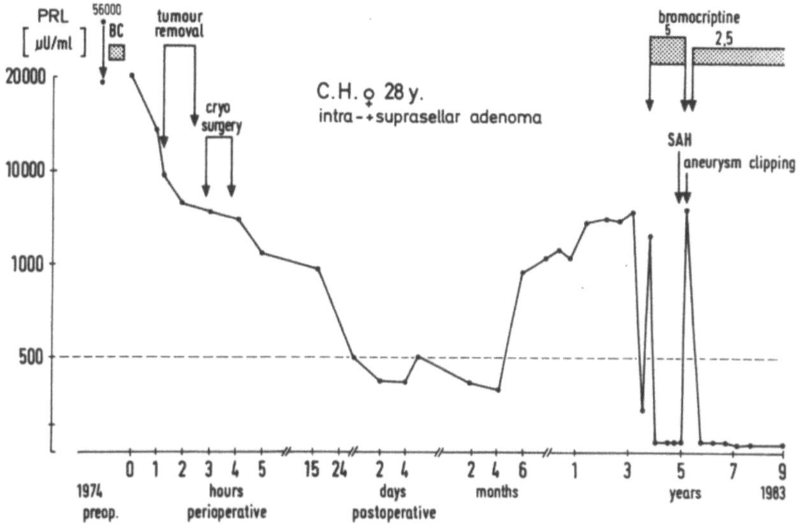

Fig. 6 Recurrence of a macroprolactinoma. In this 28-year-old patient prolactin-levels were normalized after adenomectomy for a prolactinoma. In recurrent hyperprolactinaemia, bromocriptine led to another normalization of basal prolactin-levels, but PRL-levels rose again, when bromocriptine was withdrawn.

prasellar tumour, who did not want to become pregnant, PRL-levels of 56000 µU/ml fell acutely after transsphenoidal adenomectomy and additional cryotherapy into the normal range. But prolactin-levels increased after 6 months to 3000 µU/ml and 7000 µU/ml. No recurrence of tumorous tissue could be observed in the CT-scan. Under bromocriptine prolactin-levels are within the normal range now. In this patient who did not have angiography before transsphenoidal surgery, clipping of an aneurysm of the anterior communicating artery was performed after subarachnoidal haemorrhage 5 years after the adenomectomy.

Management of macroprolactinomas

How can persisting hyperprolactinaemia, which occurs in the majority of surgically treated macroprolactinomas be prevented? Two operations in order to remove large prolactinomas totally can no longer be recommended. We have performed them in a 16-year-old male patient with a suprasellar tumour and prolactin-levels about 10000 μU/ml in 1973 (fig. 7). He was operated on by the transsphenoidal

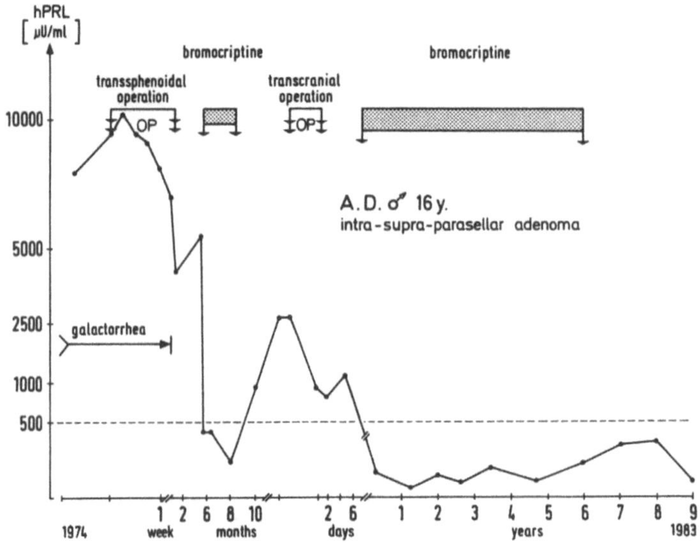

Fig. 7 Combined medical and surgical therapy in a 16-year-old male patient with a suprasellar prolactinoma. Surgery performed by transphenoidal and transcranial approaches did not lead to a normalization of the prolactin-excess. After the second operation medical treatment was given for several years. Now, PRL-levels are still normal, 3 years after withdrawal of bromocriptine.

approach but PRL-levels fell only to 3800 μU/ml. A normalization of basal PRL-levels could be achieved by additional bromocriptine therapy. At that time we did not have experience with longterm bromocriptine treatment and therefore decided to perform a second operation, which was indicated because the visual disturbances had not improved satisfactorily. After the transcranial tumour resection prolactin-levels fell to 1050 μU/ml and could be normalized again by additional bromocriptine therapy. Now, 3 years after withdrawal of bromocriptine, prolactin-levels remained in the normal range. There is no pituitary insufficiency, testosterone-levels are within the normal range.

The long-term treatment effects of dopamine-agonists can also be demonstrated in a 23-year-old male patient (fig. 8), in whom transsphenoidal resection of an intra-

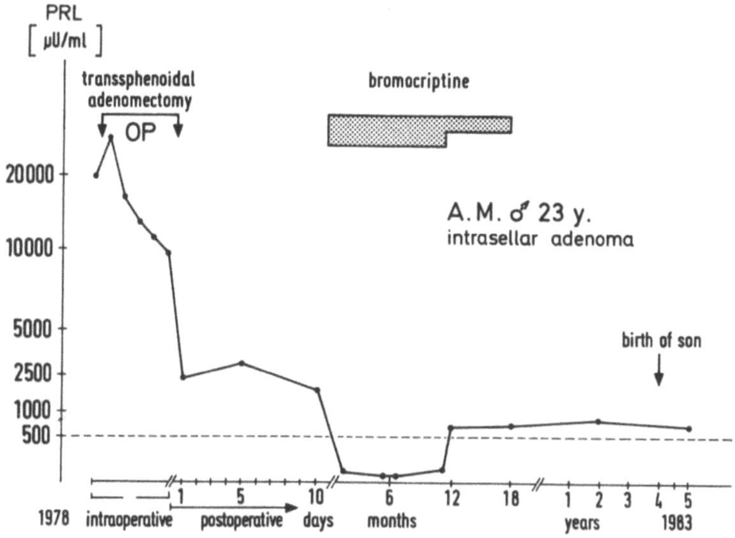

Fig. 8 Fertility of a 27-year-old male patient with a macroprolactinoma treated by surgery and bromocriptine. His fertility after treatment is documented by a normal spermiogram and the birth of a son, however, 4 years after withdrawal of bromocriptine PRL-levels are still slightly elevated.

sellar microadenoma was performed, but hyperprolactinaemia still persisted. His fertility after long-term bromocriptine-treatment and withdrawal is documented by a normal spermiogram and the birth of a son, although prolactin-levels are still slightly elevated (about 550 μU/ml).

In contrast to the long-term treatment with dopamine-agonists over a period of 3–6 years we know from short-term treatment (over a period of weeks and months) that there is an immediate re-expansion of the shrunken adenoma after withdrawal of the drugs [30]. Therefore, our present management for macroprolactinomas will be illustrated by the following case-history: In a male patient with a large supra-, para- and retrosellar prolactinoma (fig. 9), rapid shrinkage could be observed within two weeks of bromocriptine treatment. Prolactin-levels fell from 241000 μU/ml to 7400 μU/ml. After transsphenoidal surgery no tumour residuals were visible in the standard CT sections. Still elevated prolactin-levels could be normalized by bromocriptine to 385 μU/ml.

Table 5 summarizes the CT-results (horizontal sections with 5 mm collimation) and prolactin-results in 14 out of 20 patients who were pre-treated with dopamine-agonists for 2 to 4 weeks on average before transsphenoidal adenomectomy was performed. Among the 6 remaining patients, 2 were also found to be responders. 4 out of 20 patients were non-responders. When the adenoma was reduced to a size

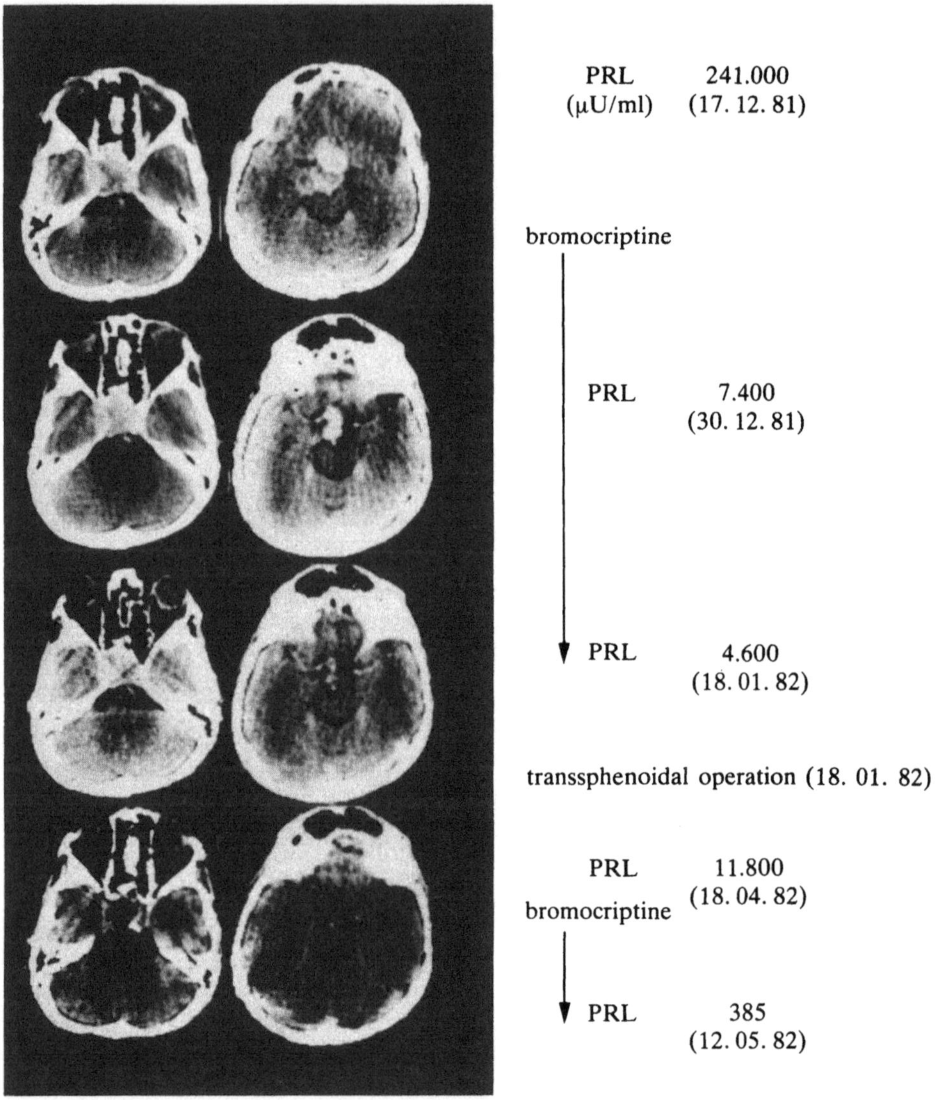

Fig. 9 Medical pre-treatment and operative result in a large supra-, para- and retrosellar macroprolactinoma (A. G.). A considerable size-reduction in the tumour and a decrease in prolactin-levels was seen within two weeks. Three months after transsphenoidal adenomectomy the CT-scan showed no tumour residuals on standard sections. PRL-levels were normalized by further administration of bromocriptine.

suitable for transsphenoidal surgery the latter was performed. Note the relatively low prolactin-levels after surgery before additional bromocriptine-treatment was started. We were able to reduce the prolactin-levels into a range between

Table 5 Preoperative treatment with dopamine-agonists in 14 patients with hyperprolactinaemia

CT-Findings				Patient	PRL			(μU/ml)	
CB	postop.	CB	pre		pre	weeks	CB	postop.	CB
–	–	S I	S II, r, p	A. G. m.	240000	4	6000	1500	normal
–	–	S I	S II	S. S. f.	27750	2	9212	3158	normal
i	i, sph.	S I, sph.	S II, r, p, sph.	L. D. m.	43400	3	7700	5300	1010
–	–	S II	S II	K. R. f.	74600	2	13250	1150	normal
–	–	i, sph.	S I, sph.	H. S. m.	106000	3	20050	63300	3060
–	–	i	S I	R. M. f.	40597	2	508	4110	1080
–	–	S I	S II	H. Z. m.	35500	3	4400	2280	normal
–	–	i, p	S I, p	A. Z. f.	15420	6	2935	3230	normal
–	–	S I	S II, sph.	T. E. m.	40350	4		800	normal
–	–	(i)	i	R. N. f.	15900	3	219	291	normal
–	–	(S II*)	S II*	J. K. m.	32200	4	1400	1513	normal
–	–	i	i, p	A. B. f.	11000	3	4800	735	normal
–	–	(S I)	S I	P. S. m.	36960	3	6390	2595	normal
–	–	i	S I	A. Z. f.	12730	4	432	648	normal

* = cystic tumour; f = female; m = male; i = intrasellar; p = parasellar; r = retrosellar; sph. = sphenoidal; S I = suprasellar adenoma (no chiasm syndrome); S II = suprasellar adenoma (chiasm syndrome); S III = suprasellar adenoma (compression of the interventricular foramen).

291 μU/ml and 5300 μU/ml in 13 out of 14 patients and normalize the CT-findings in 13 out of 14 patients postoperatively before starting additional therapy with dopamine-agonists.

Exceptional findings were observed in the following patients: In the patient H. S. prolactin-levels decreased only to 63000 μU/ml. He had a large adenoma with invasive extension into the skull base. In the patient J. K. the major part of the suprasellar tumour grade II was cystic and therefore only a moderate shrinkage of the smaller, solid tumour part could be observed by the CT during pre-treatment with bromocriptine.

Such results could not be attained, when macroprolactinomas were treated medically only. According to Chiodini et al. [3] shrinkage of the adenoma could be documented in about 2/3 of the patients though there never was a complete disappearance of the tumour in the CT-scan. This occurred in 75% of our stage-II-tumours after adenomectomy without pre-treatment, but in 13 out of 14 patients after medical pre-treatment and surgery. Furthermore vision could be improved or normalized in only 60% after medical treatment alone [3, 29, 30] but in 80% of pituitary adenomas after surgery [12].

Conclusions

In prolactin-secreting adenomas of the pituitary, the aim of surgical intervention is the resection of the tumour and a normalization of the hormone-excess. Dopamine-agonists in combination with surgery can facilitate or jeopardize this objective. Prolactinomas have to be regarded as a heterogenious biological group. The indications for surgical therapy, surgical therapy in combination with medical therapy and medical therapy alone have therefore to be related to the different groups of patients.

From the surgical point of view, the postoperative medical treatment of persisting hyperprolactinaemia is undisputed. Medical pre-treatment with dopamine-agonists in the patients with macroprolactinomas has led to great advantages for surgical therapy. The postoperative results, documented by prolactin-levels and CT-findings could be considerably improved. But in larger microprolactinomas preoperative administration of dopamine-agonists obviously impairs the results of later surgery.

Acknowledgements

The authors would like to express their gratitude for the helpful cooperation of Drs. A. Lierheimer (Neurochirurgische Klinik Großhadern, München), E. Adams, K. Mashiter (Endocrine Unit, Hammersmith Hospital, London), J. Pichl (Medizinische Klinik der Universität Erlangen), H. K. Rjosk (1. Frauenklinik der Universität München), U. Schrell (Neurochirurgische Klinik der Universität Erlangen) and K. v. Werder (Medizinische Klinik Innenstadt der Universität München) and their collaborative efforts.

References

[1] Bonneville, J. F., F. Cattin, K. Moussa-Bacha et al.: Dynamic computed tomography of the pituitary gland: "The tuft-sign". Radiology **149** (1983) 145.
[2] Buchfelder, M., I. Baer, Th. v. Poschinger et al.: Preoperative evaluation of pituitary microadenomas by CT reconstructions and operative findings. In: 3rd European Workshop on Pituitary Adenomas. Amsterdam 1983 (in press).
[3] Chiodini, P. G., A. Liuzzi, R. Cozzi et al.: Size reduction of macroprolactinomas by bromocriptine or lisuride therapy. J. Clin. Endocr. **53** (1982) 737.
[4] Derome, P. J.: Personal communication. 1983.
[5] Derome, P. J., F. Peillon, R. H. Bard et al.: Adenomes a prolactine: Results du traitement chirurgical. Nouv. Presse Med. **8** (1979) 577.
[6] Derome, P. J. (after R. Fahlbusch): Surgical failures in prolactinomas. In: Second european workshop on pituitary adenomas (P. J. Derome, C. P. Jedynac, F. Peillon, eds.), p. 273. Asclepios France, Paris 1980.
[7] Derome, P. J., J. Radacot: Preoperative shrinkage with bromocriptine. In: 3rd European Workshop on Pituitary Adenomas. Amsterdam 1983 (in press).
[8] Faglia, G., M. A. Giovanelli, according to R. Fahlbusch: Surgical failures in prolactinomas. In: Second european workshop on pituitary adenomas . p. J. Derome, C. P. Jedynac, F. Peillon, eds.), p. 273. Asclepios France, Paris 1980.

[9] Faglia, G., P. Moriondo, P. Travaglini et al.: Influence of previous bromocriptine therapy on surgery for microprolactinomas. Lancet **1** (1983) 133.
[10] Fahlbusch, R.: Surgical failures in Prolactinomas. In: Second european workshop on pituitary adenomas (J. P. Derome, C. P. Jedynac, F. Peillon, eds.), p. 273. Asclepios France, Paris 1980.
[11] Fahlbusch, R., M. Giovanelli, P. G. Crosignani, et. al.: Differentiated therapy of microprolactinomas: Significance of transsphenoidal adenomectomy. In: Pituitary Microadenomas (G. Faglia, M. A. Giovanelli, R. McLeod, eds.), p. 443. Academic Press, London 1980.
[12] Fahlbusch, R., F. Marguth: Optic nerve compression by pituitary adenomas. In: The Cranial Nerves (M. Samii, P. J. Janetta, eds.). Springer, Berlin–Heidelberg–New York 1981.
[13] Fahlbusch, R., F. Marguth: Tumoren der Hypophyse. In: Klinische Neurochirurgie, Bd. II, Klinik und Therapie (H. Dietz, W. Umbach, R. Wüllenweber, eds.), p. 86. Thieme Verlag, Stuttgart 1984.
[14] Flückiger, E., E. del Pozo, K. v. Werder: Prolactin; physiology, pharmacology and clinical findings. Springer, Heidelberg–New York 1982.
[15] Guibout, M., P. Jaquet, J.-C. Lissitzky et al.: Résultats de l'exérèse transsphenoidale des adenomes hypophysaires sécrétants. Ann. Endocrinol. (Paris) **39** (1978) 95.
[16] Hardy, J.: Le prolactinome. Neurochirurgie **27** (1981) Suppl. 1, 41.
[17] Landolt, A. M.: Personal communication, 1983.
[18] Landolt, A. M., P. J. Keller, E. R. Froesch et al.: Bromocriptine: Does it jeopardise the result of later surgery for prolactinomas? Lancet **2** (1982) 657.
[19] Laws, E. R., E. B. Kern: Complications of Transsphenoidal Surgery. In: Clinical management of Pituitary Disorders (G. T. Tindall, W. F. Collins, eds.), p. 435. Raven Press, New York 1979.
[20] Lüdecke, D. K., H. D. Hermann, C. Hörmann et al.: Comparison of effects of dopamine agonists and microsurgery in GH- and PRL-secreting adenomas. In: Lisuride and other dopamine agonists (D. B. Calne, R. Horowski, R. MacDonald, W. Wuttke, eds.), 271. Raven Press, New York 1983.
[21] Mashiter, K.: Role of culturing pituitary adenomas in clinical decision making. In: 3rd European Workshop on Pituitary Adenomas. Amsterdam, 1983 (in press).
[22] Nillius, S. J., T. Bergh, S. G. Larsson: Pituitary tumours and pregnancy. In: Second european workshop on pituitary adenomas (P. J. Derome, C. P. Jedynak, F. Peillon, eds.). Asclepios France, Paris 1980.
[23] Rjosk, H. K., R. Fahlbusch, K. v. Werder: Spontaneous development of hyperprolactinaemia. Acta endocrinol. **100** (1982) 333.
[24] Rjosk, H. K., R. Fahlbusch, K. v. Werder: Hyperprolactinaemia and pregnancy. In: Prolactin and Prolactinomas (G. Tolis, T. Stefanis, T. Mountokalakis, F. Labrie, eds.), p. 193. Raven Press, New York 1983.
[25] Schrell, U., M. Buchfelder, R. Fahlbusch et al.: Hormone secretion in cell cultures of microprolactinomas, periadenoma tissue and capsules. This volume.
[26] Serri, O., E. Rasio, H. Beauregard et al.: Recurrence of hyperprolactinaemia after selective transsphenoidal adenomectomy in women with prolactinomas. N. Engl. J. Med. **309** (1983) 280.
[27] Teasdale, G., J. A. Thompson, J. A. Ratcliffe et al.: Hyperprolactinaemia: results of operation in patients selected on the basis of dynamic endocrine tests. In: Modern Neurosurgery (M. Brock, ed.), p. 152. Springer Verlag, Berlin 1982.
[28] Teasdale, G., A. Richards, R. Bullock et al.: Fertility after operation for hyperprolactinaemia. In: 3rd European Workshop on Pituitary Adenomas. Amsterdam 1983 (in press).

[29] Thorner, M. O., J. A. Burdmann, M. T. Calabrese, et al.: Dopamine agonists and prolactinomas; Clinical and basic considerations of the mechanisms of action. In: Lisuride and other dopamine agnonists (D. B. Calne, R. Horowski, R. McDonald, W. Wuttke, eds.), p. 213. Raven Press, New York 1983.
[30] Werder, K. v., R. Fahlbusch, H. K. Rjosk: Macroprolactinomas: Clinical and therapeutical aspects. In: Prolactin and Prolactinomas (G. Tolis, C. Stefanis, T. Mountokalakis, F. Labrie, eds.), p. 415. Raven Press, New York 1983.

Prolactinomas: surgical results in 96 cases

G. Maira, G. F. Rossi, C. Anile, R. Roselli, A. Barbarino, L. De Marinis, A. Mancini, E. Menini

Introduction

Transsphenoidal surgery seems to be an efficacious treatment for patients with prolactin (PRL) secreting pituitary adenoma. PRL levels frequently return to normal and normal menstrual cycles are restored [1]. However disrupted pituitary-hypothalamic relationships may persist after surgery and/or a recurrence of the PRL secreting tumour can occur [2, 6].

The aim of the investigation reported here is to analyze the results of the transsphenoidal microsurgical treatment on the pituitary-hypothalamic function in 96 consecutively operated women with PRL secreting adenomas. In particular we have studied the responses of PRL to dynamic tests and the hypothalamic dopaminergic (DA) tone.

Material and methods

Ninety-six patients with a PRL secreting pituitary adenoma underwent selective transsphenoidal microsurgery for removal of the tumour. In all cases the adenoma was histologically verified. The grade of the lesions, according to the anatomic-radiological classification of Hardy and Vezina [3], and the range of the presurgical PRL basal levels are reported in figure 1.

The surgical results are analyzed considering: 1. the PRL basal levels (upper normal range: 20 ng/ml); 2. the PRL dynamics, as evaluated on the basis of the response of PRL to TRH and Metoclopramide (MCP) [2]; the response is defined as positive when at least a twofold increase of the PRL baseline values is reached. Note that all patients, before surgery, showed an absent or blunted response of PRL to both TRH and MCP [5]; 3. the DA tone as studied by analyzing the TSH response to MCP. The response was regarded to be positive when an increase in the TSH levels of more than 0.5 μUI/ml occurred [4]; this last analysis was performed only in 24 patients. Other pituitary functions were also studied using standard procedures [2].

Results

PRL basal levels

An immediate normalization of basal PRL levels was obtained in 53 patients (55%) following the removal of the adenoma. The relationships between early postoperative PRL normalization, grade of the lesion, and preoperative PRL basal levels are reported in figure 1.

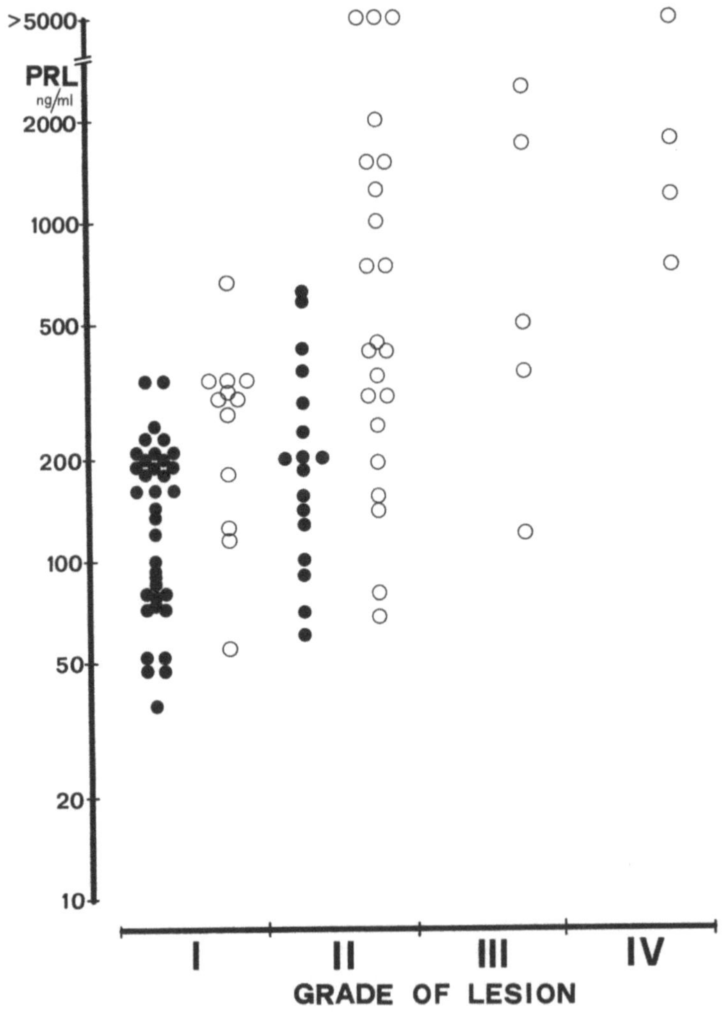

Fig. 1 Relationships between grades of the adenoma, presurgical PRL levels and early surgical results. Normal ● and high ○ immediate postoperative basal PRL levels.

The follow-up of the post-surgical normalized patients is reported in figure 2. In four of these 53 patients a late abnormal increase in the hormonal level occurred; their early postoperative PRL basal levels ranged from 11 to 15 ng/ml (fig. 2). None of these patients were pharmacologically treated. In all the 49 remaining patients with persistently normal PRL basal levels menstrual cycles resumed and galactorrhoea, when previously present, disappeared. 18 of them became pregnant without medical treatment.

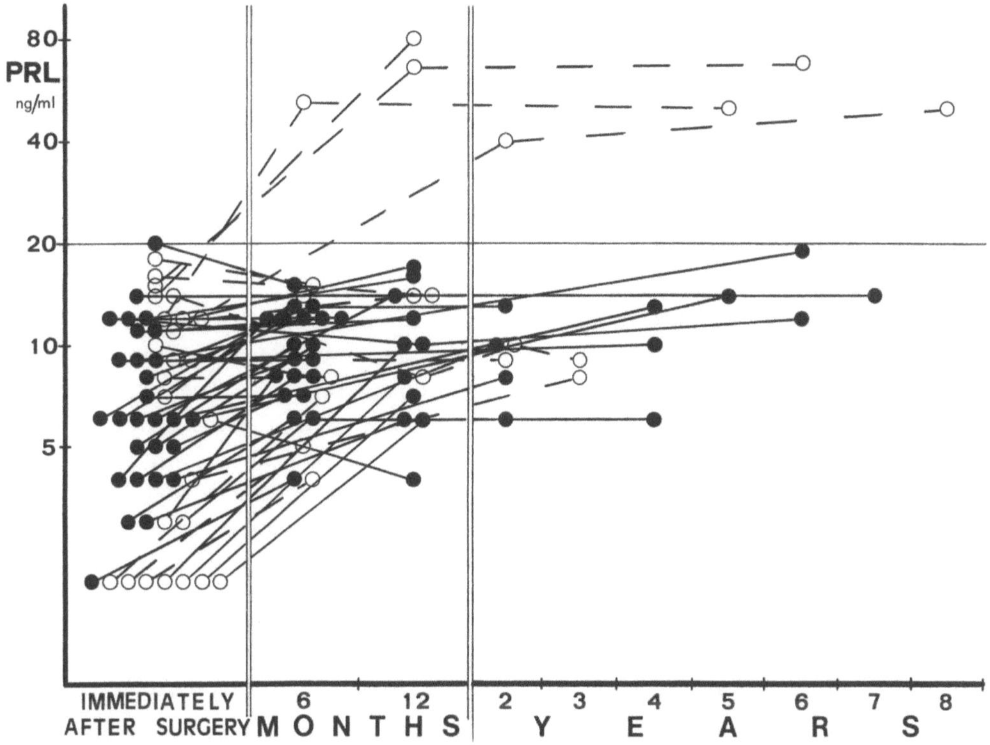

Fig. 2 Post-surgical follow-up of the 53 patients showing immediate normalization of basal PRL levels. Positive ● and negative ○ responses of PRL to TRH and MCP.

In the other 43 patients postoperative PRL levels, though decreased with respect to presurgical values, were not normalized. They ranged from 21 to 4000 ng/ml. Clinical normalization occurred in only one of them (see below).

PRL responses to TRH and MCP

A positive PRL response to provocative tests was obtained in 39 of the 53 patients with postoperative normalization of their basal PRL levels. In 29 of them this result was achieved immediately after surgery; in 10 a few weeks or months later. The positive responses to the tests persisted with the passage of time (fig. 2). In the remaining 14 patients the negative responses to both stimuli persisted postoperatively in spite of the early normalization of the basal PRL levels. To this group belong the 4 patients mentioned above (fig. 2) in whom the PRL levels became normal after surgery, but subsequently showed a progressive increase.

In 42 of the 43 patients in whom surgical treatment failed to normalize the PRL basal levels, the PRL response to TRH and MCP remained negative. In the remaining one of this group the PRL response, which was negative in the immediate postoperative period, became positive one year later, even if the PRL basal levels persisted slightly elevated (about 25 ng/ml); at the same time ovulatory cycles reappeared.

TSH response to MCP

A positive TSH response after MCP administration was found preoperatively in 18 of the 24 examined patients. In 8 of these cases, after the removal of the adenoma, normalization of PRL basal levels and the appearance of PRL responses to TRH and MCP, the TSH response to MCP disappeared and remained absent on follow-up studies [4]. The disappearance of theTSH response to MCP in the early postoperative period was found also in 4 other patients from the group in which surgery led to an immediate decrease in basal PRL levels to the normal or slightly above normal range (21 and 22 ng/ml) but not positive PRL responses to TRH and MCP stimulation; 12–24 months after surgery an increase in the basal PRL level with reappearance of the TSH response to MCP was observed. In the remaining six patients from the same group, surgery failed to normalize PRL levels and PRL responses to TRH and MCP: the positive response to MCP persisted. In six out of the 24 studied patients, the MCP failed preoperatively to elicite a significant increase in THS basal levels. In five of them a macroadenoma with extrasellar expansion was present, and in the remaining one surgery disclosed a microadenoma located close to the pituitary stalk. In three of the patients harbouring a macroadenoma, the removal of the tumour led to a decrease in the PRL basal level which, however, remained above the normal range: a positive TSH response to MCP was observed. In the other two macroadenoma patients who also showed postoperative elevated PRL values, the TSH responses to MCP remained negative after surgery.

In all patients no disorders of the other pituitary functions studied were found after surgery [5].

Discussion

Immediate normalization of basal PRL levels is obtained in the majority of patients suffering from a PRL secreting pituitary tumour and treated with selective trans-sphenoidal microsurgery. In the remaining cases, though a decrease in basal PRL levels is reached, normalization does not occur. In these cases the surgical failure is probably related to the incomplete removal of the adenoma, mainly due to its size and/or infiltrating character.

Early postoperative normalization of basal PRL levels, however, does not necessarily imply that the patient has been cured: recurrence is possible in particular in patients with post-surgical PRL levels in the upper normal range [6]. Basing on our experience, the response of PRL to provocative tests is, at present, the most reliable index of the effect of the surgery. The reappearance of the response of the lactotrophs to direct (TRH) and indirect (MCP) stimuli seems to indicate not only the complete removal of all adenomatous cells, but also the re-establishment of normal pituitary-hypothalamic relationships. In our series, so far, when this condition was present, there was no recurrence. Worth mentioning, in this connection, is the only case in whom, one year after surgery, while the postoperative PRL basal level was still slightly elevated, its responses to TRH and MCP became positive. This combination, in our experience (unpublished data), can be found also in several patients suffering from different pathologies of the sellar region (empty sella, craniopharyngioma, Rathke's cyst, non-secreting adenomas, other intracranial tumours, etc.) in whom damage of the pituitary stalk can be assured. In these cases, PRL levels slightly or moderately elevated (ranging from 20 to 200 ng/ml) can be associated either to positive or to negative responses to provocative stimuli. In the single patient here discussed, at surgery the adenoma was found to be located in the medial part of the gland near to the neurohypophysis, and its total removal required the surgical manipulation of the pituitary stalk. The patient showed diabetes insipidus for some months after operation; the reappearance of positive PRL responses to TRH and MCP and ovulatory cycles followed concurrently to the normalization of this sign.

Our data also show that an increase in the DA tone is frequently found in the presence of a PRL secreting adenoma, as documented by the preoperative positive TSH responses to MCP observed in 18 of the 24 studied cases in our series. In the six remaining patients (five of whom had a macro adenoma and one a microadenoma which was located near the stalk) the lack of the TSH response to MCP could be consequent to compression of pituitary tissue and/or the pituitary stalk. Under these conditions a high DA tone could be masked and become patient only if, after surgical removal of the adenomatous mass, restoration of the integrity of the pituitary-hypothalamic relationship is obtained.

The postoperative finding of a negative response of PRL to provocative stimuli coupled with a normalization of basal PRL levels is difficult to explain. In the cases showing a tendency of basal PRL level to increase after the immediate post-surgical normalization (4 patients), one might suggest that the removal of the secreting adenoma was extensive but incomplete. The reappearance, in two of these patients studied by the TSH response to MCP, of an increase in the DA tone in the late postoperative period seems to confirm such a hypothesis. In the other cases in this group showing the persistence with time of the combination of negative PRL responses to TRH and MCP with normal basal PRL levels (see fig. 2) one might suggest, alternatively, the occurrence of a disorder of the pituitary-hypothalamic functional connections. Whether such a disorder was pre-existing to or is a consequence of surgical procedure cannot be established by our data.

References

[1] Hardy, J.: Transsphenoidal microsurgery of prolactinomas: report on 355 cases. In: Prolactin and Prolactinomas (G. Tolis et al., eds.), pp. 431–440. Raven Press, New York 1983.

[2] Barbarino, A., L. De Marinis, C. Anile et al.: Dopaminergic mechanisms regulating prolactin secretion in patients with prolactin-secreting pituitary adenoma. Long-term studies after selective transsphenoidal surgery. Metabolism **31** (1982) 1100–1104.

[3] Hardy, J., J. L. Vezina: Transsphenoidal neurosurgery of intracranial neoplasm. In: Advances in Neurology (R. A. Thompson, J. R. Greene, eds.), pp. 261–264. Raven Press, New York 1976.

[4] De Marinis, L., A. Mancini, G. Maira et al.: Postoperative evaluation of dopaminergic tone in prolactinoma patients. II. Plasma thyrotropin response to Metoclopramide. J. C. E. M. **58** (1984) 405–409.

[5] Barbarino, A., L. De Marinis, E. Menini et al.: Pre- and postoperative pituitary function tests in patients with prolactin-secreting pituitary adenoma. In: Pituitary Hyperfunction: Physiopathology and clinical aspects (F. Camanni, E. E. Müller, eds.), pp. 333–342. Raven Press, New York 1984.

[6] Serri, O., E. Rasio, H. Beauregard et al.: Recurrence of hyperprolactinaemia after selective transsphenoidal adenomectomy in women with prolactinoma. New England Journal of Medicine **309** (1983) 280–283.

Effect of transsphenoidal surgery on pituitary function

M. Ohta, T. Uozumi, K. Sakoda, M. Gen, S. Shinohara, M. Yamanaka, K. Mukada

Introduction

We have now two effective methods for the treatment of prolactinoma, namely surgery, bromocriptine, alone and their combination. Recently, Serri et al. [2] reported the recurrence of hyperprolactinaemia after selective transsphenoidal adenomectomy in women with prolactinoma. This paper attempts to evaluate the effect of transsphenoidal surgery on pituitary function in postoperatively normalized cases.

Materials and methods

From 1978 to 1983, eighty-two patients with prolactinoma underwent transsphenoidal surgery in the Department of Neurosurgery, Hiroshima University. They consisted of fourty-five micro, twenty-four expansive, and thirteen invasive prolactinomas. The surgical procedure is a slightly modified version of the Hardy method, and any reagents such as alcohol which some neurosurgeons use to destroy the remaining adenoma cells are not used. A systematic pituitary function test (ITT, TRH test, LHRH test) is routinely scheduled before surgery, and repeated on the 7th to 10th day, 1st month, 3rd month, 6th month, and, thereafter, once a year after surgical intervention.

Results

A postoperative normalization of blood prolactin (PRL) level (less than 25 ng/ml) was observed in 69.2% of micro-, 28.6% of expansive, and none of the invasive prolactinomas, which were estimated immediately after operation. In bromocriptine-pretreated cases, the postoperative normalization rate was lower because only 52.6% of microprolactinoma were normalized (tab. 1). Among 34 postoperatively normalized cases, 25 cases (73.5%) showed less than 10 ng/ml of blood PRL levels, while 9 cases (26.5%) had levels greater than 10 ng/ml (fig. 1).

Table 1 Postoperative normalization of blood PRL level (less than 25 ng/ml)

	micro		expansive		invasive	
bromocriptine pretreatment	+	−	+	−	+	−
no. of patients	19	26	3	21	3	10
normalization	52.6%	69.2%	0%	28.6%	0%	0%

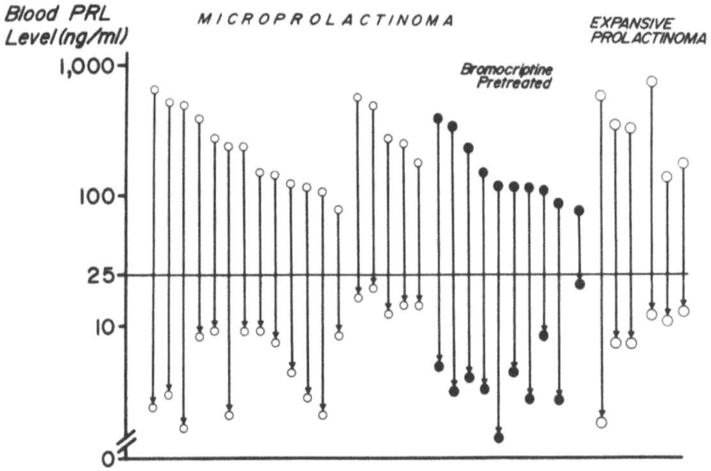

Fig. 1 Effect of transsphenoidal surgery on blood PRL levels in normalized prolactinomas.

A preoperative disturbance of GH, cortisol, TSH, FSH and LH responses was observed in 7 (20.6%), 4 (11.8%), 2 (5.9%), 3 (8.8%) and 1 (2.9%) of 34 cases. Immediately after surgery, the disturbed responses of the anterior pituitary hormones were improved in 2 (28.6%) of GH and all of the other hormones (tab. 2), and a newly impaired response of these anterior pituitary hormones, which was considered to be due to the operative manoeuver, was observed in 5 (14.7%), 3 (8.8%), 3 (8.8%), 2 (5.9%) and 1 (2.9%) of 34 cases respectively. However, this impairment was mild and transient, because it progressively improved at least within 6 months and none of the cases showed panhypopituitarism requiring hormone replacement therapy (tab. 3).

Table 2 Postoperative improvement of anterior pituitary function

GH	Cortisol	TSH	FSH	LH
29%	100%	100%	100%	100%

Table 3 Postoperative impairment of anterior pituitary function

GH	Cortisol	TSH	FSH	LH
14.7%	8.8%	8.8%	5.9%	2.9%

The recurrence of hyperprolactinaemia was observed in 3 microprolactinoma cases. Two of them were pretreated with bromocriptine. One who had a postoperative blood PRL level of 21.0 ng/ml showed a level of 50.0 ng/ml 3 months later. This means that this case might have been affected by bromocriptine even immediately after the operation and the cessation of its effect caused an elevation in blood PRL level to 50.0 ng/ml, which might be obtained purely by surgery alone. Another patient whose postoperative blood PRL level was 2.9 ng/ml showed a level of 75.0 ng/ml 3 months later but 2.1 ng/ml 6 months later. This case was considered to be normalized by surgery, while the reason for the fluctuation in blood PRL level is obscure. The last case who received only surgical treatment showed a level of 16.2 ng/ml immediately after surgery, 29.7 ng/ml 3 months later, 46.9 ng/ml 6 months later, but 18.8 ng/ml one year after surgery (fig. 2). These data are purely postoperative without any postoperative supplementary therapy, such as irradiation or bromocriptine.

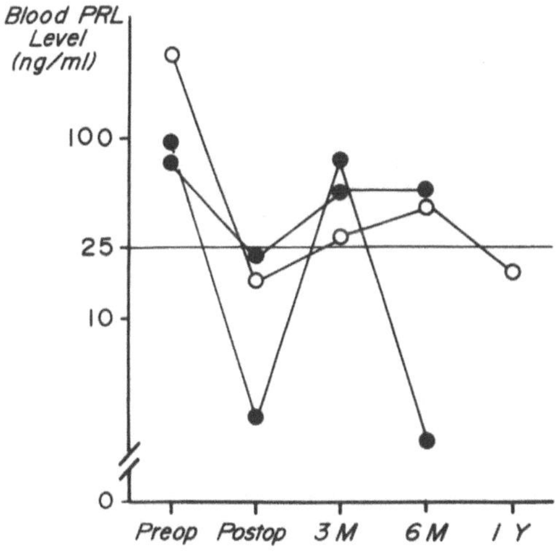

Fig. 2 Recurrence of hyperprolactinaemia.

Discussion

A purely postoperative normalization of blood PRL level was obtained in 69.2% of micro-, 28.6% of expansive and none of the invasive prolactinomas. The pretreatment with bromocriptine worsened these figures.

Pituitary hypofunction may be caused by either the growth of the adenoma leading to compression and destruction of the normal paraadenomatous tissue or the metabolic influence of the excessively secreted hormone [1]. Among anterior pituitary hormones, the gonadotropin response varies considerably in long-standing hyperprolactinaemia but other hormones are not influenced by hyperprolactinaemia itself. From our pre- and postoperative evaluation of pituitary function, transsphenoidal surgery per se did not cause permanent impairment of anterior pituitary function; on the contrary, it improved the preoperative disturbance.

The recurrence of hyperprolactinaemia was observed also in 3 microprolactinomas. One of bromocriptine-pretreated cases should not be included in the postoperative normalized group, because the decision regarding postoperative normalization should be made after the effect of bromocriptine has completely disappeared. The other two cases had fluctuations in blood PRL levels, but the reason is obscure.

Therefore, systematic pituitary function test is required and is important for the postoperative evaluation of pituitary function and follow-up of the prolactinoma.

References

[1] Fluckiger et al.: Prolactin: Physiology, pharmacology and clinical findings, p. 165. Springer-Verlag, Berlin–Heidelberg–New York 1982.

[2] Serri et al.: Recurrence of hyperprolactinaemia after selective transsphanoidal adenomectomy in women with prolactinoma. N. Engl. J. Med. **309** (1983) 280–283.

Transsphenoidal microsurgical treatment of 77 prolactinomas

K. Watanabe, T. Fukushima

Introduction

Advances in endocrinological diagnosis and neuroradiology have greatly facilitated the early detection of pituitary adenomas, particularly functioning microadenomas. Among various endocrine types of pituitary adenomas, prolactin-producing adenoma (prolactinoma) comprises the largest group and yet the clinical management of this tumours has been most controversial [4, 16, 28, 43]. Since Jules Hardy of Montreal revived the classical transsphenoidal approach to the pituitary and established the technique of microsurgery with fluoroscopic control [18]. The excision of pituitary adenomas has become one of the most successful procedure in neurosurgery with extreme safety and accuracy [12]. In the management of prolactinomas, we believe that the transsphenoidal microsurgery plays a major role and in fact we have been constantly stressing the importance of early surgical treatment (surgery first policy) [11, 12, 13]. However, some reports [2, 3, 4, 32, 37, 38, 39] recommend the medical therapy with bromocriptine as the first step. In this paper, we present the results of transsphenoidal microsurgery in our personal series of 77 prolactinomas and discuss the issues of controversies between surgical and medical managements.

Clinical materials

During the past 7 years, 104 cases of PRL-secreting pituitary adenomas were operated upon in our institutes. In 27 cases with large or giant invasive prolactinoma, transcranial or combined transcranial-transsphenoidal operations were performed. The rest of 77 patients with micro-, macro-, or some large prolactinomas underwent rhinoseptoplastic transsphenoidal microsurgery. This series of 77 prolactinomas represents the subject of investigation in this report. There were 64 females and 13 males. The age ranged from 17 to 52 years with the average of 31 years. Only one case of 13 male patients had micro-prolactinoma presented with hypogonadism and the other 12 male cases presented with visual disturbances. Among 64 female patients, 44 had microadenoma. 17 had macroadenoma and 3 had large tumour.

Fifty-seven of 64 female cases (89%) presented with typical amenorrhoea-galactorrhoea syndrome, 6 presented with amenorrhoea only and 1 case had galactorrhoea with preserved menstruation. The symptom duration ranged from 1 to 18 years with the mean of 7 years. Serum PRL levels were fairly well correlated with the adenoma size. As shown in table 1. PRL values were 83 to 1460 ng/ml (mean, 327) in 45 cases of microadenoma. 133 to 2970 ng/ml (mean, 1104) in 18 with macroadenoma and 1300 to 8600 (mean, 3760) in 14 large adenomas. It should be noted that patients in our series revealed much higher PRL values as compared to those reported in other literature.

Neurodiagnostic examinations

Complete neurodiagnostic evaluation was done in all cases, including hypocycloidal polytomography and computerized tomographic reformat studies using the updated GECT/T 8800 or 9800 scanners. Although simple lateral skull x-rays remain a very useful diagnostic test, the hypocycloidal polytomography has been shown to be much more sensitive to demonstrate subtle changes of the sella turcica. In 45 microadenomas, polytomography detected abnormality in 80% of the cases. High-resolution enhanced CT was positive in 70% of the cases with microadenoma. A half of the tumour-positive cases on CT showed low density adenomas and the other half demonstrated enhanced high density tumours. Larger microadenomas or diffuse type adenomas tended to be visualized as a high density tumour and smaller or localized microadenoma were often visualized as a low density nodule. Bromocriptine pretreated cases (9 patients) were either not visualized or detected as a low density nodule. Typical examples of micro-prolactinomas are illustrated in figure 1.

Operative technique

Our operative technique [11] consists of a unilateral dissection of the nasal mucosa and retraction of the nasal septum through an L-shaped osteotomy (fig. 2a). A specially designed U-shaped knife is used to perform a horizontal osteotomy along the base of the septum and a curved chisel to perform a vertical osteotomy in front of the anterior wall of the sphenoid sinus (fig. 2b). With this method, the entire septal structures are preserved and retracted with the nasal mucosa on the right side toward the right nasal chamber, exposing the sphenoid sinus keel bone widely. In approaching the tumour, the surface of the pituitary gland is first meticulously examined. Then, the pituitary gland is incised both horizontally and vertically. The pituitary tissue is thouroughly examined and the adenoma is totally removed. To achieve the curative resection of the tumour, the boundaries between the tumour and the normal gland are carefully cleaned up and any suspicious area for tumour invasion is resected. The dura and the pituitary capsule at the fundus and over the

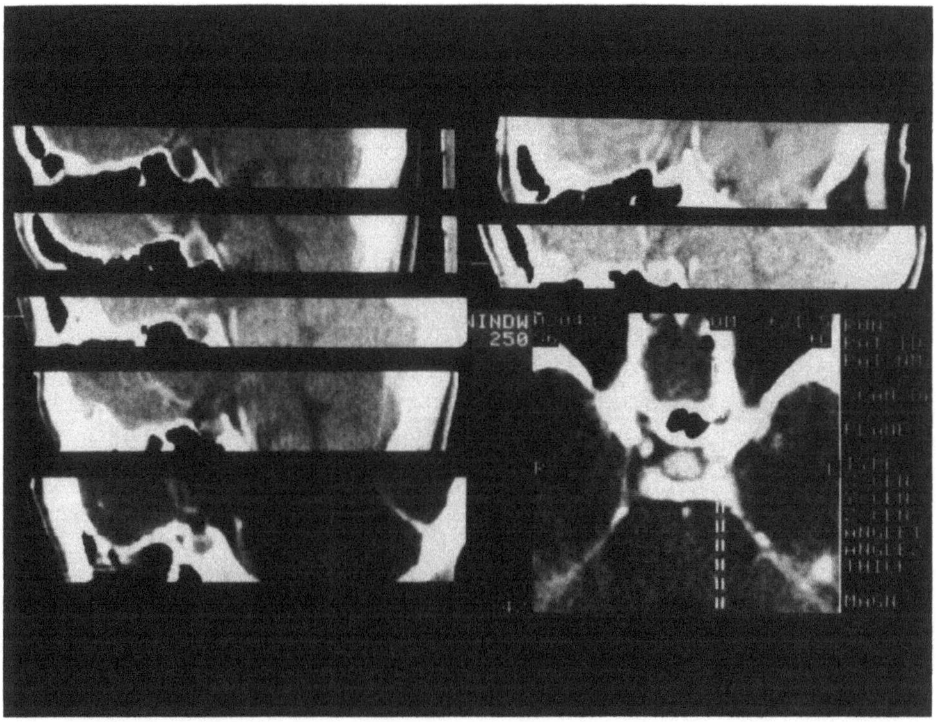

Fig. 1: Typical examples of microprolactinomas on high-resolution reformat CT examination, 5 cases of low density adenoma (left) and 3 instances of enhanced microadenoma (right).

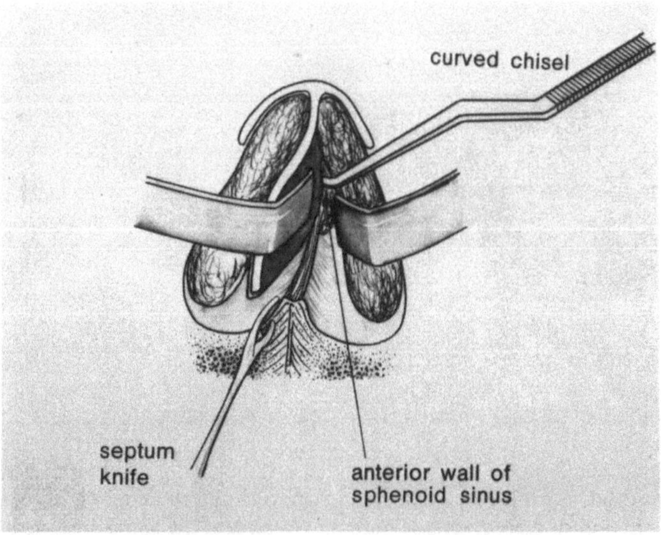

Fig. 2a Schematic drawings of our operative technique. Unilateral dissection of the nasal mucosa and retraction of the nasal septum toward the right nasal chamber.

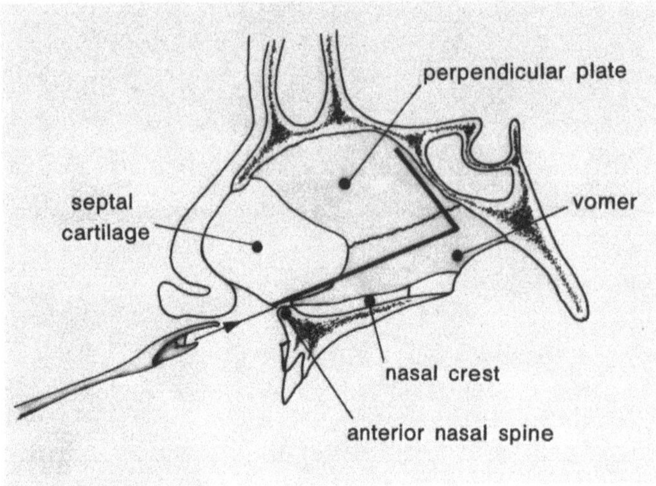

Fig. 2b Demonstration of L-shaped osteotomy with a U-shaped knife and a curved chisel.

tumour side should be resected as much as possible. The detail of our radical selective tumour resection is illustrated in figure 3. Absolute alcohol solution is applied for 5 to 10 minutes into the tumour bed before closure.

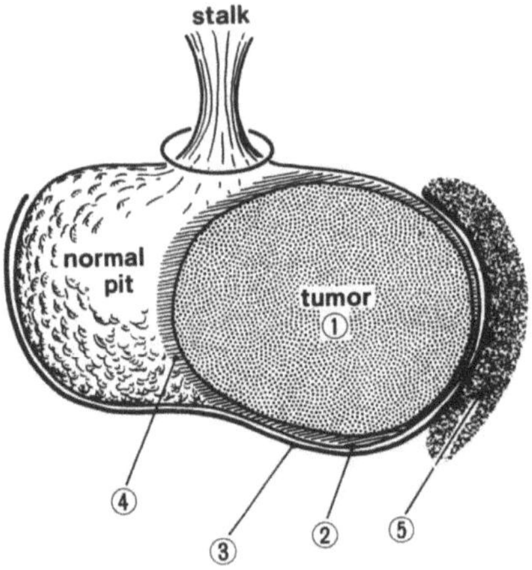

Fig. 3 The operative technique of radical-selective resection of prolactinoma.
(1) careful total excision of tumor mass; (2) removal of the pituitary capsule over the tumor; (3) resection of the dura at the fundus and the tumor side; (4) meticulous clean-up of the tumor bed which is often resected in 0.5 to 1 mm thickness; (5) generous curettage and suction of the cavernous dura and even into the sinus in cases of invasive adenoma.

Results

The operative results in the earlier series of 27 patients treated during the first 2 years were disappointing. Of 15 patients who had the preoperative PRL levels below 1000 ng/ml, only 6 (40%) gained the PRL normalization (fig. 4, right). None of the 12 cases with higher PRL values than 1000 ng/ml showed satisfactory results (fig. 4, left). However, with the increasing surgical experience and the better

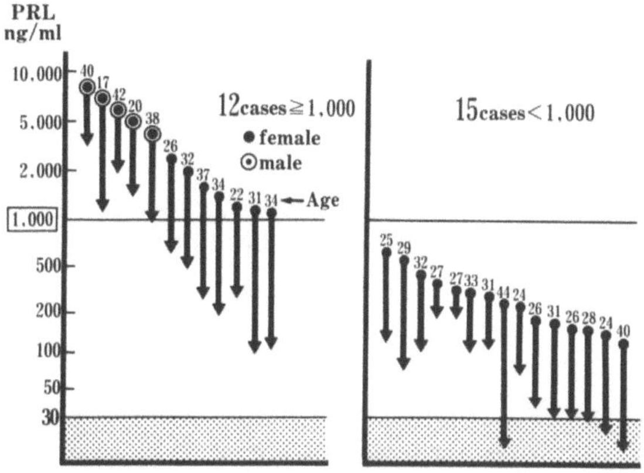

Fig. 4 Operative results in the first 2 years series. None of the 12 cases with PRL values over 1000 ng/ml showed hormonal normalization. In 15 cases with PRL levels below 1000 ng/ml, 6 (40%) showed satisfactory results. Pre- and postoperative PRL levels are shown for each patient. Black dots indicate female cases and dots with a circle indicate male patients.

Table 1 Correlation between adenoma size and serum prolactin (PRL) level in 77 prolactinomas

	♂	♀	total	PRL	(mean)
micro	1	44	45	83~1460	(327)
macro	1	17	18	133~2970	(1104)
large	11	3	14	1300~8600	(3760)

recognition of tumour tissues, and with the finer resection technique, remarkable improvement was noted in the second series of 50 cases treated for the last 5 years. Of 38 cases whose PRL were below 1000 ng/ml (83 to 954, mean 305) 34 patients (90%) had normal postoperative PRL value (fig. 5). One of 12 cases with higher PRL levels over 1000 ng/ml gained the endocrinological cure (fig. 6).

In 58 female patients aged below 40 years (22 to 38 years, mean age = 30) who were determined to be of childbearing age, 47 (81%) gained the ovulatory menses

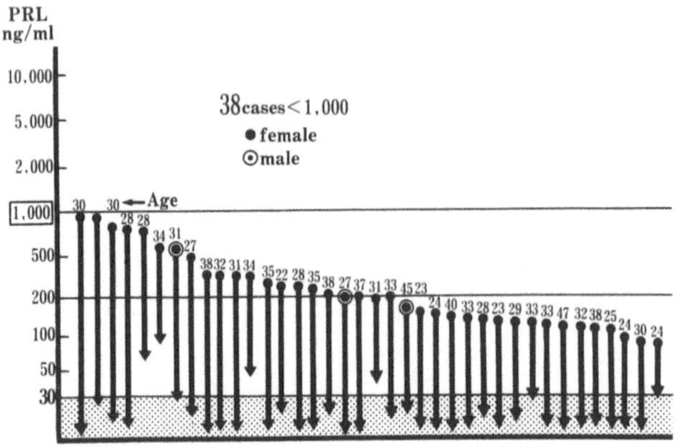

Fig. 5 Operative results in the second 5 years' series. In 38 cases with PRL levels below 1000 ng/ml, 34 (90%) showed normalization of PRL below 30 ng/ml.

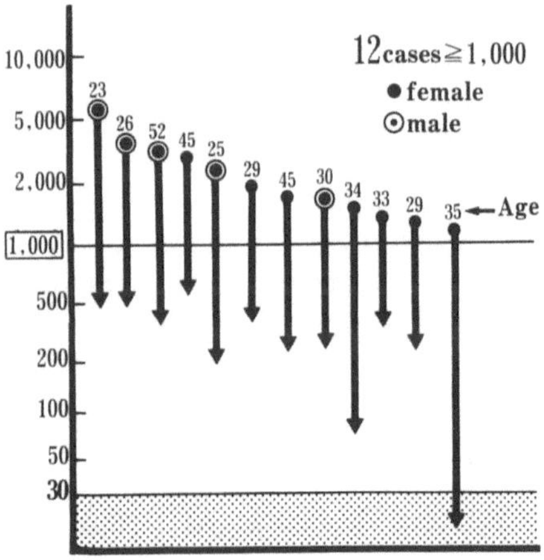

Fig. 6 Operative results in the second 5 years' series. In 12 patients with PRL values over 1000 ng/ml, one case gained the endocrinological cure with restoration of menstrual cycle.

after surgery: 26 (45%) by surgery alone, 12 by surgery und supplementary bromocriptine and 9 by the combination of surgery plus radiation or bromocriptine with or without addition of Clomid, HCG-HMG (tab. 2). Fourty patients wanted fertility and up to the present time, 27 became pregnant and 24 (60%) delivered.

Regarding operative complications, we have encountered neither mortality nor any serious morbidity. There were 5 cases with minor complications: one case of CSF-rhinorrhea with meningitis, another case with postoperative nasal musocal bleeding that was controlled by reoperation, and 3 patients showed postoperative hypopituitarism. Prolonged diabetes insipidus was noted in 2 of 3 cases with hypopituitarism (tab. 3).

Table 2 Restoration of ovulatory menses (47 cases = 81%) and achievement of pregnancies in 58 female patients with prolactinoma in the childbearing age

	micro	macro	total
Op. only	23	3	26
Op. + CB	6	6	12
Op. + CB + Clo	1	1	2
Op. + CB + HMG	1	0	1
Op. + Rad. + CB	1	2	3
Op. + Rad. + HMG	2	1	3

Pregnant 27 (delivery 24)

Table 3 Operative complications in a series of 77 prolactinomas

Mortality	0
Morbidity (minor)	5 cases (6.5%)
CSF-leak and meningitis	1
nasal mucosal trouble	1
postop. hypopituitarism	1
hypopit. + prolonged DI	2

Discussion

Our results clearly indicate that the transsphenoidal microsurgery is safe, accurate and beneficial. In recent years, even in giant adenomas, we approach the tumour first with the transsphenoidal route. Considering the fact that we have been treating patients with rather long history of symptoms and with much higher PRL levels, our operative results are to be judged as excellent. A number of reports have been published regarding the results of transsphenoidal microsurgery for prolactinomas [1, 5, 9, 10, 19, 24, 40, 43]. The success rate for postoperative normalization of PRL level has been diverse from one report to another in 40 to 70% range. The wide differences in operative results have been shown to be due to tumour size, patients' age and symptom duration [10, 28, 29, 30, 33, 34]. Nelson et al. [28] demonstrated that the patients who were below 26 years of age and had symptom duration shorter than 6 years and whose PRL levels below or around 200 ng/ml had significantly better surgical outcomes. With our current operative technique (see fig. 3, radical selective resection), patients with PRL levels below 1000 ng/ml can be cured in 90% confidence.

Recently, Serri et al. [35] reported a paper on the postoperative recurrence of hyperprolactinaemia. They described 85% initial success in microadenomas and 31% in macroadenomas. According to their follow-up study (range, 5 to 10 years), recurrent hyperprolactinaemia was noted in 50% of the cases with microadenoma and in 90% of the patients with macroadenoma. We have seen slightly elevated PRL values in 40 to 50 ng/ml range in several patients at follow-up, however, we have not yet experienced any real recurrence in cured patients for the past 7 years. During the past decade, medical management with bromocriptine has been a great appeal and used extensively to treat patients harbouring prolactinomas [16, 30, 32, 38, 39]. Although this drug normalizes hyperprolactinaemia in a majority of cases with prolactinoma and in fact reduces the tumour size in many patients [6, 14, 15, 17, 21, 25, 26, 36, 38], it can never be the curative treatment. A significant number of patients are unable to take the drug in therapeutic dosis due to side effects. Any possible harm by long-term administration has not yet been fully scrutinized [31]. Our experience with bromocriptine disclosed the development of tolerance in some cases, particularly in patients who did not take the medicine on regular basis (unpublished data). In fact, it is not practical nor easy for patients to visit hospital and to take medicine regularly life-long. Landolt [22] published a paper entitled "Bromocriptine, does it jeopardise the result of later surgery for prolactinomas". He stated at the 4th Workshop on pituitary tumours held in February, 1984 in Japan that the intraadenomatous fibrosis causes a rubber-like consistency of the adenomas which are more difficult to remove in this stage because they adhere more to the surrounding normal tissue [23]. This has been also our experience and we are confident that the preoperative manipulation with bromocriptine makes the clean total resection of prolactinoma very difficult. We have found that the adenoma tissue became degenerated, shrunk and sticky to the adjacent normal pituitary structures. The pituitary adenoma is, although slowly growing, essentially a neoplasm and a significant number of adenomas, especially prolactinomas, behave invasively. The risk of pituitary apoplexy during the conservative treatment has been estimated as 10 to 15% [42, 44]. Another risk of rapid tumour growth in pregnancy or higher incidence of abortion is not insignificant [7, 8, 20, 27, 41]. Our principle in treating prolactinomas is illustrated in figure 7. A patient with amenorrhoea and/or galactorrhoea whose PRL level constantly exceeds 80 ng/ml without other evidence for hyperprolactinaemia should be explored surgically. If any case, usually the patient with high PRL level, presents residual elevated PRL value after surgery, then, bromocriptine can help the patient in much smaller dosis than that needed without surgery. In conclusion, we strongly emphasize the importance of transsphenoidal microsurgical radical-selective resection as the primary management of prolactinomas since the surgery in experienced hands offers high chance of one-time cure with negligible risk.

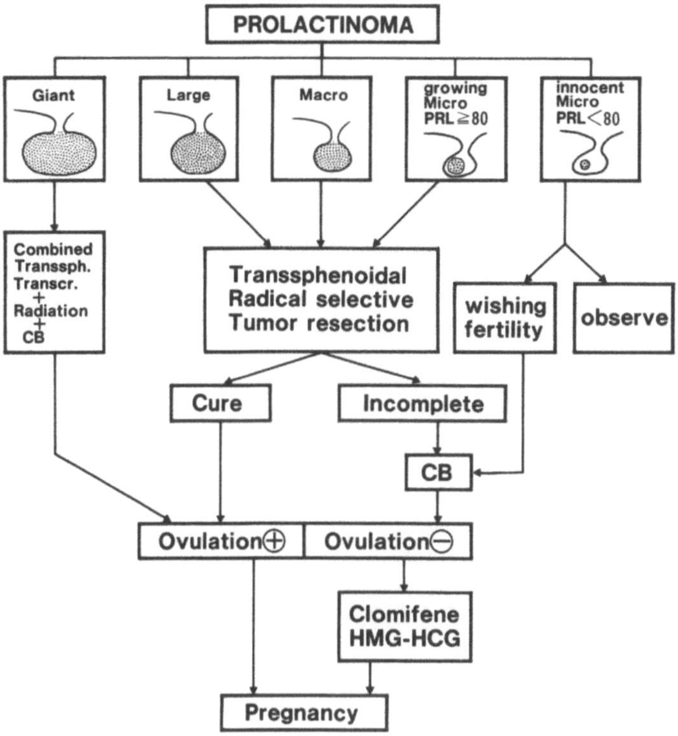

Fig. 7 Management flow chart for prolactinomas in the author's institutes. The principle is 'surgery first' policy. The possible tiny microadenomas with PRL levels below 80 ng/ml are arbitrarily designated as 'innocent micro'.

References

[1] Aubourg, P. R., P. J. Derome, F. Peillon, et al.: Endocrine outcome after transsphenoidal adenomectomy for prolactinoma: Prolactin levels and tumour size as predicting factors. Surg. Neurol. **14** (1980) 141–143.

[2] Baskin, D., C. B. Wilson: Bromocriptine treatment of pituitary adenomas. Neurosurgery, **8** (1981) 741–744.

[3] Besser, G. M., L. Parke, C. R. W. Edwards, et al.: Galactorrhea: Successful treatment with reduction of plasma prolactin levels by bromergocryptine. Br. Med. J. **3** (1972) 669–672.

[4] Bucy, P. C.: Special article, Bromocriptine. Surg. Neurol. **13** (1980) 81–83.

[5] Chang, R. J., W. R. Keye Jr., J. R. Young, et al.: Detection, evaluation, and treatment of pituitary microadenomas in patients with galactorrhea and amenorrhea. Am. J. Obstet. Gynecol. **128** (1977) 356–363.

[6] Corenblum, B., B. R. Webster, C. B. Mortimer, et al.: Possible anti-tumor effect of 2 bromoergocriptine (CB-154, Sandoz) in 2 patients with large prolactin-secreting pituitary adenomas. Clin. Res. **23** (1975) 614A.

[7] Dietemann, J. L., C. Portha, F. Cattin, et. al.: CT follow-up of microprolactinomas during bromocriptine-induced pregnancy. Neuroradiology **25** (1983) 133–138.

[8] Divers, W. A., S. S. C. Yen: Prolactin-producing microadenomas in pregnancy. Obstet. Gynecol. **62** (1983) 425–429.

[9] Domingue, J. N., I. L. Richmond, C. B. Wilson: Results of surgery in 114 patients with prolactin-secreting pituitary adenomas. Am. J. Obstet. Gynecol. **137** (1980) 102–108.

[10] Faria, M. A. Jr., G. T. Tindall: Transsphenoidal microsurgery for prolactin-secreting pituitary adenomas. J. Neurosurg. **56** (1982) 33–43.

[11] Fukushima, T., K. Sano: Sublabial rhinoseptoplastic technique for transsphenoidal pituitary surgery by a hinged-septum method. Technical note. J. Neurosurg. **52** (1980) 867–870.

[12] Fukushima, T., K. Takakura, K. Sano: Results of transsphenoidal microsurgery for hyperfunctioning pituitary adenomas: subcapsular removal versus radical excision. 7th International Congress of Neurological Surgery, July 1981, Munich.

[13] Fukushima, T., A. Teramoto, K. Takakura, et al.: Surgical treatment of prolactin-producing pituitary adenomas. Proceedings of the 2nd Workshop on Pituitary Tumors **2**, 65–83, Tokyo 1981.

[14] Goorge, S. R., G. N. Burrow, B. Zinman, et al.: Regression of pituitary tumors, a possible effect of bromoergocriptine. A. J. Med. **66** (1979)697–702.

[15] Gonzalez, E. R.: Update: Pituitary tumor regression with bromocriptine therapy. JAMA **244** (1980) 1535–1536.

[16] Gonzalez, E. R.: To treat or not to treat: Hyperprolactinaemia. JAMA **248** (1982) 513–514.

[17] Hancock, K. W., J. S. Scott, J. T. Lamb, et al.: Conservative management of pituitary prolactinomas; evidence for bromocriptine-induced regression. Br. J. Obstet. Gynaecol. **87** (1980) 523–529.

[18] Hardy, J., S. M. Wigser: Transsphenoidal surgery of pituitary fossa tumors with televised radiofluoroscopic control. J. Neurosurg. **23** (1965) 612–619.

[19] Hardy, J., H. Beauregard, F. Robert: Prolactin-secreting pituitary adenomas: transsphenoidal microsurgical treatment. In: Progress in Prolactin, Physiology and Pathology (C. Robyn, M. Harter, eds.), pp. 361–370. Elsevier North-Holland Biomedical Press, Amsterdam–New York 1978.

[20] Lamberts, S. W. J., H. J. Seldenrath, H. G. Kwa, et al.: Transient bitemporal hemianopsia during pregnancy after treatment of galactorrhea-amenorrhea syndrome with bromocriptine. J. clin. Endocr. **44** (1977) 180–184.

[21] Landolt, A. M., R. Wuthrich, H. Fellmann: Regression of pituitary prolactinoma after treatment with bromocriptione. Lancet **1** (1979) 1082–1083.

[22] Landolt, A. M., P. J. Keller, E. R. Froesch, et al.: Bromocriptine: does it jeopardise the result of later surgery for prolactinomas? Lancet **2** (1982) 657–658.

[23] Landolt, A. M.: Prolactinomas, structure, ultrastructure and bromocriptine-induced changes. Proceedings of the 4th Workshop on Pituitary Tumors, Osaka 1984 (in press).

[24] Laws, E. R., N. C. Fode, R. V. Randall, et al.: Pregnancy following transsphenoidal resection of prolactin-secreting tumors. J. Neurosurg. **58** (1983) 685–688.

[25] McGregor, A. M., M. F. Scanlon, K. Hall, et al.: Reduction in size of a pituitary tumor by bromocriptine therapy. N. Engl. J. Med. **300** (1979) 291–293.

[26] McGregor, A. M., M. F. Scanlon, R. Hall, et al.: Effects of bromocriptine on pituitary tumour size. Br. Med. J. **2** (1979) 700–703.

[27] Nelson, P. B., A. G. Robinson, D. F. Archer, et al.: Symptomatic pituitary tumor enlargement after induced pregnancy. Case report. J. Neurosurg. **49** (1978) 283–287.

[28] Nelson, P. B., M. Goodman, J. C. Maroon, et al.: Factors in predicting outcome from operation in patients with prolactin-secreting pituitary adenomas. Neurosurgery **13** (1983) 634–641.

[29] Rawe, S. E., H. O. Williamson, J. H. Levine, et al.: Prolactinomas: surgical therapy, indications and results. Surg. Neurol. **14** (1980) 161–167.

[30] Reichlin, S.: The prolactinoma problem. N. Engl. J. Med. **300**; 313–315, 1979.

[31] Rinne, U. K.: Pleuropulmonary changes during long-term bromocriptine treatment for Parkinson's disease. Lancet, No. 8210 (Jan. 1981) 44.

[32] Robinson, A. G., P. B. Nelson: Prolactinomas in women, current therapies. Ann Int. Med. **99** (1983) 115–118.

[33] Schlechte, J., B. Sherman, N. Halmi, et al.: Prolactin-secreting pituitary tumors in amenorrheic women: A comprehensive study. Endocr Rev. **1** (1980) 295–308.

[34] Schlechte, J., J. van Gilder, B. Sherman: Predictors of the outcome of transsphenoidal surgery for prolactin-secreting pituitary adenomas. J. Clin. Endocrinol. Metab. **52** (1981) 785–789.

[35] Serri, O., E. Rasio, H. Beauregard, et al.: Recurrence of hyperprolactinemia after selective transsphenoidal adenomectomy in women with prolactinoma. New Engl. J. Med. **309** (1983) 280–283.

[36] Sobrinbo, L. G., M. C. P. Nunes, M. A. Santos, et al.: Radiologic evidence for regression of prolactinoma after treatment with bromocriptine. Lancet (July 1978) 257–258.

[37] Thorner, M. O., G. M. Besser, A. Jones, et al.: Bromocriptine therapy of female infertility – A report of 13 pregnancies. Br. Med. J. **4** (1975) 694–697.

[38] Thorner, M. O., W. H. Martin, A. D. Rogol, et al.: Rapid regression of pituitary prolactinomas during bromocriptine treatment. J. Clin. Endocrinol. Metab. **51** (1980) 438–445.

[39] Thorner, M. O., R. L. Perryman, A. D. Rogol, et al.: Rapid changes of prolactinoma volume after withdrawal and reinstitution of bromocriptine. J. Clin. Endocrinol. Metab. **53** (1981) 480–483.

[40] Tindall, G. T., C. S. McLanahan, J. H. Christy: Transsphenoidal microsurgery for pituitary tumors associated with hyperprolactinemia. J. Neurosurg. **48** (1978) 849–860.

[41] Dalen, J. T. W. van, E. L. Greve: Rapid deterioration of visual fields during bromocriptine-induced pregnancy in a patient with a pituitary adenoma. Br. J. Ophthalmol. **61** (1977) 729–733.

[42] Wakai, S., T. Fukushima, A. Teramoto, et al.: Pituitary apoplexy: its incidence and clinical significance. J. Neurosurg. **55** (1981) 187–193.

[43] Weiss, M. H.: Medical and surgical management of functional pituitary tumors. Clin. Neurosurg. **28** (1981) 374–383.

[44] Yamaji, T., M. Ishibashi, K. Kosaka, et al.: Pituitary apoplexy in acromegaly during bromocriptine therapy. Acta Endocrinol. **98** (1981) 171–177.

Review of 56 prolactin-secreting pituitary adenomas

M. Pérez-Alvarez, J. M. Roda, F. Alvarez, J. Ordás, A. Cerdán, J. M. Alfonso

Introduction

Prolactin secreting pituitary adenomas have become the most frequent tumours of the hypophysis due to advances in the methods of radioimmunoassay and neuroradiological techniques. The authors present the results of transsphenoidal microsurgery in pituitary adenomas associated with hyperprolactinaemia operated in our neurosurgical department of the "Ciudad Sanitaria La Paz" of Madrid.

Material

Between the end of 1977 and December 1983 we have operated on 56 prolactin adenomas, this representing 52.3% of the total number of pituitary adenomas. The patients were admitted to the Departments of Gynecology and Endocrinology in our hospital. Fifty two cases were females whose ages ranged between 19 and 38 years, with an average of 26.2 years. Four of the patients treated were men with ages of 22, 32, 36, and 56 years respectively. 92% of the women presented with galactorrhoea and all of them amenorrhoea and anovulatory cycles. We observed partial loss of visual acuity and other visual disturbances in 8.8% of the cases. In two cases a complete bitemporal hemianopsia was found. The clinical presentation in 3 men was impotence and sterility.

Classification of the tumours

We have classified our series according to the radiological criteria suggested by Vezina and Sutton in 1974 [18]. We found two cases harbouring a grade 0 sella tumour, 17 cases a grade I, 31 cases a grade II, 5 a grade III, and 1 a grade IV tumour.

Endocrine evaluation

Determinations of the levels of serum prolactin (PRL) pre and post operatively were performed within a formal protocol of testing for pituitary function. We have related the radiological grade of tumour to the preoperative PRL levels. In the two grade 0 cases the PRL levels were 47 and 97 ng/ml respectively. The PRL levels of grade I tumours ranged between 32 and 165 ng/ml; the 31 grade II cases ranged between 65 and 1776 ng/ml; 5 grade III cases had PRL levels between 132 and 528 ng/ml and in the single grade IV tumour of our series the PRL level before operation was 5800 ng/ml.

Table 1

Radiological grade	No. of cases	Range of PRL-level	Prolactin normal Postop. N = 20 ng/ml	
			No.	Percentage
Grade 0	2	47–97	2	–
Grade I	17	32–165	14	82.3
Grade II	31	65–1766	13	41.9
Grade III	5	200–528	1	20.0
Grade IV	1	5880	0	–

Neuroradiology

All patients were studied with hypocycloidal polytomography. Since the computer-tomograph (CT) in our hospital is of the older generation, selective pneumoencephalography with tomography and cisternography either with air or metrizamide was also performed in the majority of our patients.

Surgical technique: All cases in this series were operated on by the rhinoseptal transsphenoidal approach.

Results

Clinical function: Menses resumed in 74% of women whose preoperative PRL levels were less than 200 ng/ml. In those women who wished to become pregnant the percentage of pregnancy was 66.6%. Of this percentage half of the pregnancies were achieved just by surgery and in the other half the pregnancies were reached by the combination of surgery and bromocriptine. Visual anomalies improved in all cases except in the two patients who presented with a complete bitemporal hemianopsia before operation.

Endocrine function: In no case did we observe alteration of the functional hypophysary reserve after surgery nor did any case improve significantly if the reserve was altered before surgery. The results of surgery were closely related to the preoperative PRL levels. In table 1 the radiological grade of sella tumours and the preoperative PRL levels are related to the normalization of post-operative PRL levels. A prognosis of normalization of PRL levels after surgery can be presumed in accordance with the preoperative PRL levels. Thus, those cases in which the preoperative PRL levels were less than 200 ng/ml reached normalization after surgery of PRL levels in 80.6% of the cases, whereas only 40% of those cases with preoperative PRL levels greater than 200 ng/ml achieved normal PRL values.

Complications

There was no mortality following 56 transsphenoidal operations for a pituitary adenoma. One of the most frequent postoperative complications we encountered was transient diabetes insipidus which appeared in 15 cases (26.7%) and normally disappeared after treatment with carbamazepine. Never was the diabetes insipidus permanent. Six patients presented with CSF leakage which appeared during surgery. Their condition was resolved through postural treatment and acetazolamide. Only one case required continuous lumbar drainage for a period of four days. Two patients have been reoperated. Both were women with grade II sella tumours who neither reached normal PRL valuers after surgery nor responded to bromocriptine. Tumoral remnants were excised during reoperation.

Discussion

As has been previously suggested in different series in the literature, there is a close relationship between the sellar size and the preoperative PRL levels, so that the larger the size of the sella turcica the higher the preoperative PRL levels [9, 10, 12, 17]. This fact is also true in our series. In grade 0 pituitary tumours the upper level of PRL was 97 ng/ml and in grade I was 165 ng/ml. In grade II tumours the preoperative PRL levels depended on whether or not there was suprasellar extension of the tumour. In those cases the levels varied from 370 ng/ml in those patients with exclusively intrasellar tumours to 1776 ng/ml in the other cases with suprasellar growth. There were closer variations in grade III tumours although the minimal level encountered was 200 ng/ml. It is interesting to note that the highest preoperative PRL level found in this group did not exceed that of those tumours with suprasellar extension and a grade II sella. According to these data one might postulate a possible relation between the existence of high PRL levels and a pituitary stalk impairment due to the suprasellar growth.

The return to normal values of PRL after surgery is closely related to the size of the tumour. Thus, in microadenomas the normalization of PRL levels was achieved in 84% of the cases, whereas in macroadenomas this figure decreased to 38%. These findings agree with those published by other authors [1, 4, 10, 12, 17]. The preoperative PRL levels are also in close relationship with the normalization of PRL levels following the operation [1, 8, 10, 12, 17]. In our series when PRL levels were less than 200 ng/ml the normalization after surgery was achieved in 80.6% of the cases whereas only 40% of them reached PRL normal values when the preoperative levels were greater than 200 ng/ml. The elevation of PRL levels after surgery has been explained by a mechanism of interference in the normal delivery of prolactin inhibitory factor due either to pituitary stalk impairment, consequence of tumoral growth or surgical action, or to the persistence of remnants of tumour [13]. In those cases periodical controls of PRL levels will be the best diagnostic method to clarify the mechanism in each particular case.

All the patients in our series have been operated on by the transsphenoidal approach with no mortality and scanty morbidity. This fact is in accordance with other publications [1, 7, 8, 10, 12, 17]. This approach is not only indicated in intrasellar tumours but also should be performed in all those cases with suprasellar growth, circumscribing the extraarachnoid space. A mixed transsphenoidal and transcranial approach would be the surgical treatment of choice in those tumours with asymmetrical extrasellar growth [5].

There is controversy in the literature about the treatment of these tumours with radiotherapy. Primary treatment of prolactinomas with conventional external radiotherapy seems to be effective for a short time, and is accompanied by slight or no modifications in PRL levels. Neither is the size of the pituitary tumour altered [15]. The results of interstitial irradiation are discouraging as well. Therefore, the main role for radiotherapy at the present time is on the basis of being an effective adjunct of surgery in some cases. Postoperative external irradiation may be considered in all those cases with pituitary tumours larger than 10 mm of diameter, with partial excision or invasive characteristics. Some authors consider that postoperative external radiotherapy of the pituitary gland is more important in relation to recurrences, than the total removal of the tumour [5, 6]. On the other hand, some others do not find a clear remission of the tumoral size or normalization of PRL levels after the administration of postoperative radiotherapy [3, 11]. In our series 6 patients received postoperative radiation therapy in an attempt to prevent recurrences and up to now none of them has presented with a recurrence.

Bromocriptine as the primary treatment in prolactinomas is controversial [2, 14, 16]. Barrow et al. [2] suggest that preoperative treatment with bromocriptine makes the surgical excision easier, while other authors do not advise it, since it causes the disappearance of the natural plane of cleavage of the tumour even earlier [5, 14].

Conclusions

We advocate combined treatment bromocriptine and surgery. This is because 64% of our patients were taking bromocriptine before surgery and those in whom surgical results were not favorable continued taking bromocriptine. We disapprove of radiotherapy except in cases of macroadenoma which could not be treated successfully either by surgery or with bromocriptine and which showed an important degree of hypophysary reserve disturbance before surgery. Radiotherapy is always necessary in grade IV tumours.

In small tumours which were not satisfactorily removed after the first operation and were unresponse to bromocriptine we suggest reoperation. If the patient does not wish to bare children and suffer a tumour grade 0 or I and does not specifically desire surgery we would suggest the use of bromocriptine. If the patient wants to be pregnant, while harbouring a sella tumour of grades II, III or IV there is no alternative but surgery.

References

[1] Aubourg, P. R., P. J. Derome, F. Peillon, et al.: Endocrine outcome after transsphenoidal adenomectomy for prolactinoma: prolactin levels and tumor size as predicting factors. Surg. Neurol. **14** (1980) 141–143.

[2] Barrow, D. L., G. T. Tindall, K. K. Kovacs, et al.: Clinical and pathological effects of bromocriptine on prolactin-secreting and other pituitary tumors. J. Neurosurg. **60** (1984) 1–7.

[3] Carter, J. N., J. E. Tyson, G. Tolis, et al.: Prolactin-secreting tumors and hypogonadism in 22 men. N. Engl. J. Med. **299** (1978) 840–852.

[4] Chang, R. J., W. R. Keye Jr., J. R. Young, et al.: Detection, evaluation and treatment of pituitary microadenomas in patients with galactorrhea and amenorrhea. Am. J. Obstet. Gynecol. **128** (1977) 356–363.

[5] Ciric, I., M. Mikhael, T. Stafford, et al.: Transsphenoidal microsurgery of pituitary macroadenomas with long-term follow-up results. J. Neurosurg. **59** (1983) 395–401

[6] Collins, W. F.: Pituitary tumor management: an overwiev. In: Clinical Management of Pituitary Disorders (G. T. Tindall, W. F. Collins, eds), pp. 179–186. Raven Press, New York 1979.

[7] Derome, P. J., F. Peillon, R. H. Bard, et al.: Adénomas a prolactine: résultats du traitement chirurgical. 120 cas féminins, 30 cas masculins. Nouv. Presse Med. **8** (1979) 577–583.

[8] Domingue, J. N., IL. L. Richmond, B. B. Wilson: Results of surgery in 114 patients with prolactin-secreting pituitary adenomas. Am. J. Obstet. Gynecol. **137** (1980) 102–108.

[9] Fahlbusch, R.: Surgical failures in prolactinomas. In: Pituitary Adenomas. Biology, Physiopathology and Treatment (P. J. Derome, C. P. Jedynak, F. Peillon, eds.), pp. 273–284. Asclepios France, Paris 1980.

[10] Faria, M. A. Jr., G. T. Tindall: Transsphenoidal microsurgery for prolactin-secreting pituitary adenomas. Results in 100 women with the amenorrhea-galactorrhea syndrome. J. Neurosurg. **56** (1982) 33–43.

[11] Grisoli, F., F. Vincentelli, P. Jaquet, et al.: Prolactin secreting adenoma in 22 men. Surg. Neurol. **13** (1980) 241–247.
[12] Hardy, J., H. Beauregard, F. Robert: Prolactin secreting Pituitary Adenomas: Transsphenoidal Microsurgical Treatment. Clin. Neurosurg. **27** (1980) 38–47.
[13] Kleinberg, D. L., G. L. Noel, A. G. Frantz: Galactorrhea a study of 235 cases including 48 with pituitary tumors. N. Engl. J. Med. **296** (1977) 589–600.
[14] Landolt, A. M., P. J. Keller, E. R. Froesch, et al.: Bromocriptine does it jeopardise the result of later surgery for prolactinomas? Lancet **2** (1982) 657–658.
[15] Nabarro, J. D. N.: Pituitary Prolactinomas. Clin. Endocrinol. 17, 129–155 (1982).
[16] Thorner, M. O., R. L. Perryman, A. D. Rogol, et al.: Rapid changes of prolactinoma volume after withdrawal and reinstitution of bromocriptine. J. Clin. Endocrinol. Metab. **53** (1981) 480–483.
[17] Tindall, G. T., S. Mc Lanahan, J. H. Christy: Transsphenoidal microsurgery for pituitary tumors associated with hyperprolactinemia. J. Neurosurg. **48** (1978) 849–860.
[18] Vezina, J. L., T. J. Sutton: Prolactin secreting pituitary microadenomas. Roentgenologic diagnosis. A. J. R. **120** (1974) 46–54.

The effect of transsphenoidal selective microadenomectomy on patients with prolactinomas

E. Bosadjieva, L. Karagiozov, A. Kechaiov, M. Andreeva, E. Platonova, K. Karagiozov, Tch. Georgiev, G. Kirilov

Introduction

The syndrome of galactorrhea and amenorrhea is more frequently encountered than was believed some years ago. D. Kleinberg et al. [4] established that in a group of 235 patients with galactorrhea, 42 female and 6 male patients (20%) were with radiological evidence for pituitary tumours. According to K. Post [5] prolactinoma is the most common pituitary tumour representing 30—70% of all hypophyseal tumours. It is well known that "if the tumour is large with neurological deficits, surgery is mandatory. The issue, however, is more complex for smaller tumours, particularly microadenomas" [3]. K. Post [5] also states that "Functional tumours secreting ACTH, GH or TSH are always considered candidates for surgery, while there is still some question regarding prolactin-secreting microadenomas".

Material and methods

Twenty-eight patients with prolactinomas underwent transsphenoidal selective adenomectomy at the Clinic of Neurosurgery in Sofia between the beginning of 1978 and the middle of 1983. The diagnosis prolactinoma was based on radiological examination, hyperprolactinemia, galactorrhea and gonadal disturbances.

The group consisted of 24 female patients, aged from 19 to 43, mean age 34 years and 4 male patients, aged from 20 to 36, mean age 29.3 years. Fourty-three percent of all the patients had microadenomas – 11 female patients aged from 18 to 39, mean age 31.2 years, and one male, 34 years old.

Sixteen patients (57%), 13 female aged from 19 to 43, mean age 29 years, and 3 male, aged 20, 27 and 36, mean age 27.7 years, had larger tumours. The female patients sought medical consultation at the Clinic of Endocrinology for the amenorrhoea-galactorrhoae syndrome or infertility and the male patients, for impotence.

Galactorrhoea was not present only in one female and in one male patient. The same technique was used and the same surgeon performed all the operations. Empty sella was found in 4 female patients who were not included in this series. In six patients prolactinoma was associated with polycystic ovarian disease, surgically proved. Along with the serum levels of the pituitary hormones, the functions of the thyroid gland, the adrenal cortex and the gonads were examined in all patients.

The results were evaluated as "good" (cured) in cases of normalisation of the gonadal function and prolactinaemia, as "transient" in cases of recurrence and "without effect" (no change).

Results

A "good" effect was established in 9 patients – 7 female aged from 24 to 41, mean age 36.3 years and in 2 male patients aged 34 and 36, mean age 35 years (tab. 1). The mean age of this group (patients with a post-operative "good" effect) was 36 years (from 24 to 41 years).

In 4 of these patients the size of the pituitary fossa was normal or in the upper limit of normal and in the other five it was slightly enlarged. The tumours were examined histologically in 6 cases. Two of them were chromophobic adenomas, 2 mixed chromophobic and acidophilic (eosinophilic) and 2 – mixed chromophobic and basophilic adenomas (tab. 2). Transient diabetes insipidus developed in one patient (11.1%) and permanent diabetes insipidus in another (11.1%). No other complications were observed (tab. 3). The specialized sensitivity was examined in 4 patients. In 2 of these evidence of central otoneurological syndrome (50%) was found. No changes were established in two patients.

Eighteen patients – 16 female, aged from 19 to 38, mean age 28 years and 2 male patients, 36 and 20 years old, mean age 28 years, were not affected by treatment (tab. 1). In 6 patients the pituitary fossa was normal or in the upper limits of normal. In the other 12 patients, the pituitary fossa was enlarged. The tumours were histologically examined in 15 patients. Chromophobic adenoma was found in 9 patients, mixed-chromophobic and acidophilic adenoma in 5 and in one patient the material sent for examination represented neurohypophyseal tissue only (tab. 2).

The specialized sensitivity was examined in 11 patients. In 9 of these evidence of central otoneurological syndrome (81.8%) was found. No changes were established in 2 patients only (tab. 2).

No improvement was ascertained in the patients with prolactinoma associated with polycystic ovarian disease (tab. 4). These patients were aged from 19 to 38 years, mean age 27 years. The pituitary fossa of 4 of these was of normal size or in the upper limits of normal and enlarged in two. In 2 patients postoperative diabetes insipidus developed (33.3%).

Table 1 Results of treatment according to the patients age and the duration of disease history

Results of treatment	Females			Males			Total group of patients		
	Number of patients	Mean age (years)	Mean duration of disease (years)	Number of patients	Mean age (years)	Mean duration of diseases (years)	Number of patients	Mean age (years)	Mean duration of disease (years)
Good (Cured)	7	36.3 (24–41)	7.1 (1–12)	2	35 (34–36)	5.75 (1.5–10)	9	36 (24–43)	6.8 (1–12)
Transient	1	25	6				1	25	6
No change	16	28.4 (19–38)	3.9 (0.25–8)	2	28 (20–36)	7.5 (5–10)	18	29.3 (19–38)	4.3 (0.25–10)

Table 2 Results of treatment according to the fossa size and to the otoneurological distrubances

	Total group of patients			Fossa size		Otoneurological syndrome				Histology of the adenoma			
Results of treatment	Number of patients	Percent	Mean age	Normal	Slightly enlarged	Normal	Central	Peri-pheral	Combi-ned	Chromo-phobic	Acido-philic	Chromo-phobic Acido-philic	Chromo-phobic + Basophilic
Good	9	32.1%	36	4 (44.4%)	5 (55.6%)	1 (25%)	2 (50%)	1 (25%)		2 (33.3%)		2 (33.3%)	2 (33.3%)
Transient	1	3.6	25	1		1				1			
No change	18	64.3	28.3	6 (33.3%)	12	2 (18.2%)	9 (81.8%)			9 (64.3%)		5 (35.7%)	

Table 3 Postoperative complications

Effect of treatment	Diabetes insipidus					
	Transient		Permanent		Total number (frequency)	
Good	1/9	11.1%	1/9	11.1%	2/9	22.2%
Transient						
No change	1/18	5.67%	5/18	27.7%	6/18	33.4%

The specialised sensitivity was examined in 3 patients and in all 3 there was found a central otoneurological syndrome. The tumours were examined histologically in 5 patients. Chromophobic adenoma was established in 2 patients, in one of whom there was cell-atypism. Two patients had mixed adenoma – chromophobic and acidophylic and the material of one patient sent for examination contained only neurohypophyseal tissue.

In this subgroup of patients the following complications were observed: 4 patients with permanent diabetes insipidus, in 2 of whom it was associated with arachnoiditis, one patient with arachnoiditis only and one with CSF rhinorrhoea and fistula. We treated the patients who showed no effect with bromocriptine.

The effect of treatment in one patient was estimated as transient. The size of the pituitary fossa in this case was normal. Histologically the tumour was a chromophobic adenoma with areas of acidophilic cells. Electronmicroscopical examination revealed lactotropic cells. After the removal of the tumour the patient had a normal pregnancy, but later galactorrhoea and amenorrhoea reappeared.

The thyroid and adrenal functions before and after the tumour removals were normal and this proves that the adenomectomy was really selective.

In the overall group of patients with prolactinomas, the incidence of postsurgical diabetes insipidus was 21.4% (6 patients). In the subgroup of the patients without treatment effect it was 27.7% and in the subgroup of patients with "good" effect it was 11%. In 4 of the patients with diabetes insipidus the tumours were small ones (microadenomas) (tab. 3).

Comments

In the series reported by G. Bertrand and G. Tolis [1] of 36 female and 5 male patients with prolactinomas there was no mortality, no serious morbidity and a success rate of 90% for small, not previously operated on tumours. The results of our

Table 4 Results of transsphenoidal adenomectomy in patients with prolactinomas associated with polycystic ovarian disease

				Plasma prolactin level (IU/l)			Otoneurological syndrome			Histology of the adenoma		
Effect of treatment	Number of patients	Mean age (years)	Mean duration of the disease (years)	Before the operation	After the operation	Normal	Central	Periphe-ral	Combi-ned	Chromo-phobic	Chromo-phobic + acidophilic	Neuro-hypo-physis
Good												
Transient												
No change	6	27 (19–38)	5.1 (1.5–12)	3080.7 ±1303.9	3931.4 ±1771.0		3			2	2	1

study do not compare favorably with these data. We established that the effect of transsphenoidal selective adenomectomy in patients with microprolactinomas is not better than the effect in patients with larger prolactinomas. According to our data, the patients' age is a very important factor (tab. 1). In younger patients the disease has a more severe course and the surgical treatment is more often without effect.

The effect of transsphenoidal adenomectomy in patients with active acromegaly is dependant for the most part on the tumour size. An otoneurological study of 26 patients with active acromegaly demonstrated a correlation between the frequency of the central otoneurological syndrome and the tumour size (tab. 5). The results of our study in patients with prolactinomas established a greater rate of frequency of the central otoneurological syndrome in patients without treatment effect, notwithstanding the size of the tumour (tab. 6). In patients with a central otoneurological syndrome the fila olfactoria, the vestibular, the auditory and the gustatory analysers are more often damaged. The audiometric curves show a retrolabyrinthic direction. The results of our study show that the disturbances are localized most often in the subtentorial structures.

Table 5 Frequency of the central otoneurological syndrome in patients with active acromegaly according to the size of the pituitary fossa

Size of pituitary fossa	Number of patients who were studied	Number of patients with central otoneurological syndrome
Normal	4	1 (25%)
Slightly enlarged	8	7 (87.5%)
Strongly enlarged	14	14 (100%)

Table 6 Frequency of the central otoneurological syndrome in patients with prolactinomas according to treatment results

Results of treatment	Number of patients who were studied	Number of patients with central otoneurological syndrome
Cured	4	2 (50%)
No change	11	9 (82%)

The course of the disease is more severe and the surgical treatment is without effect also in the patients with prolactinomas associated with polycystic ovarian disease. According to G. Tucker and coworkers [6] a persistent defect in the regulation of prolactin secretion after successful pituitary tumour removal in women with the galactorrhoea-amenorrhoea syndrome suggests a hypothalamic defect. This suggestion is supported also by the high rate of disturbances of the specialized sensitivity in the patients in whom there was no treatment effect, some of whom had microadenomas, as well as the high rate of postoperative diabetes insipidus in patients with microprolactinomas which shows that in these cases the adenoma mass is not a factor. Our study also points to the very complex pathogenesis of the hyperprolactinaemia in patients with prolactinomas.

Most authors are of the opinion that surgery or irradiation, or both, are still indicated in most patients to relieve the mass effects of the adenoma and to prevent further tumour growth [2]. K. Post [5] stated that "with microadenomas the cure rate by selective adenomectomy is very high, the morbidity extremely low and mortality zero and that there is no evidence to date that radiation therapy is effective enough against prolactin-secreting tumours to consider radiation as the primary form of therapy". In a previous study we established that in patients with acromegaly, under the influence of conventional radiation therapy, the disturbances of the specialized sensitivity increased, proving that radiation therapy is damaging to brain tissue.

Although our results are not as good as the results of J. Bertrand and G. Tolis [1] we agree that selective adenomectomy is the treatment of choice for the microprolactinomas and that "it is logical to offer the patient a surgical exploration as soon as the diagnosis is established".

References

[1] Bertrand, G., G. Tolis et al.: Surgical treatment of prolactinomas. In: Clinical Endocrinology, pp. 449–453. Raven Press, New York 1979.

[2] Goodman, R. H., M. Molitch, K. Post, et al.: Prolactin-secreting adenomas in the males. In: The pituitary adenoma, 91–108. Plenum Med. Book Company, New York and London 1980.

[3] Hardy, J. et al.: Trans-sphenoidal microsurgical removal of pituitary adenoma. In: Progress in neurological surgery, p. 86. Excerpta Medica, Amsterdam 1974.

[4] Kleinberg, D. L., G. L. Noel, A. Frantz: Galactorrhea: A study of 235 cases, including 48 with pituitary tumours. N. Engl. J. Med. **296** (1977) 589–600.

[5] Post, K. D.: General considerations in the surgical treatment of pituitary tumours. In: The pituitary adenoma, pp. 341–363. Plenum Med. Book Company, New York and London 1980.

[6] Tucker, G. H., V. Lankford, F. Gardner, et al.: Persistent defect in regulation of prolactin secretion after succesful pituitary tumour removal in women with the galactorrhea-amenorrhea syndrome. J. Clin. Endocrinol. Metab. **51** (1980) 968–971.

Surgical results and long-term follow-up in female and male prolactinomas

L. M. Auer, G. Clarici, G. Leb, G. Tscherne, G. F. Walter, G. Schneider, W. Urdl, H. Warnkross, H. Höfler

Introduction

Ever since the introduction of microsurgical techniques and pharmacotherapeutic approach for the treatment of prolactin-producing pituitary adenomas, the indication for operation or medication or combination of therapeutic possibilities has been a matter of considerable debate. Transsphenoidal microsurgery for pituitary adenomas has been justifiably considered as a great improvement neurosurgery regarding the surgical risk, rate of recurrencies and cure of the clinical symptoms. The experience of several years has, however, shown that normalization of the clinical symptoms in patients with prolactinomas cannot be generally expected [2, 10, 16, 18, 26, 34, 38, 39, 42, 54, 58]. On the contrary, the rate of complete cure, probably depending on the selection of patients, was maximally in a range of 40 to 70%, and probably less in unselected patient groups. This gave rise to considerations of generally replacing surgery by medical treatment with bromocriptine in well defined groups of patients. However, definitions never became uniform until recently and some groups favour surgery for microadenomas [15, 21, 29, 38], others for macroadenomas [61]. Similarly, bromocriptine has been proposed mainly for microadenomas [56, 61] and large tumours [33, 52]. Especially in the light of recent reports about failure with bromocriptine treatment [6] of non-responding prolactinomas – preoperatively undistinguishable from responding tumours – one may suggest careful indication criteria and timing of surgery assessed with the help of experience so far available.

The aim of our patient study was to determine factors of importance in the indication for surgical treatment. Furthermore, to specify the place for medical treatment with bromocriptine and its combination with surgery and radiation therapy. Therefore, a follow-up investigation was performed including systematic endocrinological, clinical, ophthalmological and radiological controls. A group-differentiation had to be made into microadenomas and macroadenomas, and special care was used to describe the different prognoses of the female and male patients. The study was designed as a prospective follow-up study for the estimation of recurrence-rates in the various groups of patients as well as cure-rates depending on the type of treatment.

Selection of patients and methods

In the Neurosurgical Unit of the University of Graz, between 1978 and 1983, 140 patients have been treated for a pathological process in the sellar region. Trans-sphenoidal operation was performed in 117 patients, a pituitary adenoma was diagnosed in 100 (tab. 1); among them were 33 prolactinomas. Twenty-one of the latter patients were female, 12 were male.

Table 1 Unselected sellar tumours 1978–1983

Adenomas		100
inactive	44	
HGH-Prod.	20	
ACTH-Prod.	3	
Prolactinomas	*33*	
other tumours		17
total		117

All women except one 60 year old patient were admitted via the Gynecology Department because of amenorrhoea. Galactorrhoea was present in 14 of these 20 women. Visual field defects were present in 2 women (10%). Acromegalic symptoms were found in 1, and nanism in 1 patient. Reduction in libido was reported in 5 women and hypogonadism was diagnosed in 2 instances. Two patients suffered from headache.

Male patients presented with disturbance of libido/potence in 7 cases, headache in 5, nausea in 3, adynamia in 3 cases and visual field defects were found in 42%. Two men had a history of epileptic fits and one of them was admitted with an apoplectic adenoma.

In all patients, endocrinological investigation was performed including serum-PRL, -HGH, -ACTH, -TSH, -LH, -FSH and -cortisol levels under resting conditions and following stimulation by insulin-induced hypoglycemia (0.15 μg/kg, TRH (200 μg i.v.) and LHRH (100 μg i.v.). Serum-levels of serum-Prolactin (s-PRL) were estimated using a commercially available radio-immunoassay test-kit (Serono).

This preoperative endocrinological test was postoperatively repeated after 1 week (except stimulation tests), 1, 3, 6, 9 and 12 months, and thereafter according to their requirement, however, at least at yearly intervals [30].

Plain skull X-ray films, sellar tomography and computerized tomography (CT) were done in all patients [44]. Postoperative CT scans were made depending on whether a micro- or macroadenoma had been found, and on the postoperative PRL-levels and clinical signs. A tumour was diagnosed as a "macroadenoma" when a diameter of more than 7 mm was estimated. On preoperative carotid angiography in 21 patients, displacement of suprasellar carotid arteries and/or proximal anterior cerebral arteries was found in 1 female and 3 male patients with macroadenoma.

Histological sections from excised tumour material and suspicious border zone areas were made intra- and postoperatively, using routine staining techniques for light microscopy as well as immunohistochemical techniques with antibodies to hCrH, PRL, ACTH, s-TSH, s-FSH, s-LH, α-submit of glycoprotein hormones and electron microscopy [22]. All patients were operated via the sublabial, transseptal, transsphenoidal approach in a supine position with the head reclined by 20–30°, under fluoroscopic X-ray control with the surgeon in the head-side position. One femal patient had a recurrent macroadenoma after subfrontal craniotomy in 1975, all others were newly diagnosed. If no tumour was apparent on opening of the dura (capsule), the pituitary gland was incised diagonally in both directions. In the first 11 patients, muscle-tissue was used for tamponade of the tumour-cavity in the sella and the sphenoid sinus. In 21 patients, fibrin-tissue-glue (Beriplast®) in combination with surgical fibrin sponge (Spongostan®) were used without muscle. In most instances, septal bone was used for reconstruction of the bottom of the bony sella and the wall of the sphenoid sinus. In one male patient with para- and retrosellar extension of the macroadenoma, subtemporal craniotomy was performed in a second session. Postoperative intensive care observation was performed over 12–24 hours. The nasal tamponade was removed after 48–72 hours.

Postoperative irradiation was performed in 2 women and 4 men, all with macroadenomas. Postoperative bromocriptine therapy was given to 13 women and 3 men. Clinical follow-up examination were performed 1, 3, 6, 9 and 12 months postoperatively, and thereafter at yearly intervals.

Results

Preoperative radiological and endocrinological findings

None of the patients had normal plain skull X-ray and/or sella tomography; a double-contoured floor of the sella was formed in 9 of the 21 women and in 2 of the 12 men, i. e. 36% of female and 9% of male microadenomas and in 8% of macroadenomas of either sex. The sellar space enlarged in 20 women and 11 men. A bony defect of the sella floor was seen in 2 female microadenomas. Preoperative CT scans were normal in 3 female microadenomas, diagnosed with a scanner of the second generation. Among microadenomas, slight suprasellar extension was found in 1 woman. From intraoperative and CT-scan findings, 15 of the 21 female tumours were diagnosed as microadenomas (71%) as well as 1 of the 12 male tumours (8%). From the 6 female macroadenomas, 3 showed suprasellar, 3 a parasellar extension. Among 11 male macroadenomas, CT exhibited suprasellar growth in 5 and parasellar in 4 patients. Preoperative s-PRL levels correlated positively with the size of the tumours (fig. 1) and negatively with the chance for pos-

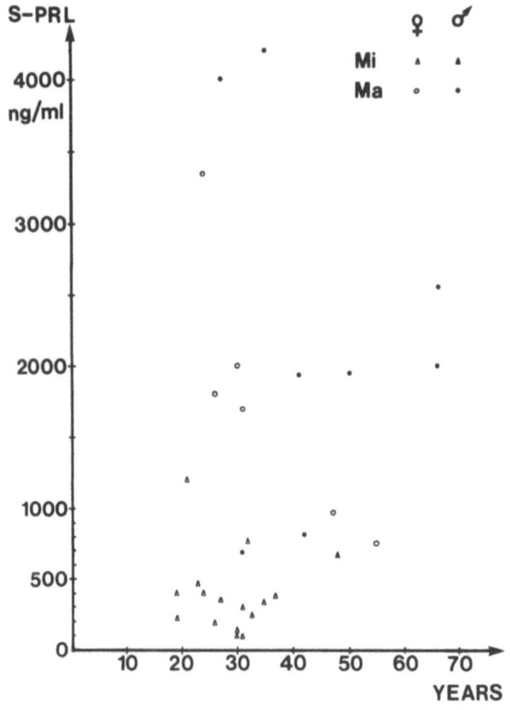

Fig. 1 Preoperative serum-prolactin levels (s-PRL) in ng/ml plotted against age at operation. Female macroadenomas (Ma) have significantly ($p<0.0005$) higher levels than microadenomas (Mi), and the latter patients were significantly younger ($p<0.05$).

toperative normalization of symptoms and s-PRL-levels. The mean levels of s-PRL preoperatively and from the first postoperative investigation are indicated in tables 2a, b. The mean age of the female patients with microadenomas was significantly lower (28 ± 1.5 years) than that of women with macroadenomas (35.5 ± 5.1 years) ($p<0.05$); However, among microadenomas, there was no correlation between age and levels of s-PRL. The difference of mean ages between female and male macroprolactinomas was statistically not significant (fig. 1). Preoperative values in women were significantly higher in macroadenomas than in microadenomas ($p<0.0005$), and in male compared to female macroadenomas. Postoperative s-

PRL levels were not significantly lower than preoperative values in male macroadenoma, however, significantly ($p<0.025$) lowered after operation of female macroadenomas. After operation of microadenomas, s-PRL also fell significantly ($p<0.005$).

Surgical complications

There was no surgical mortality among the patients with prolactinoma. The transsphenoidal operation as a first step in the total series of 100 patients with pituitary adenomas operated during the same observation period also had no mortality. Rhinoliquorrhoea occurred in 1 male patient with a macroadenoma 5 months after operation during bromocriptine treatment. The fistula was closed by transsphenoidal reoperation. Transient polyuria was observed in 3 female patients, all with microadenomas and preoperative s-PRL levels between 140 and 350 ng/ml. One patient had transitory pituitary insufficiency, 3 further patients required continuous sustitution therapy; all patients had macroadenomas. One patient had oculomotor palsy following subtemporal craniotomy. Intraoperatively, an unremovable parasellar rest of the tumour was thought to have been left behind in 6 patients, all with macroadenomas, 2 women and 4 men. This suspicion was confirmed by CT in

Table 2a Mean preoperative S-prolactin levels (ng/ml) in 28 patients (range)

	Female	Male
Microadenomas	377 (100–1202)	671
	*	
Macroadenomas	1760 (760–3300)	2474 (688–4200)

* significant difference, p < 0.0005

Table 2b Mean postoperative S-prolactin levels (ng/ml) in 28 patients (range)

	Female		Male
Microadenomas	124 (5.6–300)		240
	*		
Macroadenomas	619 (31.8–2000)	*	1808 (100–4000)

* significant difference

the 4 male patients. All 4 patients had postoperative s-PRL levels between 1500 and 2300 ng/ml; however, similar postoperative values were also observed in 2 patients without residual tumour.

Clinical and endocrinological follow-up results

The follow-up period ranges from 5 months to 5 years in the female and from 8 months to 5 years in the male patients with an average of 3.8 years and 3.1 years, respectively.

The main preoperative symptoms (tab. 3) of amenorrhoea-galactorrhoea improved in 17 out of 19 women below 40 years of age. Seven women with microadenomas had 12 pregnancies and delivered healthy children, one woman with a macroadenoma. A flattened or absent HGH-response in 14 patients had been preoperatively observed in 13 macroadenomas and a microadenoma with s-PRL of 466 ng/ml; none of the patients was spontaneously cured by surgery alone [23]. Postoperative normalization of s-PRL without and with bromocriptine treatment in micro- and macroadenoma is indicated in table 4.

Table 3 Postoperative clinical course in 19 women of child-bearing age

	Micro	Macro
Spont. menstr.	3	0
Menstr. under bromocriptine	12	2
No menstr. despite bromocriptine	0	2
Pregnancy – Delivery (Children)	7 (10)	1 (2)

Table 4 Postoperative S-prolactin levels

	Micro	Macro	Total
Normal without bromocriptine	3	1	4
Patholog, without bromocriptine	1	6	7
Normal with bromocriptine	12	8	20
Patholog, despite bromocriptine	0	2	2
Total	16	17	33

From the 16 patients with microadenomas, only 3 women had spontaneously normalized s-PRL levels (10 ng/ml) in the early postoperative period and remained so during follow-up. Preoperative levels ranged between 70 and 390 ng/ml. In a fourth woman, s-PRL normalized spontaneously after 2 months, early postoperative values were around 200 ng/ml; one year later, the patient became pregnant and delivered. All other postoperative values ranged from 44 to 708 ng/ml; the latter value was measured in a patient with a preoperative level of 384 ng/ml. In 12 women, s-PRL normalized during postoperative bromocriptine treatment, 7 became pregnant and delivered. In 1 woman with a microadenoma, s-PRL remained elevated after surgery, without bromocriptine.

Early postoperative s-PRL was still elevated in all except one patient with macroadenoma, but could be normalized with bromocriptine in 8 patients and reduced to levels around or below 100 ng/ml in 2 patients. Six patients did not take bromocriptine and remained with elevated s-PRL levels.

Visual field defects in 7 patients with macroadenoma were normalized within one week postoperatively in 2 patients, improved and thereafter stabilized in 1; in 4 patients normalization occurred after observation periods of two to three years. Improvement of libido/potence and/or cephalea was reported from 4 out of the 12 male patients.

Routine histological investigation revealed chromophobe adenomas in 16 patients, eosinophilic adenomas in 4 and *mixed* adenomas in 2 instances. In 3 cases, only normally appearing pituitary tissue from the tumour's border zone was found; in 1 patient, nodular hyperplasia was present. Histochemical analysis in 22 patients revealed a prolactin immunoreactivity in 18 cases; in 4 cases of chromophobe adenomas no immunohistochemical prolactin-reaction was found despite s-PRL levels of 140, 760, 2020 and 4000 ng/ml; elevated postoperative levels in 3 patients responded well to bromocriptine treatment.

Tumour recurrence was observed in a male patient with macroadenoma; reoperation was not performed because of a poor general condition at the age of 72 years; but the patient is asymptomatic under bromocriptine treatment. Of the 3 other patients with postoperative residual tumours in the CT, one was treated with irradiation and bromocriptine, and the tumour disappeared completely (fig. 2). The third patient has so far remained free from clinical symptoms without irradiation, and the residual tumour portion has not shown any tendency to grow on CT follow-up (fig. 3). The fourth patient with the diffusely invasive macroadenoma at the skull base was irradiated and treated with bromocriptine after transsphenoidal operation and subtemporal craniotomy. The tumour shows no tendency to grow and the patient has no new symptoms.

Discussion

As reported previously from other series [13, 34, 38], the surgical treatment of prolactinomas via the transsphenoidal approach is combined with a very low rate of complications. Small sellar abnormalities in the skull X-ray and tomography are

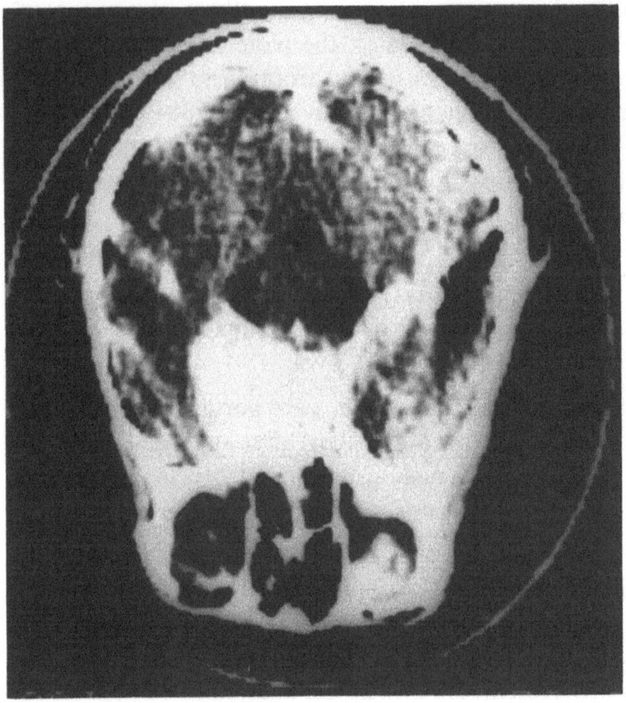

Fig. 2 CT scan after transsphenoidal operation of intra-, supra- and parasellar invasive prolactinoma.

found in the vast majority of patients with suspected microprolactinoma. It appears, however, not reliable to trust too much in this finding alone, since healthy normal volunteers also show abnormalities in two thirds of cases [57]. Sellar tomography will therefore probably become an unnecessary diagnostic routine [16], especially with third-generation CT scanners available.

S-PRL level as well as tumour size were found to be potent factors in the prediction of a postoperative cure without bromocriptine-treatment, and there is a high correlation between the two factors [16, 24, 27, 32, 43]. Moreover, the age was an important factor in women, as it also correlated with s-PRL and tumour size. This held true for comparison between the groups of patients with micro- and macroadenomas, however, not regarding an absolute threshold of age for individual patients [34].

In contrast to other reports [9, 34, 42, 53], s-PRL levels – found to be spontaneously normalized in the early postoperative period – were not observed to rise again at a later stage, although patients were not treated with bromocriptine. In part, data of recurrent s-PRL elevation might be an artifact of the level called "normal" in the early postoperative period which was below 10 ng/ml in our 3

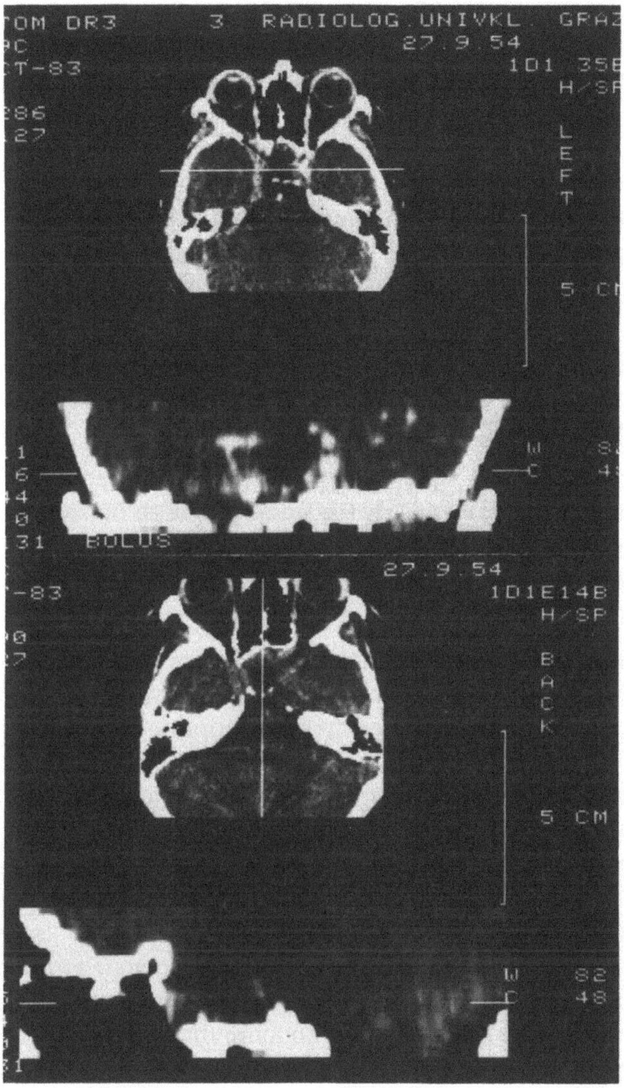

Fig. 3 After radiation therapy and during bromocriptine treatment the extrasellar tumour is no longer visible.

patients, however, was fixed e. g. at a level of 30 ng/ml by Nelson et al. [34]. An abnormal HGH-response in 14 patients of the present series turned out to be a prognostic sign against immediate cure by surgery alone, as previously reported by others [23, 34].

The likelihood for spontaneous postoperative normalization of s-PRL and clinical signs appears practically restricted to patients with microadenomas and lower s-

PRL values [2, 3, 5, 10, 16, 18, 26, 29, 34, 35, 38, 39, 42, 50, 53, 54] although an absolute threshold for the latter seems less reliable from our material. Comparison of incidence of postoperatively normal s-PRL – indicated in other publications with up to 60–70% in patients with microadenomas [17, 36] – between different series does not appear very helpful, since the mean values of important prognostic factors like s-PRL level for such postoperative normalization are not always comparable. Thus in our series, only 3 patients had preoperative s-PRL lower than 200 ng/ml and values ranged up to 1200 ng/ml.

The mean age of patients with microadenomas and their mean preoperative s-PRL level of the present group of patients is in exact accordance with a recent report from Nelson et al. [1]. Interestingly, all 3 cases of transient diabetes insipidus occurred in patients with microadenomas with low preoperative serum-PRL [10, 16]. This observation has already been made by Bosadjieva et al. [8].

The fact that only one of the patients with macroadenoma in the present series had normalized s-PRL postoperatively indicates clearly the worse prognosis of patients with macro-versus micro-prolactinomas [37, 39]. High postoperative s-PRL could be observed both together with residual tumour found in the CT-control and with a quasi normal CT.

Bromocriptine treatment alone can reduce tumour size [47], however, it does not have a tumoricidal action, and a rise in s-PRL must be expected on withdrawal of the drug [62]. Moreover, a group of non-responders to bromocriptine is known [7, 11] where s-PRL levels can be lowered, despite the tumour continuing to grow. It has recently been described and specified [6], that these patients habour tumours which lack immuno-histochemical display of PRL-granules, as seen in 4 patients of our series. Since this group of patients can only be identified from histological material, it appears still not without risks to recommend only bromocriptine therapy to higher risk patients such as women who want pregnancy, without interdisciplinary discussion prior to the start of treatment. In fact, further tumour growth and complications during pregnancy and bromocriptine have been observed [7, 19, 20, 25, 40], and tumour shrinkage can be expected in no more than 60 to 70% of patients with macroadenomas [45, 55]. After long-term treatment with bromocriptine [59], fibrosis [28] may turn a macroadenoma into a tough structure that becomes practically unmanageable via the transsphenoidal approach, thus narrowing therapeutic possibilities; a very important point which should be considered before deciding on the first therapeutic step. On the other hand, bromocriptine has proven valid for preoperative treatment to improve the rate of cures by surgical treatment [60]. Moreover, bromocriptine has been considered as the primary step of treatment in patients with large invasive adenomas, where surgery alone often fails, with the decision about surgery or irradiation as a second step, depending on the responsiveness of the tumour [52]. A rapid reduction in tumour size has been reported from single patients [51]. Postoperative supportive bromocriptine has proven helpful to normalize values in about 80% of patients with still elevated s-PRL levels and to normalize symptoms which cannot be cured by surgery alone, as seen from the present series and others [49, 61].

Reports on spontaneously regressing microprolactinomas are interesting, however, not of importance for the decision for one type of treatment, as long as a preoperative differentiation from other prolactinomas is not possible. Moreover, rapid growth of microprolactinomas in the spontaneous course has been observed, which can end with the early surprise of a macroadenoma with its higher risk [59]. Surgical as well as medical treatment seem to be advisable for microadenomas with high s-PRL levels. Medical treatment alone with bromocriptine may be indicated in very small adenomas with low s-PRL, also in elderly patients with large invasive tumours and a high surgical risk.

The problem of early diagnosis remains difficult in male patients. As seen from the present data ands other results, maximally 10–20% of men [12, 14, 37, 46, 48] present with a microadenoma, all others have larger tumours [27, 46] mostly already causing visual field defects. Surgery regularly improved visual field defects, however, the problem of sexual impotence was rarely altered [41, 46].

As shown from our own material, postoperative radiation therapy and treatment with bromocriptine seem to influence the prognosis favourably. All cases of postoperative residual tumours in complicated locations in the CT were men, none of them has so far required repeated surgery. Nonetheless, adequate information of the population and practitioneers on a broader basis is required to clarify that impotence can be caused by a pituitary tumour, and should accordingly be investigated with adequate care.

It is important to stress that any decision on medical or surgical treatment or a combination of both needs to be taken individually for each patient, considering reports on dopamine-agonist intolerance in up to 30% of patients [31], considering also the patient's own decision to undergo or refuse surgery.

Our data do not support the assumption from other studies [1], that recurrence is more frequent in patients with prolactinomas compared with those with endocrinologically inactive adenomas [4].

In summary, the present data support previous statements [34] regarding the importance of earliest possible diagnosis and treatment of prolactin-producing pituitary adenomas in order to increase the chance of curing the disease of amenorrhoea-galactorrhoea in women, and impotence in men, with or without bromocriptine therapy, with or without surgery, and in order to lower the risk for recurrence to a minimum. The earlier the treatment starts, the higher is the chance of a complete cure. Each of the two types of treatment can fail under above described circumstances. Therefore, it is still important and advisable to discuss findings and to plan treatment for each individual patient on an interdisciplinary basis.

References

[1] Aleshire, S. L., V. E. Cruz, C. A. Bradley, et al.: Long term follow-up prolactinomas. Clinical and morphologic correlation. This volume, pp. 295–300.
[2] Aubourg, P. R., P. J. Derome, F. Peillon, et al.: Endocrine outcome after transsphenoidal adenomectomy for prolactinoma: Prolactin levels and tumor size as predicting factors. Surg. Neurol. **14** (1980) 141–143.
[3] Aubourg, P. R., P. J. Derome, F. Peillon, et al.: Endocrine prognosis of PRL-secreting adenomas in 90 female cases. Ann. Endocrinol. **41** (1980) 57–58.
[4] Auer, L. M., in preparation 1984.
[5] Barbarino, A., L. De Marinis, E. Menini, et al.: Prolactin-secreting pituitary adenomas: Prolactin dynamics before and after transsphenoidal surgery. Acta Endocrinol. **91** (1979) 397–409.
[6] Barrow, D. L., G. T. Tindall, K. Kovacs, et al.: Clinical and pathological effects of bromocriptine on prolactin-secreting and other pituitary tumors. J. Neurosorg. **60** (1984) 1–7.
[7] Bergh, T., S. J. Nillius, P. Enoksson, et al.: Bromocriptine-induced pregnancies in women with large prolactinomas. Clin. Endocrinol. **17** (1982) 625–631.
[8] Bozadjieva, E., L. Karagiosov, A. Kehaiov, et al.: The effect of transsphenoidal selective microadenectomy on patients with prolactinomas. This volume, pp. 253–260.
[9] Buchfelder, M., A. Lierheimer, U. Schrell, et al.: Recurrence of hyperprolactinemia detected in long term follow-up of surgically normalized microprolactinomas. This volume, pp. 183–187.
[10] Chang, R. J., W. R. Keye Jr., J. R. Young, et. al.: Detection, evaluation, and treatment of pituitary microadenomas in patients with galactorrhea and amenorrhea. Am. J. Obstet. Gynecol. **128** (1977) 356–363.
[11] Crosignani, P. G., C. Ferrari, A. Liuzzi, et al.: Treatment of hyperprolactinemic states with different drugs: A study with bromocriptine, metergoline, and lisuride. Fertil. Steril. **37** (1982) 61–67.
[12] Derome, P. J., F. Peillon, R. H. Bard, et al.: Prolactin secreting adenomas: Surgical treatment and results. Nouv. Presse Med. **8** (1979) 577–583.
[13] Domingue, J. N., I. L. Richmond, C. B. Wilson: Results of surgery in 114 patients with prolactin-secreting pituitary adenomas. Am. J. Obstet. Gynecol. **137** (1980) 102–108.
[14] Eversmann, T., R. Eichinger, R. Fahlbusch, et al.: Hyperprolactinemia in man: Clinical features and treatment. Schweiz. Med. Wochenschr. **111** (1981) 1782–1789.
[15] Fahlbusch, R., P. Stass: Hypophysenadenome. Stand der Diagnostik und Therapie. Münch. Med. Wschr. **123** (1981) 549–555.
[16] Faria, M. A. Jr., G. T. Tindall: Transsphenoidal microsurgery for prolactin-secreting pituitary adenomas. J. Neurosurg. **56** (1982) 33–43.
[17] Ferrari, E., F. Agrimonti, P. A. Bossolo: Rhythmometric study of the circadian profile of plasma prolactin in patients with prolactinoma or empty sella syndrome. This volume, pp. 131–139.
[18] Franks, S., J. D. N. Nabarro: Prolactin secretion in patients with chromophobe adenomas of the pituitary: Incidence and presentation of hyperprolactinaemia: Results of surgical treatment. Ann. Clin. Res. **10** (1978) 17–163.
[19] Griffith, R. W., I. Turkalj, P. Braun: Pituitary tumours during pregnancy in mothers treated with bromocriptine. Br. J. Clin. Pharmacol. **7** (1979) 393–396.
[20] Hammond, C. B., A. F. Haney, M. R. Land, et al.: The outcome of pregnancy in patients with treated and untreated prolactin-secreting pituitary tumors. Am. J. Obstet. Gynecol. **147** (1983) 148–157.

[21] Hardy, J., H. Beauregard, F. Robert: In: Progress in Prolactin in Physiology and Pathology (C. Robin, M. Harter, eds.), pp. 361–370. North Holland Biomedical Press, Amsterdam 1978.
[22] Höfler, H., G. F. Walter, H. Denk: New immunocytochemical observations in prolactinomas. Proc. 1st Int. Symp. on Prolactinomas, Graz 1984.
[23] Jungmann, E., P. H. Althoff, G. J. Hermann, et al.: Evidence for functional impairment of growth hormone secretion in prolactinoma. This volume, pp. 147–153.
[24] Keye, W. R. Jr., R. J. Chang, S. E. Monroe, et al.: Prolactin-secreting pituitary adenomas in women: II. Menstrual function, pituitary reserves, and prolactin production following microsurgical removal. Am. J. Obstet. Gynecol. **134** (1979) 360–365.
[25] Lamberts, S. W. J., H. J. Seldenrath, H. G. Kwa, et al.: Transient bitemporal hemianopsia during pregnancy after treatment of galactorrhea-amenorrhea syndrome with bromocriptine. J. Clin. Endocrinol. Metab. **44** (1977) 180–184.
[26] Landolt, A. M.: Biology of pituitary microadenomas. In: Pituitary Microadenomas (G. Faglia, M. A. Giovanelli, R. M. MacLeod, eds.), pp. 107–122. Academic Press, New York 1980.
[27] Landolt, A. M.: Surgical treatment of pituitary prolactinomas: postoperative prolactin and fertility in seventy patients. Fertil. Steril. **35** (1981) 620–625.
[28] Landolt, A. M.: Structure and ultrastructure of prolactinomas. This volume, pp. 3–13.
[29] Laws, E. R. Jr., N. C. Fode, R. V. Randall, et al.: Pregnancy following transsphenoidal resection of prolactin-secreting pituitary tumors. J. Neurosurg. **58** (1983) 685–688.
[30] Leb, G., H. Warnkross, G. F. Walter, et al.: Impairment of pituitary hormone secretion in patients with prolactinoma. This volume, pp. 189–196.
[31] Lüdecke, D. K., H. D. Herrman, C. Hörmann, et al.: Comparison of effects of dopamine agonists and microsurgery in GH- and PRL-secreting adenomas. In preparation.
[32] McComb, D. J., K. Kovacs, E. Horvath, et al.: Correlative ultrastructural morphometry of human prolactin-producing adenomas. Acta Neurochir. **53** (1980) 217–225.
[33] Muhr, C., P. O. Lundberg, A. L. Hulting, et al.: Pituitary adenomas with hyperprolactinemia in males. This volume, pp. 169–178.
[34] Nelson, P. B., M. Goodman, J. C. Maroon, et al.: Factors in predicting outcome from operation in patients with prolactin-secreting pituitary adenomas. Neurosurgery **13** (1983) 634–641.
[35] Nicola, G. C., G. P. Tonnarelli, A. Griner: One hundred and ten prolactin secreting adenomas: Results of surgical treatment. In: Pituitary Microadenomas (G. Faglia, M. A. Giovanelli, R. M. MacLeod, eds.), pp. 91–105. Academic Press, New York 1980.
[36] Ohta, M., T. Uozumi, K. Sakoda, et al.: Effect of transsphenoidal surgery on pituitary function. This volume, pp. 231–234.
[37] Randall, R. V., E. R. Laws Jr., C. F. Abboud, et al.: Transsphenoidal microsurgical treatment of prolactin-producing pituitary adenomas. Result in 100 patients. Mayo Clin. Proc. **58**, (1983) 108–120.
[38] Rawe, S. E., H. O. Williamson, J. H. Levine, et al.: Prolactinomas: Surgical therapy, indications and results. Surg. Neurol. **14** (1980) 161–167.
[39] Reichlin, S.: The prolactinoma problem. N. Engl. J. Med. **300** (1979) 313–315 .
[40] Rjosk, H. K., R. Fahlbusch, J. H. Greite, et al.: 2nd European Workshop on Treatment of Pituitary Adenomas, Paris 1979.
[41] Schellen, T. M. C. M., A. Declercq: Hyperprolactinemia, male impotence, oligozoospermia and the treatment with bromocriptin. Dermatol. Monatsschr. **164** (1978) 568–570.
[42] Schlechte, J., B. Sherman, N. Halmi, et al.: Prolactin-secreting pituitary tumors in amenorrheic women: A comprehensive study. Endocr. Rev **1** (1980) 295–308.

[43] Schlechte, J., J. VanGilder, B. Sherman: Predictors of the outcome of transsphenoidal surgery for prolactin-secreting pituitary adenomas. J. Clin. Endocrinol. Metab. **52** (1981) 785–789.
[44] Schneider, G. H.: CT-findings in pituitary adenomas. This volume, pp. 91–103.
[45] Scotti, G., G. Scialfa, S. Pieralli, et al.: Macroprolactinomas: CT evaluations of reduction of tumor size after medical treatment. Neuroradiology **23** (1982) 123–126.
[46] Serri, O., M. Somma, E. Rasio, et al.: Prolactin-secreting pituitary adenomas in males: transsphenoidal microsurgical treatment. CMA J. **122** (1980) 1007–1013.
[47] Sobrinho, L. G., M. C. Nunes, C. Calhaz-Jorge, et al.: Effect of treatment with bromocriptine on the size and activity of prolactin producing pituitary tumours. Acta Endocrinol. **96** (1981) 24–29.
[48] Somma, M., H. Beauregard, E. Rasio: Prolactinoma in men: Clinical and biological study. Neuro-Chir. **27** (1981) Suppl 1, 37–39.
[49] Spark, R. F., C. A. Wills, G. O'Reilly, et al.: Hyperprolactinaemia in males with and without pituitary macroadenomas. Lancet **2** (1982) 129–132.
[50] Spence, J. T., B. S. Underwood, J. W. Cotton: Elementary Statistics. Appleton Century Croft, New York 1968.
[51] Thorner, M. O., W. H. Martin, A. D. Rogol, et al.: Rapid regression of pituitary prolactinomas during bromocriptine treatment. J. Clin. Endocrinol. Metab. **51** (1980) 438–445.
[52] Thorner, M. O., I. S. Ciric: Treatment of prolactinomas (letter to the editor). Surg. Neurol. **19** (1983) 303–304.
[53] Tindall, G. T., C. S. McLanahan, J. H. Christy: Transsphenoidal microsurgery for pituitary tumors associated with hyperprolactinemia. J. Neurosurg. **48** (1978) 849–860.
[54] Tucker, H. S. G., D. P. Becker: Microsurgical removal of pituitary tumors with "cure" and retention of pituitary function. In: Pituitary Microadenomas (G. Faglia, M. A. Giovanelli, R. M. MacLeod, eds.), pp. 473–481. Academic Press, New York 1980.
[55] Wass, J. A. H., J. Williams, M. Charlesworth, et al.: Bromocriptine in management of large pituitary tumours. Br. Med. J. **284** (1982) 1908–1911.
[56] Watanabe, K., T. Fukushima: Transsphenoidal microsurgical treatment of 77 prolactinomas. This volume, pp. 235–245.
[57] Weinstein, D., S. L. G. Rothmann, R. B. Geehr, et al.: Sella erosions in a series of 50 normal women. The place of tomography in the diagnosis of prolactin secreting pituitary microadenomas. Eur. J. Obstet. Gynecol. Reprod. Biol. **13** (1982) 169–175.
[58] Weiss, M. H.: Comment to the paper of Nelson, P. B. et al "Factors in predicting outcome from operation in patients with prolactin-secreting pituitary adenomas. Neurosurgery **13** (1983) 640–641.
[59] Weiss, M. H., J. Teal, P. Gott, et al.: Natural history of microprolactinomas: Six-year follow-up. Neurosurgery **12** (1983) 180–183.
[60] Weiss, M. H., R. R. Wycoff, R. Yadley, et al.: Bromocriptine treatment of prolactin-secreting tumors: Surgical implications. Neurosurgery **12** (1983) 640–642.
[61] Werder, K. v., R. Fahlbusch, R. Landgraf, et al.: Treatment of patients with prolactinomas. J. Endocrinol. Invest. **1** (1978) 47–58.
[62] Werder, K. v., C. Brendel, T. Eversmann, et al.: Medical therapy of hyperprolactinemia and Cushing's disease associated with pituitary adenomas. In: Pituitary Microadenomas (G. Faglia, M. A. Giovanelli, R. M. MacLeod, eds.), pp. 383. Academic Press, London 1980.

Otoliquorrhoea in large prolactinomas. Pathomechanism and surgical management

M. Bobest, A. Perneczky

Introduction

In cases of untreated pituitary adenomas nasal CSF leakage is a seldom but not exceptional finding [4]. We have not found any report in the literature about spontaneous otoliquorrhoea due to expanding pituitary lesions.

Patients and methods

First case report

Sz., Gy., a man aged 46 was first admitted on 2. 12. 1981. His pituitary tumour, a secreting adenoma was diagnosed one year earlier, but the patient resisted surgical treatment. The serum prolactin was 170 ng/ml. One month previous to his admission he noticed a continuous discharge of colourless watery clear fluid from his left ear. The patient related: "I had to wring out the cotton-wool tampon every other minute." Some days later he had fever but he refused hospitalisation. At last he was admitted in a drowsy, irritable state with signs of severe meningitis. In the CSF the protein reactions were highly positive, WBC's per cmm were 12,500, 95% of polymorphs. Repeated cultures were negative. Spontaneous vestibular signs were absent, there was a reaction to sound on both sides. Rhinological findings were normal, but otologically the central part of the left tympanic membrane was thinner, its normal glaze was lost, and it seemed to be wet.

At puncture some drops of watery clear fluid were obtained. Parenteral and intrathecal Gentamycin administration was introduced. On the next day profuse CSF otorrhoea was confirmed so an emergency mastoidectomy was performed. At operation the considerably enlarged mastoid cell system was found filled with liquor. At revision of the cavity the fistula was found.

The mastoid cavity was filled with a piece of muscle. Postoperatively – continuing the antibiotic treatment – the meningitis healed, he showed a rapid improvement, and the otorrhoea ceased.

The tomography revealed a paper-thin sheet of dorsum with erosion in the direction of the clivus (fig. 1, a, b). In the a–p view there were extremely large air cells of petrous apex on the left side (Fig. 1, c). In the angiograms and encephalograms there were no signs of suprasellar extension.

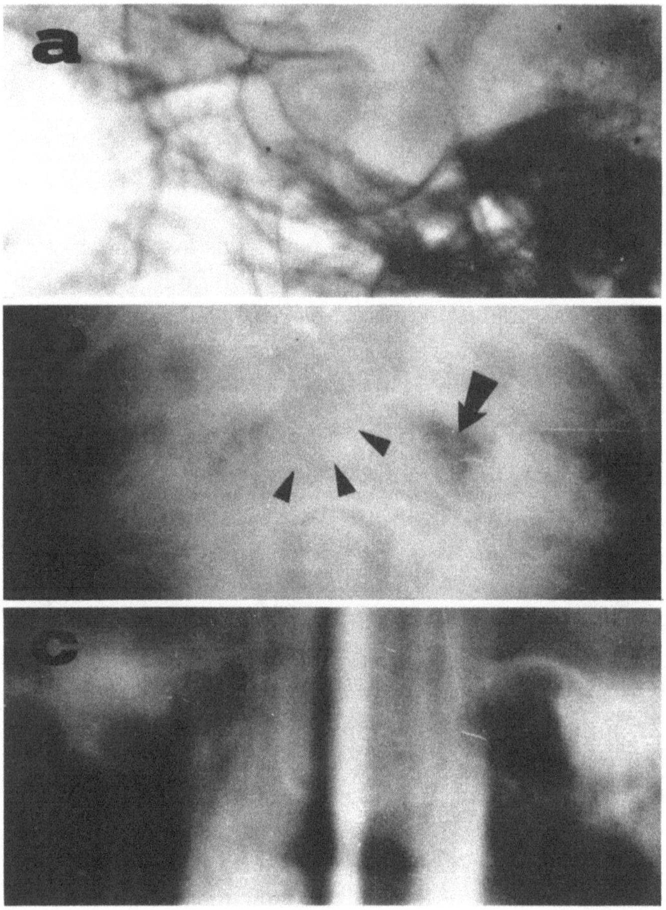

Fig. 1

Following an uneventful period the sella was explored through the transseptal-transsphenoidal approach and the adenoma was microsurgically removed. The sella and partly the sphenoid sinus were packed with muscle sealed with Tissucol. There was no postoperative complication, the prolactin level normalized, and the patient has remained well since, with normal otological, ophthalmological and neurological findings. On our schematic drawing (fig. 2) we show the possible pathway of the cerebrospinal fluid.

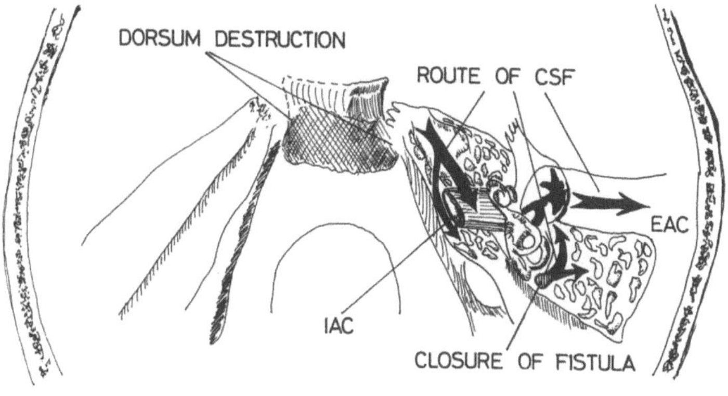

Fig. 2

Second case report

Sch., J., a 58 year old man was first transethmoidally operated in 1973. Clinically he had a panhypopituitarism with slightly elevated serum prolactin (under 100 ng/ml). He remained well for several years but during the last two years the prolactin level moderately elevated. At Xmas 1982 he noticed the discharge of watery fluid from his right ear, his pillow became wet during the night. After some weeks he went to a Physician. The fluid from the ear was identical with CSF. He had neither headache, nor meningitis. The visual fields were normal. The most impressing finding was seen in the CT (fig. 3). The sphenoid sinus was filled with a tumour mass. On the right the adenoma had invaded the petrous bone and had eroded the cavity of the middle ear.

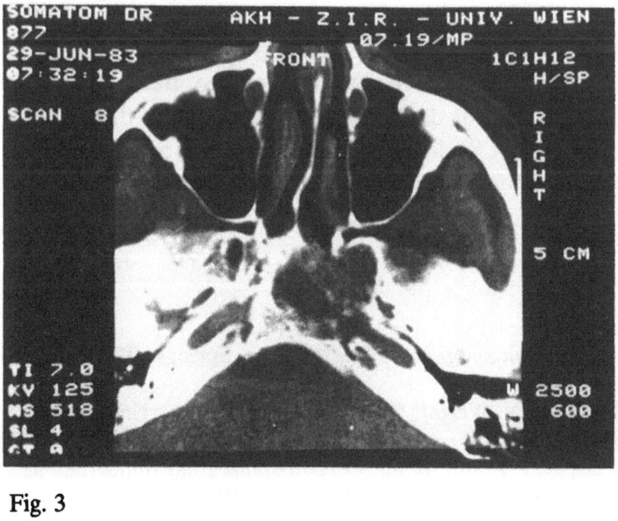

Fig. 3

Audiologically he had moderate loss of hearing on that side. On the first July, 1983 by the transseptal-transsphenoidal route a large adenoma was microsurgically removed. It revealed that the adenoma had penetrated the arachnoidea. The cavity was packed with muscle and nasal cartilage using fibrin sealant (Tissucol, Immuno-Wien). The patient was discharged on the sixth postoperative day. At a control investigation in February 1984, he had no complaints. There was no CSF leakage, neither from the ear, nor in the nasopharynx. Serum prolactin normalized at 21 ng/ml, otologically there were no complaints, with a slight improvement in hearing.

Comments

A spontaneous otoliquorrhoea can be due to a congenital defect [5], or the result of petrosal i.e. parapetrosal pathological processes. Tumours may cause CSF otorrhoea by eroding the temporal bone, either in an intracranial or extracranial location [2]. In the first case it was a predisposing factor, namely the extremely enlarged petrosal tip. Denecke [1] reported on the basis of postmortem examinations on skulls that in 9–10 percent a well developed continuous aircell system is to be found connecting the petrous apex with the mastoid antrum.

According to Taveras [6] the large expanding growing pituitary adenomas can produce erosion of petrous bone. The erosion of the large tumour mass posteriorly through the dura may be sufficient to produce a fistula between the arachnoid space and the mastoid cells. In the second case the pathomechanism of CSF otorrhoea is obvious; the tumour penetrated directly into the middle ear causing an arachnoidal lesion.

In both cases the prolactinomas had grown, expanding on the basis without suprasellar extension. Nutkiewicz et al. [3] suggested that a strongly competent sellar diaphragm may resist tumour extension superiorly and – as in our cases – may direct the growth posteriorly. There is another common feature, namely in both cases the function of Eustachian canals was damaged so it developed – through the lesion in the tympanic membrane – a CSF leakage via the external auditory canal. In the first case the surgical management was performed in two steps. In the second one the transsphenoidal intervention was succesful alone.

References

[1] Denecke, H. J.: Die oto-rhino-laryngologischen Operationen. Springer-Verlag, Berlin–Göttingen–Heidelberg 1953.

[2] Hicks, G. W., J. W. Wright Jr., J. W. Wright: Cerebrospinal fluid otorrhea. Laryngoscop. Supplement. No. 25. **90** (1980) 1.

[3] Nutkiewicz, A., D. R. DeFeo, R. I. Kohut, et al.: Cerebrospinal fluid rhinorrhea as a presentation of pituitary adenoma. Neurosurgery. **6** (1980) 195.

[4] Rothrock, J. F., J. F. Laguna, A. F. Reynolds: CSF rhinorrhea from untreated pituitary adenoma. Arch. Neurol. **39** (1982) 442.
[5] Pimontel-Appel, B., J. Vignaud: Cerebrospinal fluid otorrhea due to a congenital defect of the petrous bone. J. Neuroradiology **6** (1979) 15.
[6] Taveras, J. M., E. H. Wood: Diagnostic Neuroradiology. Second Edition. Williams and Wilkins Company, Baltimore 1976.

Invasive prolactinomas in adolescents

A. D. Parent

Introduction

In 1955, Sir Geoffrey Jefferson first coined the term, *invasive* adenoma [8]. Fifteen years earlier, he had scrutinized the criteria for pituitary malignancy, recognizing that "size is not an index, ... unless there is either invasion or metastasis" [7]. The term *invasive adenoma* specifically refers to tumors with extrasellar extension, including dural sinuses, bone, and even cranial nerves while the term *pituitary carcinoma* is reserved for tumors that demonstrate metastasis. The usual characteristics of cellular pleomorphism, mitotic activity, necrosis, vascularity, and nuclear atypia cannot reliably predict the clinical growth of adenomas. Ultrastructurally and immunocytologically, no distinguishing features have allowed a dichotomy to be made between these adenomas.

In the past decades, several authors [10, 13, 18] have commented on the unusual invasiveness of pituitary tumors in children. Prolactin secreting adenomas appear to be the most common of these tumors, but a low surgical curability has been reported [1, 9] with this pediatric hypersecretory endocrinopathy. This observation differs, however, from the results of Hardy [6] and Wilson [15], where the cure rate approximated the results seen in adults.

Because of our concern with this variance, we have studied our series of 32 prolactinomas to compare tumor invasiveness in adults and adolescents. There were 7 males and 25 females in the entire series, but all three adolescent patients were females. Ten invasive prolactin tumors were identified and only one case was found in the adolescent group. Illustrative examples of noninvasive and invasive macroadenomas are presented from the adolescent patients.

Patients and methods

Case 1

A 19-year-old white female had a normal menarche at the age of 11 but ceased having menstrual periods at age 13. Two years later, she noted the spontaneous onset of a thin white discharge from her breast. She also complained of dull frontal headaches, but had no problems with visual difficulties. Her examination demonstrated normal pubic hair development and normal breast. Bilateral galactorrhoea was noted.

Her fasting prolactin level was 2578 ng/ml with no response to a thyrotropin releasing hormone (TRH) stimulation test. The remainder of the endocrinologic studies were normal. The preoperative CT scan demonstrated an intrasellar tumor that appeared to destroy the sella floor (fig. 1). At transsphenoidal surgery, tumor tissue was encountered extruding through the sella into the sphenoid sinus mucosa.

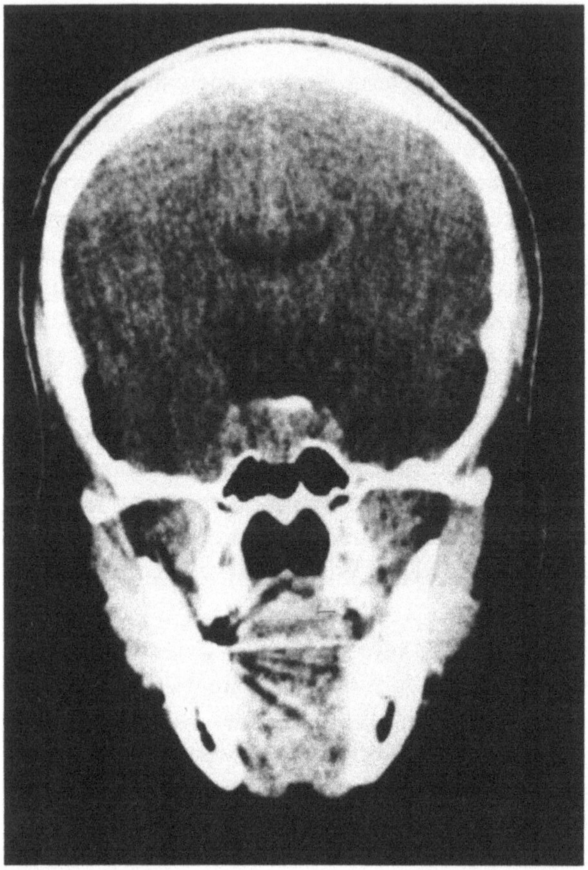

Fig. 1 Coronal section of CT scan demonstrating intrasellar enhancing lesion with erosion of the sellar floor.

Histologically, by Hemotoxylin and Eosin stain, a rather benign appearing pituitary tumor was identified. Immunoperoxidase stains revealed that 70–80% of the cells were positive for prolactin. Sections of the tissue initially removed from the sella floor showed tumor cells infiltrating between collagen bundles of the dura and mucosa (fig. 2).

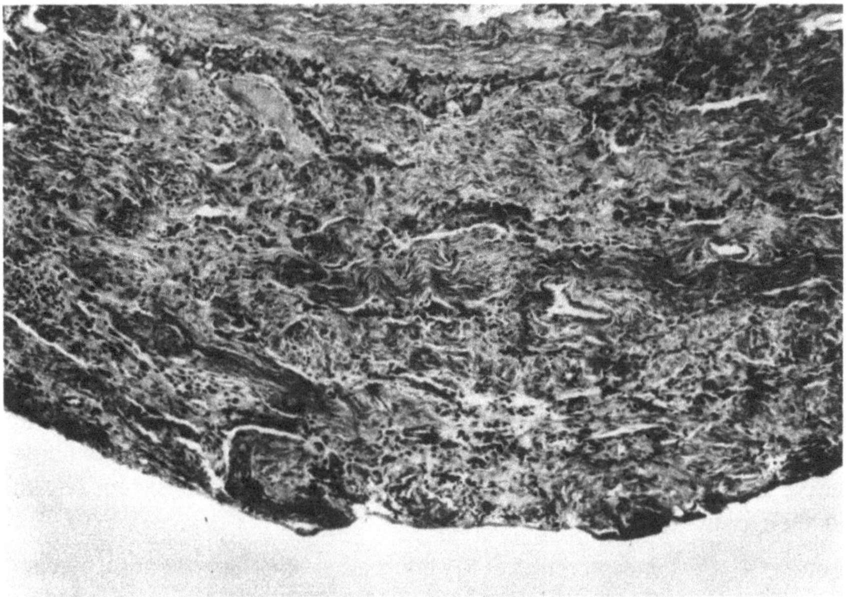

Fig. 2 Low power (×10) histologic section (*trichrome stain* of tissue) from the sella floor with tumor cells interspersed with collagenous tissue.

Her postoperative fasting prolactin level was 268 ng/ml. Although the galactorrhoea resolved, she remained amenorrhoeic. LH, FSH, and serum oestradiol levels were normal. Two years later, bromocriptine therapy was discontinued and the prolactin level initially remained normal. When the symptoms of galactorrhoea and headaches recurred at two months, her prolactin level was 46.6 ng/ml. Her symptoms resolved with the reinstitution of medical therapy.

Case 2

A 15-year-old black female with galactorrhea and primary amenorrhea was evaluated in December 1983. She had noted an increase in the size of her breasts with the recent onset of lactation and weight gain of 60 pounds. She had no history of headaches nor of visual disturbances. With the exception of galactorrhea, she had an unremarkable physical examination. Her preoperative prolactin level was 92 ng/ml with a minimal response to TRH stimulation. The CT scan demonstrated a hypodense lesion, extending into the suprasellar cistern, measuring approximately 1.5 cm. At transsphenoidal surgery, a noninvasive prolactinoma was excised. Her postoperative prolactin was 6.5 ng/ml and clinically her galactorrhoea abated and she menstruated spontaneously two months later.

This tumor was characterized by a dense fibrous stroma and a uniform cell population. In some areas, haemosiderin was seen within the fibrotic tissue. All tumor cells stained positive for prolactin in this case.

Discussion

The lack of correlation between clinical findings and pituitary tumor invasiveness was noted by Martin et al. [10] as well as the propensity for tumors to occur in the younger age groups. Two of their five patients were less than twenty years of age, but the series was limited to young military men. Complaints of impotence and galactorrhea suggestive of the pituitary prolactinoma syndrome was noted in two cases. In a series of 115 patients, Ortiz-Suarez and Erickson [13] reported that all four of their adolescent patients presented with an invasive pituitary adenoma. Cranial nerve palsies due to extrasellar tumor extension was a consistent clinical feature in their patients.

Hyposecretory [4] and hypersecretory [15] endocrinopathies have been recognized with at least 80% of pediatric pituitary tumors. Richmond and Wilson [15] in a group of 25 children and adolescents, found 15 prolactinomas. Postoperatively, 12 of these patients had normal prolactin levels. However, Barrio et al. [1], in a similar adolescent series of eight macroprolactinomas treated by transsphenoidal surgery, had only three patients with diminished prolactin levels and none had normal prolactin values. Lucas et al. [9] encountered 12 adolescent cases in a series of 110 prolactin secreting pituitary adenomas. Despite an apparent total excision, hyperprolactinaemia persisted in 9 of 12 patients. Cystic and haemorrhagic changes were commonly seen in these tumors and evidence of lactotropic hyperplasia was absent, but no specific comments about tumor invasiveness were made.

Prolactin secreting adenomas in adolescents with primary amenorrhoea, as reported by Coulam et al. [3], may be associated with a poor rate of resolution of hyperprolactinaemia. Only one of four microadenoma patients had normalized prolactin levels after surgery in their series. In reviewing the Mayo Clinic [14] series of 100 prolactinomas, six adolescent cases were identified, with four microadenomas and two invasive adenomas. The surgical results were directly related to tumor size and invasiveness, as well as preoperative prolactin values.

Faria and Tindall [5] reported on 100 prolactinomas in women with galactorrhoea and amenorrhoea. There were twelve adolescents in this series [20] with excellent surgical results in patients with microadenomas and preoperative prolactin levels less than 200 ng/ml. Prolactinomas in their adolescent group did not appear to be more invasive or less curable than at other age groups.

Complete surgical extirpation of macroadenomas is less certain than in cases of microadenomas. Classically, pituitary tumors were categorized by tumor size and suprasellar extension. With newer neuro-diagnostic techniques, the tumor relationship to surrounding structures can be appreciated. Hardy's tumor classification [6] differentiates between enclosed and invasive tumors regardless of tumor size.

Intraoperative frozen section biopsies are important to determine the completeness of tumor extirpation. Fibrous trabeculae and capsular tissue may harbour tumor cells that should be recognized and excised. Extra-adenoma biopsies are particularly useful to identify diffuse adenomas, cellular hyperplasia, as well as tumor invasiveness. The transsphenoidal route provides an excellent opportunity to study tumor dural interphase for evidence of tumor invasion.

In our small series of 32 patients, invasive prolactin adenomas do not appear to be more frequent in adolescents than in adults (fig. 3). Dural invasion was surgically

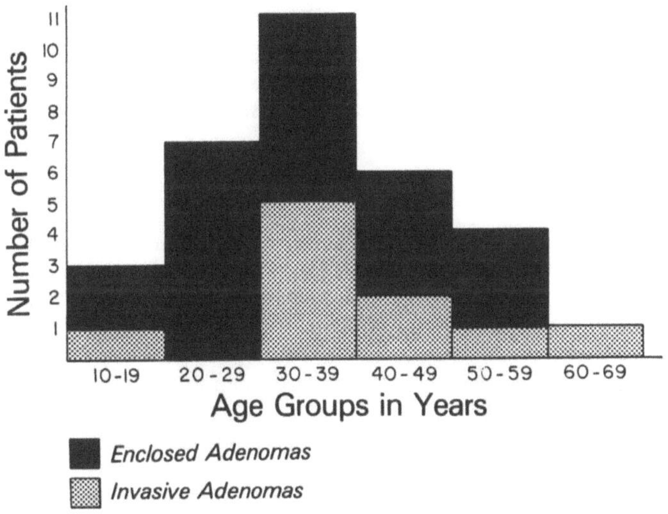

Fig. 3 Histogram of non-invasive and invasive pituitary tumors graphed by decades.

recognized and histologically verified in six adults and one adolescent. All of these patients have persistent, albeit diminished hyperprolactinemia. Four patients with markedly elevated prolactin levels have elected to be treated with chronic bromocriptine therapy.

Bromocriptine, especially in adolescents [2, 9, 16], is advocated to correct persistent hyperprolactinemia. The incidence of gonadotropic and somatotropic insufficiency, due to radiation therapy, has prompted us to delay radiation until after puberty in children. Furthermore, since prolactinomas have been considered relatively insensitive to radiation, chronic bromocriptine therapy should be considered an acceptable alternative to radiation.

Summary

Persistent hyperprolactinemia after the excision of a prolactinoma could be explained by hypothalamic-portal vessel dysfunction, lactotroph cell hyperplasia, or residual tumor. Tumor size, preoperative prolactin level, and radiologic evidence of tumor invasion have been utilized as predictors of surgical outcome [17]. In our patients tumor invasiveness was not consistently associated with suprasellar tumor extension. However, Shaffi et al. [19] have noted invasion of the diaphragma sella by tumor cells in 5 of the operative cases in their series of invasive adenomas. We believe that greater attention to dural invasiveness by prolactinomas may be a useful predictor of surgical outcome.

Acknowledgements

I wish to acknowledge assistance from Dr. Robert R. Smith and Dr. John P. Kapp for reviewing this manuscript and to Dr. Edward Smith for assisting with the neuropathologic study. I also wish to thank Ms. Lucia Griffin for secretarial assistance.

References

[1] Barrio, R., M. Roger, J. L. Chaussain, et al.: Les adénomes hypophysaires à prolactine de l'enfant et de l'adolescent. Arch. Fr. Pediatr. **36** (1979) 785–793.
[2] Bergh, T., S. J., Willins, L. Wide: Bromocriptine treatment of seven women with primary amenorrhea and prolactin secreting pituitary tumors. Clin. Endocrinol. **10** (1979) 145–154.
[3] Coulam, C. B., E. R. Laws, C. F. Abboud, et al.: Primary amenorrhea and pituitary adenomas. Fertil. Steril. **36** (1981) 615–619.
[4] DiRocco, C., G. Maira, P. Borelli: Pituitary microadenomas in children. Child's Brain **9** (1982) 165–178.
[5] Faria, M. A., G. T. Tindall: Transsphenoidal microsurgery for prolactin-secreting pituitary adenomas. J. Neurosurg. **56** (1982) 33–43.
[6] Hardy, J., G. Mohr: Le Prolactinome-Aspects. Chirurgicaux Neurochirurgie 27 (suppl. 1), 41–60 (1981).
[7] Jefferson, G.: Extrasellar extensions of pituitary adenomas: President's address. Proc. R. Soc. Med. **33** (1940) 433–458.
[8] Jefferson, G.: The invasive Adenomas of the Anterior Pituitary. The Sherrington Lectures, No. 3. University of Liverpool press, Liverpool 1955.
[9] Lucas, C., M. Guibout, P. Jaquet, et al.: Aspects diagnostiques et évolutifs de l'adénome à prolactine chez l'enfant. Arch. Fr. Pediatr. **37** (1980) 79–86.
[10] Martin, A. N., G. J. Hayes, L. G. Kempe: Invasive pituitary adenomas. J. Neurosurg. **22** (1965) 268–276.
[11] Nabairo, J. D. W.: Pituitary prolactinomas. Clin. Endocrinol. **17** (1982) 129–155.
[12] Nelson, P. B., M. Goodman, J. C. Maroon, et al.: Factors in predicting outcome from operation in patients with prolactin-secreting pituitary adenomas. Neurosurgery **13** (1983) 634–641.
[13] Ortiz-Suarez, H., D. L. Erickson: Pituitary adenomas of adolescents. J. Neurosurg. **43** (1975) 437–439.

[14] Randall, R. V., E. R. Laws, C. F. Abboud, et al.: Transsphenoidal microsurgical treatment of prolactin producing pituitary adenomas. Mayo Clin. Proc. **58** (1983) 108–121.
[15] Richmond, I. L., C. B. Wilson: Pituitary adenomas in childhood and adolescence. J. Neurosurg. **49** (1978) 163–168.
[16] Sadeghi-Nejad, A., J. I. Wolfsdorf, B. J. Biller, et al.: Hyperprolactinemia causing primary amenorrhea. J. Pediatr. **99** (1981) 802–804.
[17] Schlechte, J., J. Vangilder, B. Sherman: Predictors of the outcome of Transsphenoidal surgery for prolactin-secreting pituitary adenomas. J. Clin. Endocrinol. Metab. **52** (1981) 785–789.
[18] Schroffner, W. G.: Prolactin-secreting pituitary tumor in early adolescence. Arch. Int. Med. **136** (1976) 1164–1168.
[19] Shaffi, O. M., P. Wrightson: Dural invasion by pituitary tumors. N. Zealand. Med. J. **81** (1975) 836–390.
[20] Tindall, G. T.: Personal communication.

Residual anterior pituitary function following transsphenoidal resection of pituitary macroadenomas

D. P. Becker, A. T. Nelson jr., H. St. G. Tucker jr.

Introduction

Transsphenoidal microsurgery has become the accepted mode of treatment for pituitary tumours. It is effective both for small tumours causing endocrinopathy and for larger tumours presenting with visual impairment or other evidence of mass effect [1, 5, 6, 7]. The purpose of this study is to examine the effects of transsphenoidal surgery for larger tumours on anterior pituitary function.

Material and methods

This study analyzed data from 84 patients who underwent a total of 88 transsphenoidal procedures for tumours greater than 1 cm in size between 1972 and 1982 at the Medical College of Virginia. This group included 38 males and 46 females, and included 36 prolactinomas, 15 growth hormone secreting tumours, and 33 non-secreting tumours. The patients ranged in age from 19 to 78 (mean 44). Tumours were grouped according to Hardy grade [3] (tab. 1). Suprasellar extension was evident in 84% of the patients. Four patients underwent repeat transsphenoidal procedures for residual tumour; endocrine outcome was evaluated after the second procedure.

Table 1 Tumour grade (Hardy)

Grade I	0
Grade II	7
Grade III	14
Grade IV	63

All patients underwent complete endocrinologic workups prior to surgery. The pituitary-thyroid axis was evaluated with baseline thyroxine, tri-iodothyronine resin uptake, and thyroid stimulating hormone (TSH) levels. TSH reserve was measured after 1977 following administration of thyrotropin releasing hormone. Pituitary-adrenal function was determined with baseline AM and PM cortisol levels and 24 hour urinary 17-hydroxycorticosteroid excretion. ACTH reserve was determined both with insulin tolerance testing and metyrapone suppression. Baseline prolactin was measured (after 1977), and chlorpromazine stimulation and 1-DOPA suppression were performed. Growth hormone baseline levels were measured along with insulin tolerance testing and glucose loading suppression. Pituitary-gonadal function was evaluated with baseline testosterone or estradiol, leutenizing hormone, and follicle stimulating hormone measurements.

All patients underwent transsphenoidal exploration as described by Hardy [2, 3], employing the operating microscope and televised intra-operative flouroscopy. A wide, boney exposure was used and aggressive curretage was employed until all visible tumour was removed.

Repeat endocrinologic evaluations were carried out at two or three month intervals postoperatively and thereafter at six month to one year intervals. Decisions regarding postoperative hormonal replacement were made on the basis of preoperative endocrine status and postoperative evaluations.

Results

Patients were categorized into three groups according to preoperative endocrine status (exclusive of prolactin and growth hormone axes). Group A patients had normal anterior pituitary function on the basis of normal pituitary-thyroid, pituitary-adrenal, and pituitary-gonadal axes on baseline and provocative testing. Group A contained 44 patients. Group B patients were deficient in one or more axes but had evidence of some anterior pituitary function. This group contained 21 patients. Group C consisted of patients without evidence of anterior pituitary function preoperatively and contained a total of 19 patients.

After surgery 33 (78%) of the 44 patients in group A continued to have normal pituitary function. Two additional patients were lost to follow-up but were felt to be endocrinologically normal on clinical grounds. Nine patients (21%) in group A lost pituitary function after surgery (6 panhypopituitary, 2 hypogonadal, 1 hypothyroid with decreased ACTH reserve but not requiring steroid), (tab. 2).

Group B contained 21 patients. Postoperatively 7 patients improved endocrinologically, 7 remained unchanged, and 7 deteriorated. The axes affected are summarized in table 3.

Group C contained 19 patients, all of whom were panhypopituitary prior to surgery. No patients in this group had any improvement in pituitary function after surgery.

Table 2 Postoperative endocrine results of group A

Remained normal		33 (78%)
Deteriorated		9 (21%)
Hypogonadal	1	
Hypothyroid	1	
↓ ACTH reserve	2	
Panhypopituitary	6	
Lost to follow-up		2 (1%)
Total		44 (100%)

Table 3 Postoperative endocrine results of group 8

Improved			7 (33%)
Preop.	*Postop.*		
↓ AR	Nml	1	
↓ G	Nml	1	
↓ T, G	Nml	1	
↓ T, G, AR	↓ G, AR	3	
↓ T, G	↓ G	1	
Deteriorated			7 (33%)
↓ G	↓ G, T	1	
↓ G	PHP	2	
↓ G, T	PHP	3	
↓ G, T, AR	PHP	1	
Unchanged			7 (33%)
↓ G		5	
↓ G, T		1	
↓ G, AR		1	
			21

↓ G = deficient pituitary-gonadal axis
↓ T = deficient pituitary-thyroid axis
↓ AR = decreased ACTH reserve but not requiring steroid therapy
PHP = panhypopituitary
Nml = normal anterior pituitary function

Loss of anterior pituitary function was analyzed with respect to tumour grade. All 7 Hardy grade II patients were in group A, and none lost pituitary function as a result of surgery. Of the 14 grade III patients, 12 were in groups A or B, i.e., preoperatively had full or partial function, and two (16%) lost some or all pituitary function. Fourteen (43%) of 32 grade IV patients in groups A or B preoperatively deteriorated after surgery. In this series 11 patients in groups A or B were rendered panhypopituitary by surgery; ten had grade IV tumours.

Early surgical results are presented in table 4. Residual tumour was felt to be present in the prolactinoma or acromegaly patients if the postoperative prolactin was above 25 or growth hormone was above 10 respectively at six months after surgery. Non-secreting tumours were considered extirpated if a total tumour removal was clearly accomplished at the time of surgery and if no residual tumour was evident clinically or radiographically on follow-up examinations.

Table 4 Early surgical results

Prolactinomas	
Normalized, PRL < 25	15
Not Normalized, PRL > 25	21
HGH-Secretors	
Normalized, HGH < 5	12
Not Normalized, HGH > 5	3
Non-Secretors	
Tumour Extirpated	28
Residual Tumour	5
	84

We conclude that transsphenoidal surgery for larger pituitary tumours is a safe procedure regarding anterior pituitary function. The risk of sacrificing pituitary function is not unlike that reported in series containing smaller tumours [1, 4]. The risk of sacrificing pituitary function is greater for patients with impaired pituitary function preoperatively and for patients with larger tumours. Patients with larger tumours should receive complete preoperative and postoperative endocrine testing so that a rational decision regarding the necessity for postoperative hormonal replacement can be made.

References

[1] Faria, M. A., G. T. Tindall: Transsphenoidal microsurgery for prolectic-secreting pituitary adenomas. J. Neurosurg. **56** (1982) 33–43.
[2] Hardy, J.: Transsphenoidal hypophysectomy. J. Neurosurg. **34** (1971) 582–584.
[3] Hardy, J.: Transsphenoidal microsurgery of the normal and pathological pituitary. Clin. Neurosurg. **16** (1969) 185–217.
[4] McLanahan, C. S., J. H. Christy, G. T. Tindall: Anterior pituitary function before and after transsphenoidal microsurgical resection of pituitary tumors. Neurosurgery **3** (1978) 142–145.

[5] Tucker, H. S. G., S. R. Grubb, J. P. Wigand, et al.: The treatment of acromegaly by transsphenoidal surgery. Arch. Intern. Med. **140** (1980) 795–802.
[6] Tucker, H. S. G., S. R. Grubb, J. P. Wigand, et al.: Galactorrhea-amenorrhea syndrome: Follow-up of forty-five patients after pituitary tumor removal. Arch. Intern. Med. **94** (1981) 300–307.
[7] Zervas, N. T., J. B. Martin: Management of hormone secreting pituitary adenomas. N. Engl. J. Med. **302** (1980) 210–214.

Long-term follow-up of prolactinomas. Clinical and morphologic correlation

S. L. Aleshire, V. E. Cruz, C. A. Bradley, F. F. Parl

Introduction

During the past decade the development of radioimmunoassays for human prolactin has led to better understanding of the galactorrhea-amenorrhea syndrome. Recognition of prolactin-secreting tumours (prolactinomas) of the pituitary now accounts for a large portion of cases of secondary amenorrhea [9]. Concomitant with this evolution has been the advent of newer surgical and medical treatment methods such as the refinement of transsphenoidal hypophysectomy and pharmaceuticals which inhibit prolactin secretion. Little information is available, however, regarding the clinical outcome of prolactin secreting tumours [10]. In order to further define the course of prolactinomas we reviewed the clinical information, biochemical data and pathologic material of patients with these tumours seen at our institution.

Materials and methods

Information on patients with clinically manifested pituitary tumours was retrieved by review of surgical pathology records at Vanderbilt University Hospital for the period 1972–1982. Radioimmunoassay for prolactin followed the method of Hwang et al. [5]. Other pituitary hormones were measured by specific radioimmunoassay [3, 7, 8]. Patients with elevated growth hormone levels were excluded from the study. Patients were initially evaluated by either pneumonecephalography or computed axial tomography. Patients who were found to have prolactin secreting adenomas were divided into two groups according to whether radiologically their tumours were microadenomas (less than 10 mm) or macroadenomas (greater than 10 mm) [6]. Hospital and out-patient clinical treatment charts were reviewed on all patients. Those patients having prolactinomas were then personally contacted and questioned for current symptoms attributable to their pituitary tumours. Tissue immunoperoxidase staining was performed on the pathologic material obtained at surgery using the peroxidase antiperoxidase (PAP) method with antibodies to human prolactin, growth hormone, and adrenocorticotrophic hormone (Dako Corp.,

Santa Barbara, California, USA). A semi-quantitative assessment using 0–4+ scale (no staining to most intense staining) of overall microscopic tumour prolactin content was made by three independent observers. Statistical analysis was performed using the paired t-test for significance of differences of means. Chi-square analysis with Yates' correction was used in comparison of dichotomous variables.

Results

During the study interval 132 patients presented to our institution who were subsequently found to have clinically manifested pituitary tumours (tab. 1). There were

Table 1 Patients with clinically manifested pituitary tumours (January 1972 – December 1982)

	Women		Men	
Tumour type	No. of patients (Percentage)	Mean age at Diagnosis (range)	No. of patients (Percentage)	Mean age at Diagnosis (range)
Prolactin	21 (29)	29.7 (19–43)	8 (14)	37.9 (13–70)
Growth hormone	11 (15)	42.8 (27–68)	20 (34)	38.6 (16–70)
ACTH	28 (38)	40.5 (17–71)	10 (17)	46.7 (17–72)
Other*	13 (18)	54.9 (50–76)	21 (35)	50.1 (17–72)
Total	73 (100)	42.0 (17–76)	59 (100)	43.3 (13–72)

* This group is composed of cases which were not reactive by immunohistochemistry.

73 women and 59 men (no prepubertal patients were seen). Acromegaly was predominant in males, while Cushing's disease and prolactinomas were more commonly seen in women. The mean age of all patients was 42.6 years. The mean duration of follow-up of all patients was 61.9 ± 6.8 months (standard error of the mean, SEM).

The 21 women with prolactinomas averaged 29.7 years of age (tab. 2), and had average durations of amenorrhea of 5.1 years and galactorrhea of 4.1 years. The mean preoperative prolactin level in females was 356 ng/ml. Thyroid stimulating hormone was normal in the twelve women assayed, however, eight women had depressed luteinizing hormone levels. Follicle stimulating hormone was normal in all but one of the women surveyed. Twelve patients had microadenomas and 9 had macroadenomas (tab. 3). The ages at diagnosis for these two groups were not statistically different, while the duration of symptoms were significantly different (p <

Table 2 Clinical and laboratory findings in 21 women with prolactinoma

Age at onset	29.7*	
Duration of amenorrhoea (N = 19)	5.1 years	
Duration of galactorrhoea (N = 18)	4.1 years	
TSH (N = 12)	2.3 (1.1–4.5)	(normal: less than 8 μU/ml)
LH (N = 12)	7.8 (2.2–19)	(normal: 8–25 mlU/ml)
FSH (N = 11)	6.1 (2.0–10.9)	(normal: 3–15 mlU/ml)

* Mean (range, where indicated); N = number of patients.

Table 3 Pre- and postoperative data in women with prolactinoma according to tumour size

	Microadenomas (N = 12)	Macroadenomas (n = 9)	Significance
Pre-operative			
Age at diagnosis (years)	28.7 ± 2.3*	30.8 ± 2.7	NS
Duration of symptoms (years)	2.7 ± 0.5	8.1 ± 1.6	p<0.01
Serum prolactin (ng/ml)	187 ± 47	937 ± 295	p<0.02
Post-operative			
No recurrence	11	0	
Recurrence	1	9	
Tumour free interval (months)	55	23.4 ± 4.9	

* Values expressed as mean ± standard error of mean; NS = not significant

0.01). The preoperative prolactin values were also significantly different ($p < 0.02$) between the groups. Ten of the twelve patients with microadenomas underwent neurosurgical removal of their tumour. Although none of these recurred, one patient treated medically with dopamine agonists had tumor recurrence after 55 months. Another patient had tumour persistence despite medical treatment. All patients with macroadenomas underwent neurosurgery as their primary therapy. Eight women experienced tumour recurrence as determined by radiologic examination at an average interval of 23.4 ± 4.9 months (SEM) postoperatively. The mean prolactin levels at relapse was 436 ng/ml. Women with microadenomas who regained menses did so at 10 months (average), while macroadenoma patients required 24 months for return of menses.

The average age at diagnosis of the men was 34.7 years (tab. 4). Five men experienced secondary sexual symptoms (diminished libido, impotence, or gynecomastia). Six men had extrasellar extension as compared to less than half the women having this finding. Thyroid stimulating hormone was normal in all men. Luteinizing hormone was low in two men, and follicle stimulating hormone was also decreased in the four men assayed.

Table 4 Clinical and laboratory findings in 8 men with prolactinoma

		Mean	
Age at onset		34.7	
Secondary sexual symptoms		5 patients	
Testosterone	(N = 4)	1.7	(normal: 2–11 ng/ml)
TSH	(N = 4)	2.3	(normal: less than 8 μU/ml)
LH	(N = 4)	8.3	(normal: 6.1–9.7 mIU/ml)
FSH	(N = 4)	3.4	(normal: 5.8–16.6 mIU/ml

Table 5 Pre- and postoperative data in men with prolactinoma according to tumour size

	Microadenomas (N = 1)	Macroadenomas (N = 7)
Pre-operative		
Age	29.5	40.1 ± 9.9*
Prolactin (ng/ml)	90	1129 ± 481
Post-operative		
No recurrence	1	3
Recurrence	0	4
Tumour free interval (months)	–	8.5 ± 1.8

* Values expressed as mean ± standard error of mean

One man had a microadenoma and seven men had macroadenomas (tab. 5). There was no significant age difference between the groups. The microadenoma patient had an initial prolactin of 90 ng/ml. The seven men with macroadenomas had mean preoperative prolactin levels of 1129 ng/ml. Four of the seven had recurrence of their tumour within 8.5 months of their surgery.

Microadenoma patients as a group (both females and males) had mean preoperative prolactin levels of 180 ng/ml, whereas those with macroadenomas had serum levels of 1021 ng/ml ($p < 0.02$). Thirteen patients (81%) with macroadenomas (combined sexes) experienced postsurgical tumour recurrence, while only one patient with a microadenoma (8%) developed clinical and radiologic evidence of recurrence, ($p < 0.01$). The tumour free interval was 55 months for the microadenoma patient, and 18.8 months for those with recurrent tumour. The mean preoperative serum prolactin level of all patients with recurrent tumour was 1006 ng/ml compared to 304 ng/ml in those without recurrence. The mean postoperative serum prolactin at the time of recurrence was 340 ng/ml.

Light microscopic examination of the pituitary tumours showed well-preserved cytoarchitecture and minimal to mild cytologic atypia [2]. Most tumours had combined patterns of sinusoidal and diffuse growth. Cellular prolactin demonstrated by PAP staining revealed that tumour prolactin content was generally proportional to preoperative serum prolactin levels. Tissue staining judged to be 0–1+ correlated with serum levels of 0–200 ng/ml; 2–3+ staining was found to represent serum levels of 200–500 ng/ml; 4+ staining ws indicative of levels greater than 500 ng/ml. Growth hormone and adrenocorticotrophic hormone staining was minimal in the neoplastic cell population.

Discussion

Recognition of prolactinomas as an important cause of the galactorrhea-amenorrhea syndrome has led to the development of a variety of contemporary treatment approaches [1, 4, 10, 12, 13]. Attention has been drawn to the re-emergence of hyperprolactinemia after therapy [10, 12], however, the frequency of frank tumour recurrence is unclear [4, 14]. Our data indicate that despite adequate therapy prolactinomas recur more frequently than has been previously recognized. Close postoperative monitoring is therefore necessary to assure prompt therapy of recurrences, a consideration of particular importance with macroadenomas [11].

The morphology of the normal and neoplastic pituitary has been exhaustively studied during the past decade [2]. The usefulness of immunohistochemistry in demonstrating tumour prolactin content is evident in our ability to closely correlate tumour antigen density with serum prolactin levels. This technique can be used in the identification and follow-up of patients with pituitary tumours in cases where serum prolactin assays may not have been performed.

Recognition of the relatively frequent rate of recurrence of prolactinomas emphasizes the need for a means of predicting tumour behaviour. Tumours which were larger than 10 mm at presentation were associated with higher serum prolactin levels and more frequent recurrence rates than smaller tumours. Serum prolactin levels exceeding 40 ng/ml very frequently were indicative of tumour recurrence within two years. These findings are in keeping with the return of hyperprolactinemia after treatment observed by other investigators [6, 10, 12] in patients having relatively higher initial prolactin values.

References

[1] Corenblum, B., P. J. Taylor: Long term follow-up of hyperprolactinemic women treated with bromocriptine. Fert. Steril. **40** (1983) 596–599.

[2] Ezrin, C., et al.: Pathology of the adenohypophysis. In: Endocrine Pathology, General and Surgical (J. M. B. Bloodworth, ed.), second edition, pp. 101–132. William and Wilkins, Baltimore 1982.

[3] Faiman, C., R. J. Ryan: Radioimmunoassay for human luteinizing hormone. Proc. Soc. Exp. Biol. Med. **125** (1967) 1130–1133.

[4] Frantz, A. G., et al.: Long-term evaluation of the results of transsphenoidal surgery and radiotherapy in patients with prolactinoma. In: Endocrinology of Human Infertility: New Aspects (P. Crosignani, B. L. Rubin, eds.), pp. 161–170. Academic Press, London 1981. (Sereno Clinical Colloquia on Reproduction No. 2).

[5] Hwang, P., et al.: A radioimmunoassay for human prolactin. Proc. Nat. Acad. Sci. **68** (1971) 1902–1906.
[6] Jaffe, R. B.: Physiologic and pathophysiologic aspects of prolactin production in humans. In: Prolactin (R. B. Jaffe, ed.), pp. 181–217. Elsevier, New York 1981.
[7] Midgley, A. R.: Radioimmunoassay for human follicle-stimulating hormone. J. Clin. Endocrinol. **27** (1967) 295–299.
[8] Powell, D. A.: Radioligand assays for pituitary gonadotropins. In: Hormones in Human Blood, Detection and Assay (H. N. Antoniades, ed.), pp. 401–422. Harvard Press, Cambridge 1976.
[9] Reichlin, S.: The prolactinoma problem (editorial). New Engl. J. Med. **300** (1979) 313–315.
[10] Serri, O., et al.: Recurrence of hyperprolactinemia after selective transsphenoidal adenomectomy in women with prolactinoma. New Engl. J. Med. **309** (1983) 280–283.
[11] Spada, A., et al.: In vitro studies on prolactin release and adenylate cyclase activity in human prolactin-secreting pituitary adenomas. Different sensitivity of macro- and microadenomas to dopamine and vasoactive intestinal polypeptide. J. Clin. Endocrinol. Metab. **56** (1983) 1–10.
[12] Tucker, H. St. G., et al.: Galactorrhea-amenorrhea syndrome: follow-up of forty-five patients after pituitary tumor removal. Ann. Int. Med. **94** (1981) 302–307.
[13] von Werder, K., et al.: Treatment of hyperprolactinemia. In: Frontiers in Neuroendocrinology (W. F. Ganong, L. Martini, eds.), vol. 7, pp. 123–159. Raven Press, New York 1982.
[14] Zarate, A., et al.: Follow-up of patients with prolactinomas after discontinuation of long-term therapy with bromocriptine. Acta Endocrinol. **104** (1983) 139–142.

Clinicopathological and neurosurgical comparative analysis of operated recurrent prolactinomas and non-secreting chromophobe pituitary adenomas

N. Roosen, W. J. Bock

Recurrence of operated pituitary adenomas is rather frequent. Its rate varies between 4.8 and 42.5% because of different reasons such as the biological nature of the tumour, the volume of the adenoma, the surgical technique, the use of the operating microscope, post-operative radiotherapy, the length of follow-up, etc. [1–10].

During the past two and a half years 107 patients with pituitary adenoma were operated in our clinic, comprising a group of 10 patients treated surgically at a previous occasion. All these cases were chromophobe pituitary adenomas. Endocrinologically, we can distinguish four prolactinomas, three cases with borderline hyperprolactinaemia and three normoprolactinaemic cases. The three patients with borderline hyperprolactinaemia were women, whereas all other patients were men. The median age at the time of the first operation was 45 years with a range between 30 and 61 years.

The four prolactinoma patients (tab. 1), who all were men, presented with visual field loss. Three of them had reduced visual acuity and one had diplopia due to a sixth cranial nerve paresis. Endocrinologically, one patient was asymptomatic, whereas the other patients had hypopituitarism. In case 1 the tumour was completely intrasellar, the others showed extrasellar expansion, so marked in case 2 that a transcranial reoperation was necessary, although the other cases could be managed very well transsphenoidally. The recurrences were heralded by reappearing neuroophthalmological signs. All recurrent tumours had suprasellar expansion, operated by a transsphenoidal approach in cases 1 and 3 and transcranially in the other two. The adenomas, recurring after five and four years, cases 1 and 2 respectively, were pathologically benign. In case 3 the recurrent adenoma showed a moderately elevated mitotic activity: this could explain the rapid regrowth with the need for a second operation after only one year. In case 4 moderate anaplasia and elevated mitotic activity were already noted at the occasion of the first operation. This patient had two recurrences: each three years after the previous operation. The last two patients were treated with radiotherapy. Cases 1, 3 and 4 were treated with bromocriptine, which has not prevented, however, a second recurrence in case 4.

Table 1 Recurrent prolactinoma in four men

	Age at 1st operation	PRL+ (ng/ml)	Pituitary insufficiency as presenting sign	Pathology	Recurrence after	Operative treatment
Case 1	30 yrs	1. 120.0 2. 2600	+	benign	5 yrs	1. TS*, radical 2. TS, radical
Case 2	37 yrs	1. 650.0 2. –	–	benign	4 yrs	1. TS, TC°, radical 2. TC, radical
Case 3	56 yrs	1. 367.6 2. 358.8	+++	mitoses	1 yr	1. TS, radical 2. TS, radical
Case 4	51 yrs	1. – 2. 1600 3. 660.0	++	mitoses anaplasia	1. 3 yrs 2. 3 yrs	1. TS, radical 2. TC, subtotal 3. TC, subtotal

+: PRL: prolactin
*: TS: transsphenoidal
°: TC: transcranial

The three cases with borderline hyperprolactinaemia are shown in table 2. These women presented with a narrowed visual field and one of them also had reduced visual acuity (case 7). Case 6 and case 7 showed hypopituitarism. In case 6 the adenoma had no extrasellar expansion, whereas in case 7 its growth was even parasellar. The tumours were radically operated by a transcranial or transsphenoidal approach. Subtotal extirpations were performed in some cases of recurrent tumours: the adenoma expanded markedly infra- and suprasellarly in case 6, and was very invasive in case 7 with infiltration of bone and nervous tissue. Pathologically, the first two cases of this group were benign. Case 7, however, showed cellular anaplasia and mitotic activity from the beginning, and even more pronounced in the following biopsy specimens. This patient was treated with two courses of radiotherapy.

The normoprolactinaemic patients are presented in the third table (tab. 3). The first patient complained of headache, whereas the other two showed typical neuroophthalmological signs such as reduced visual acuity and loss of visual field. No presenting signs of pituitary insufficiency were found. Cases 8 and 10 presented with an intrasellar adenoma, whereas the recurrent tumours had suprasellar expansion in the three patients and the second recurrence in Case 10 was even parasellar. The tumours were removed by transcranial or transsphenoidal operative proce-

Table 2 Recurrent chromophobe pituitary adenoma with borderline hyperprolactinaemia in three women

	Age at 1st operation	PRL⁺ (ng/ml)	Pituitary insufficiency as presenting sign	Pathology	Recurrence after	Operative treatment
Case 5	61 yrs	1. – 2. 26.0	–	benign	10 yrs	1. TC°, radical 2. TC, radical
Case 6	34 yrs	1. – 2. – 3. 27.0 4. 20.5	+	benign	1. 2 yrs 2. 5 yrs 3. 1 yr	1. TC, radical 2. TS*, radical 3. TS, subtotal 4. TC, subtotal
Case 7	56 yrs	1. – 2. – 3. 35.2 4. –	+	mitoses anaplasia	1. 4 yrs 2. 1/2 yr 3. 2 yrs	1. TC, radical 2. TC, TS, radical 3. TC, subtotal 4. TC, subtotal

⁺: PRL: prolactin
*: TS: transsphenoidal
°: TC: transcranial

Table 3 Recurrent chromophobe pituitary adenoma with normoprolactinaemia in three men

	Age at 1st operation	PRL⁺ (ng/ml)	Pituitary insufficiency as presenting sign	Pathology	Recurrence after	Operative treatment
Case 8	37 yrs	1. 7.5 2. 1.7	–	benign	5 yrs	1. TS*, radical 2. TS, subtotal
Case 9	48 yrs	1. – 2. 8.6	–	benign	7 yrs	1. TC°, radical 2. TC, subtotal
Case 10	41 yrs	1. – 2. 1.5 3. 2.5	–	benign	1. 7 yrs 2. 7 yrs	1. TC, radical 2. TS, subtotal 3. TC, subtotal

⁺: PRL: prolactin
*: TS: transsphenoidal
°: TC: transcranial

dures, radically at the occasion of the first operation and subtotally in the case of recurrence. All of these adenomas were pathologically benign.

In reviewing these 10 patients, we can separate the pituitary adenomas with borderline hyperprolactinaemia: they constitute an individual group with a very late recurrence in case 5 and marked dedifferentiation in case 7. Borderline hyperprolactinaemia can be caused by prolactinoma, but by impairment of prolactin inhibiting factor as well. Whether any of our three cases is a prolactinoma is not clear because immunocytochemical studies were not performed. For that reason no valid conclusions can be made about these three patients.

The first four patients, however, have prolactinomas and the last three patients have non-secreting chromophobe adenomas. Corresponding with previous findings, which suggested a worse overall cure rate for prolactinomas in men than in women [11–14], all these patients are men. The prolactinomas recurred earlier than the normoprolactinaemic adenomas (tab. 1 and 3). Because all adenomas were radically extirpated at the time of their first operation, other reasons for this difference must be sought. Maybe the known propensity of pituitary adenomas for the invasion of mesodermal tissues [15] is more pronounced in prolactinomas. This is particularly obvious in patients 3 and 4, in whom the adenomas were dedifferentiated and in whom they were invasive, according to Hardy and Vezina's criteria [16, 17]. This parallels Robert's findings, who reported mitoses in 27% of prolactinomas in a series of 40 men, occurring exclusively in large or diffusely infiltrating prolactinomas [18]. On the other hand, Lundberg et al. could not find any cytological difference between invasive and non-invasive adenomas [19].

All of these features contrast the recurrent prolactinomas with the recurrent normoprolactinaemic chromophobe adenomas, and support the hypothesis that prolactinomas are more malignant and more invasive in their biological behaviour than non-secreting chromophobe pituitary adenomas, and are recurring earlier. Recurrence in pituitary adenomas should be studied further to clarify these points.

References

[1] Henderson, W. R.: The pituitary adenomata. A follow-up study of the results in 338 cases (Dr. Harvey Cushing's series). Br. J. Surg. **26** (1939) 811–912.
[2] Ray, B., R. H. Pattersson, jr.: Symposium on pituitary tumors. I. Surgical treatment of pituitary adenomas. J. Neurosurg. **19** (1962) 1–8.
[3] Martins, A. N., L. G. Kempe, G. J. Hayes: Pituitary adenomas. Concepts based on twelve years experience at Walter Reed General Hospital. Acta Neurochir. **13** (1965) 469–494.
[4] Elkington, S. G., W. McKissock: Pituitary adenoma. Results of combined surgical and radiotherapeutic treatment of 200 patients. Br. med. J. **i** (1967) 263–266.
[5] Olivecrona, H.: The surgical treatment of intracranial tumours. In: Handbuch der Neurochirurgie (H. Olivecrona, W. Tönnis, eds.), Vol. IV/4, pp. 1–301. Springer Verlag, Berlin–Heidelberg–New York 1967.

[6] Svien, H. J., M. Y. Colby, jr.: Treatment for chromophobe adenomas. C. C. Thomas (Publisher), Springfield (Illinois) 1967.
[7] Wirth, F. P., H. G. Schwartz, P. R. Schwetschenau: Pituitary adenomas. Factors in treatment. Clin. Neurosurg. **21** (1974) 8–25.
[8] Muhr, C., K. Bergström, R. Hugosson et al.: Pituitary adenomas: computed tomography and clinical evaluation in a follow-up after surgical treatment. Eur. Neurol. **19** (1980) 171–179.
[9] Salmi, J., B. Grahne, S. Valtonen et al.: Recurrence of pituitary adenomas after operation and postoperative radiotherapy. Acta. Neurol. Scand. **66** (1982) 681–689.
[10] Symon, L., V. Logue, S. Mohanty: Recurrence of pituitary adenomas after transcranial operation. J. Neurol. Neurosurg. Psychiatry. **45** (1982) 780–785.
[11] Carter, J. N., J. E. Tyson, G. V. Tolis et al.: Prolactin secreting tumors and hypogonadism in men. New. Engl. J. Med. **299** (1978) 847–852.
[12] Hardy, J., H. Beauregard, F. Robert: Prolactin secreting adenomas: transsphenoidal microsurgical treatment. In: Progress in prolactin physiology and pathology (C. Robyn, M. Harte, eds.), pp. 361–370. Elsevier/North Holland Biomedical Press, Amsterdam 1978.
[13] Nabarro, J. D. N.: Pituitary surgery for endocrine disorders. Clin. Endocrinol. **13** (1980) 285–298.
[14] Pelkonen, R., B. Grahne, E. Hirvonen et al.: Pituitary function in prolactinoma. Effect of surgery and postoperative bromocriptine therapy. Clin. Endocrinol. **14** (1981) 335–348.
[15] Russell, D. S., L. J. Rubinstein: Pathology of tumours of the nervous system. 4th ed., p. 313. Edward Arnold (Publishers) Ltd., London 1977.
[16] Hardy, J., J. L. Vezina: Transsphenoidal neurosurgery of intracranial neoplasms. Adv. Neurol. **15** (1967) 261–274.
[17] Vezina, J. L.: Le prolactinome. Aspects radiologiques de la selle turcique. Neurochirurgie **27** (1981) Suppl. 1, 19–28.
[18] Robert, F.: Le prolactinome. Aspects pathologiques. Neurochirurgie **27** (1981) Suppl. 1, 61–73.
[19] Lundberg, P. O., B. Drettner, A. Hemmingsson et al.: The invasive pituitary adenoma. A prolactin-producing tumor. Arch. Neurol. **34** (1977) 742–749.

V Pharmacotherapy

New aspects of medical treatment of prolactinomas

K. von Werder, T. Eversmann, R. Landgraf, H. K. Rjosk

Hyperprolactinaemia, the most common hypothalamic-pituitary disorder in man may be caused by three different mechanisms [1].

1. Autonomous prolactin (PRL) secretion by a pituitary adenoma (prolactinoma).
2. Reduced or absent dopamine effect on the lactotroph cell.
3. Stimulation of the lactotroph cell overriding physiological inhibition.

All hyperprolactinaemic patients in whom drug induced elevation of PRL-levels, renal failure or hypothyroidism has been excluded most likely harbour a prolactinoma. The latter is supported by the findings of Jung et al. [2] who demonstrated microadenomas with high resolution CT in 15 out of 16 hyperprolactinaemic women with a normal or equivocal radiological sella turcica. Though there may be patients with what is called "functional hyperprolactinemia", we are still unable to make the differential diagnosis between these two entities [3]. For clinical purposes the latter is of no importance since the management of both clinical situations is identical.

Spontaneous development of hyperprolactinaemia

There is very little difference in the morphology of small adenomas and invasive macroprolactinomas [4]. However, the spontaneous clinical course may be very different, which has to be considered if the decision about management of these patients is to be made. Thus, the majority of patients with hyperprolactinaemia and a normal sella turcica or proven microprolactinoma have prolactin levels which remain within the same range over an observation period of up to 10 years [5]. This is in obvious contrast to the development of large invasive macro-prolactinomas which often have only a short history of symptoms related to hyperprolactinaemia [1].

Medical therapy of prolactinomas

Egot derivatives with long-lasting dopaminergic activity have been used for the treatment of hyperprolactinaemia. The greatest experience has been obtained with bromocriptine which belongs to the lysergic acid amides and contains a tripeptide [1]. Lisuride and mesulergin (Cu 32-085) belong to the 8α-aminoergoline family whereas pergolide, a very potent prolactin inhibitor, belongs to the clavines family [1].

All these substances lead to dopamine receptor stimulation and inhibition of PRL-secretion without uterotonic and vascular effects which are found in other ergot alkaloids [1]. Moderately elevated PRL-levels in patients with normal sella turcica or a radiologically apparent microprolactinoma are generally normalized with moderate DA-agonist dosages [1, 5]. Though the PRL lowering efficacy of DA-agonists can be even more pronounced in patients with very high prolactin levels [5], PRL-levels are not always normalized if they are above 1000 ng/ml, even if bromocriptine dosages up to 40 mg and more per day are used [1, 5]. This great variability in the responsiveness of PRL-secretion to dopaminergic suppression is also demonstrated during acute dopamine infusion [6]. Evidence has been presented, that the addition of tamoxifen, an estrogen antagonist, may improve the responsiveness to bromocriptine in selected cases [7]. However, this treatment has not been tried yet in a larger number of patients.

In addition to normalization of PRL-secretion, a reduction in tumour mass is an important therapeutical goal in patients with microprolactinomas. Since it has been shown that DA-agonists may lead to a dramatic reduction in tumour volume in the majority of patients with macroprolactinomas and extensive suprasellar extension [8, 9, 10, 11], primary medical therapy has become generally accepted in patients with prolactinomas.

Tumour shrinking effect of DA-agonists

Eight years ago reports describing a reduction in adenoma size after DA-agonist therapy documented by conventional X-ray have been published (for review see [1, 5]). The tumour shrinking effect of DA-agonists in humans became more clear, when the regression of suprasellar adenoma extension could be shown by CT [8]. DA-agonist induced tumour reduction may occur within days [12]. Initially, the rapidity of the tumour shrinkage suggested that tumour apoplexy may be responsible for this phenomenon. However, it could be shown, that bromocriptine leads to a reduction in lactotroph cell volume and decrease in cytoplasmic structures responsible for prolactin synthesis [13, 14]. Whether the morphometrically demonstrated reduction in cell volume is the only mechanism of tumour shrinkage is still open, since cell size reduction was also observed in those patients who had no demonstrable adenoma reduction [15]. It would explain however, that prolactinomas can reexpand after DA-agonist withdrawal and shrink again in a rapid fashion after reinstitution of DA-therapy (fig. 1), which cannot be explained by a cytotoxic effect of DA-agonists. However, persisting suppression of PRL-secretion after long-term treatment with dopamine agonists has been observed [16]. Recently, Winkelmann et al. reported persistent normalization of PRL-levels after long-term bromocriptine treatment and withdrawal in patients with microprolactinomas [17].

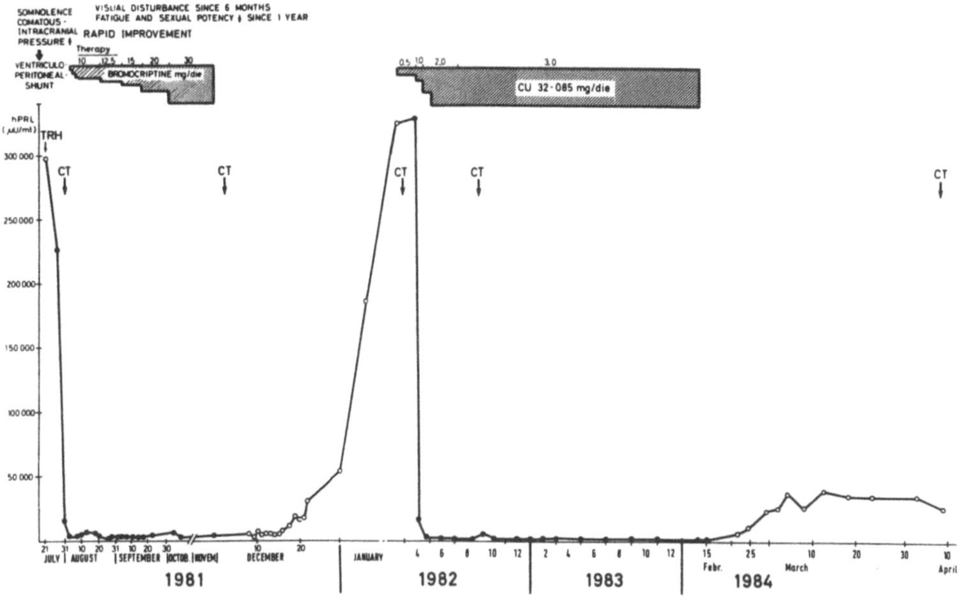

Fig. 1 DA-agonist therapy in a patient with a macroprolactinoma. After bromocriptine withdrawal, within one month a rapid increase in the PRL-levels up to the level before therapy is observed. After the administration of another dopamine agonist (CU 32-085) normalization of PRL-levels is achieved. The second withdrawal of DA-agonist treatment, which had been persued for two years, leads to a less rapid increase in PRL-level, which does not reach the pretreatment range during the observation period. Tumour shrinkage and tumour expansion was parallel to the prolactin levels (modified after von Werder et al., Raven Press, New York, 1984).

Adenoma shrinkage is also observed in those patients in whom PRL-secretion has not normalized during DA-agonist therapy (fig. 2). On the other hand, even complete normalization of prolactin levels in patients with macroprolactinomas does not imply changes in adenoma volume [18]. Several series have been published reporting the outcome of primary medical therapy of macroprolactinomas [8, 9, 10, 11], demonstrating that between 50 and 80% of all patients with macroprolactinomas will respond to DA-agonist therapy with adenoma shrinkage. However, until now it cannot be predicted which patient will respond and which patient will not benefit from medical therapy reducing the adenoma volume.

The recent report that DA-agonist therapy of longer duration may jeopardize the outcome of later neurosurgical intervention [19] has not been confirmed [20]. Proliferation of prolactinomas during DA-agonist therapy occurs very rarely [21]. We have observed one female patient who after neurosurgery, developed a spinal metastasis of her prolactinoma which was indicated by increasing PRL-levels despite increasing dosages of DA-agonists. This spinal metastasis turned out to be almost

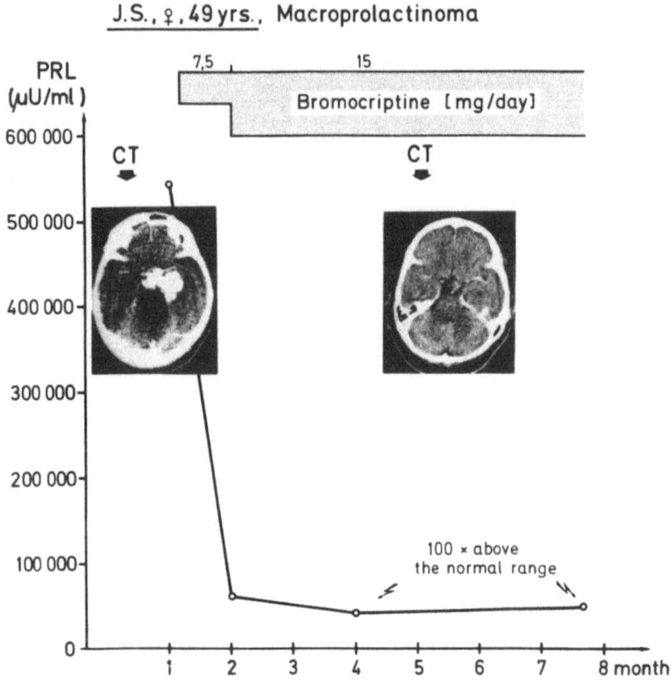

Fig. 2 Disappearance of suprasellar prolactinoma extension during bromocriptine therapy without normalization of PRL-levels. Though PRL-levels remain around 50,000 μU/ml during therapy (upper normal range 500 μU/ml) there is dramatic reduction in supra- and parasellar tumour extension documented by CT-scan during bromocriptine treatment.

completely unresponsive to DA-agonist therapy (fig. 3). Two further patients with documented prolactinoma metastases in the central nervous system have been reported [22, 23].

Operative treatment and radiotherapy

Though in patients with small microadenomas transsphenoidal surgery leads to normalization of PRL-levels in the majority of patients, very few patients with large prolactinomas have normal prolactin levels after operation [1, 5]. In addition, in patients with normalized PRL-levels after transsphenoidal surgery recurrences in up to 50% of the patients may occur [24].

Radiotherapy with 4500 rad has been applied to patients with hyperprolactinaemia. However, the efficacy of this treatment in lowering PRL-levels is poorly documented and varies in individual patients [1, 5]. Complete normalization of PRL-secretion after radiotherapy in patients with macroprolactinomas is rarely ob-

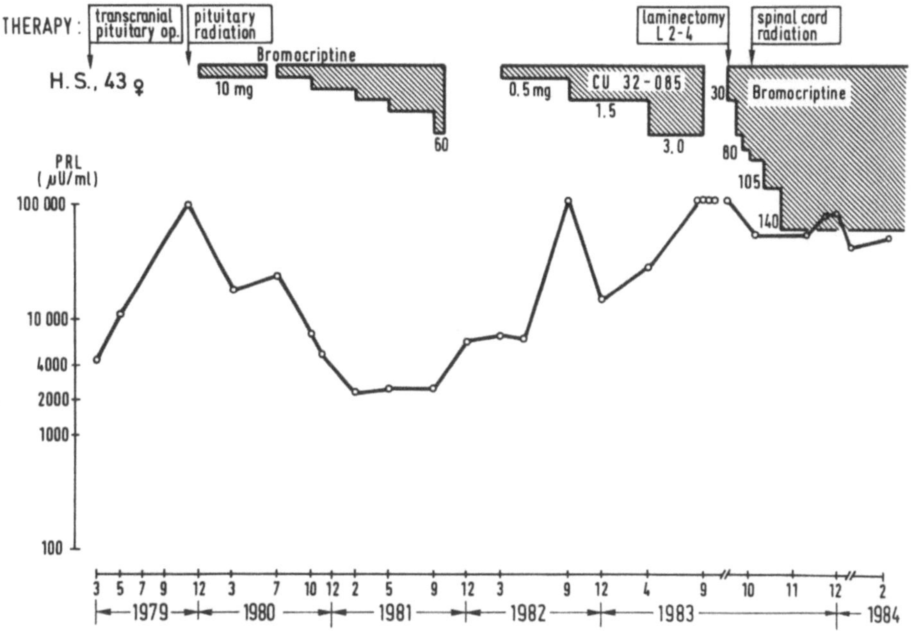

Fig. 3 Spinal metastasis of a pituitary prolactinoma after surgery and radiotherapy. Despite high dosages of bromocriptine PRL-levels remain elevated indicating the loss of dopamine receptors of the spinal tumour. The latter was shown to be a prolactinoma by immunohistochemistry. There was no adenoma recurrence detectable at cranial CT (R. Landgraf).

served [1]. Therefore, this therapy should be reserved for those patients who are inoperable and do not respond to DA-agonist treatment (tab. 1).

Table 1 Clinical appearance of prolactinomas

Parameter	Small adenoma ("microadenoma")	Large invasive macroadenoma
Sex distribution	mainly females	females/males
Proliferation rate	slow	rapid
Elevation of prolactin level	moderate	excessive
Visual field defects	none	frequent
Neurosurgery	mostly successful	no hPRL-normalization
DA-agonist therapy (normalization of hPRL-levels)	effective	effective
DA-agonist therapy (adenoma shrinkage)	?	50–80%
Persistent suppression after cessation of DA-agonist therapy	none	frequent

Pregnancy in prolactinoma patients

Pregnancy is an important therapeutical goal in hyperprolactinaemic females which can be achieved in the majority of cases with DA-agonist treatment [5, 25]. Those females, who do not show normalization of PRL-levels during DA-agonist therapy may be treated with pulsatile GnRH-administration. The latter has been shown to facilitate uneventful pregnancies in persistently hyperprolactinaemic patients [26]. Even in patients with large prolactinomas after surgery and radiotherapy and after a long-term treatment with bromocriptine who still have elevated prolactin levels and have severe hypogonadotropic hypogonadism, may respond to pulsatile GnRH treatment with restoration of follicular maturation (fig. 4).

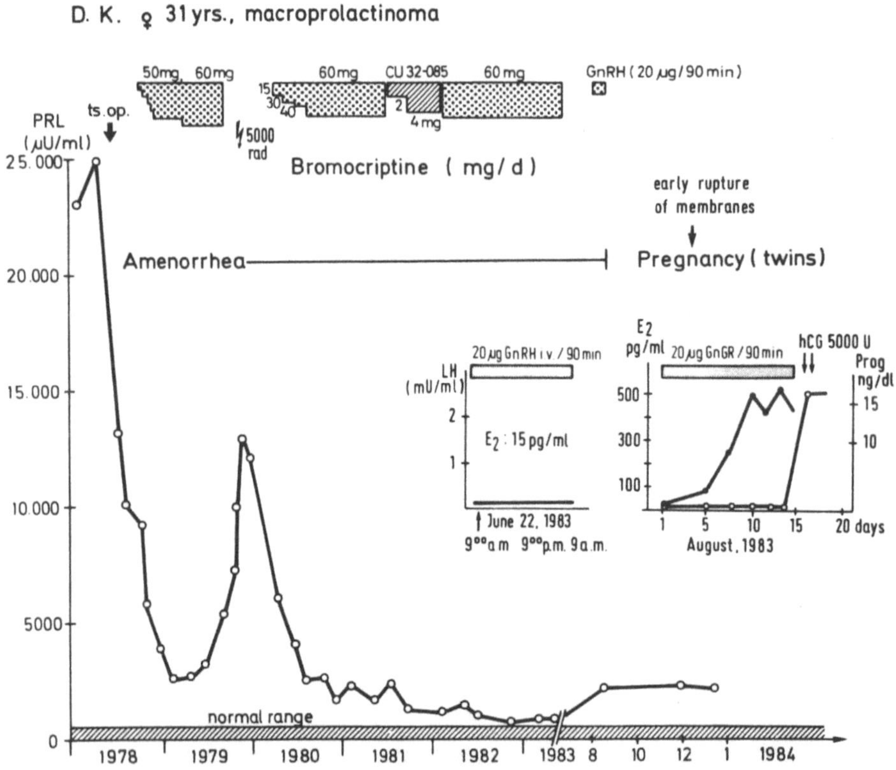

Fig. 4 Prolactin levels and gonadal function in a 31 year old patient with macroprolactinoma after transsphenoidal surgery, radiotherapy and long-term DA-agonist treatment. Since PRL-levels could not be normalized with the various forms of antiprolactinoma treatment, pulsatile administration of GnRH in order to restore gonadal function was performed. Though GnRH treatment in a dosage of 20 μg i.v. every 90 min did not lead to pulsatile LH-secertion in the presence of low oestrogens (June 22, 1983) continuous pulsatile treatment led to an increase in oestradiol and normal ovulation documented by a subsequent twin pregnancy (August, 1983).

However, women with prolactinomas may develop complications during pregnancy. Haemorrhagic phenomena inside the adenoma may lead to a sudden increase in adenoma size, leading to blindness, cranial nerve palsy or fatal intracranial haemorrhage (for review see [1]).

Magyar and Marshall [27] reported 91 pregnancies occurring in 73 women harbouring an untreated pituitary adenoma. In 14 patients symptoms like visual field disturbances or headaches were so severe that surgical intervention during pregnancy became necessary. However, only 4 patients who were operated and received radiotherapy later developed permanent mild visual field defects. This is in contrast to the rate of complications observed in females who had previous treatment directed towards the prolactinoma. In this group only 4% developed headaches and 5% visual field disturbances and only one patient required treatment during pregnancy.

Gemzell and Wang [28] reviewed the outcome of 217 pregnancies in 178 patients with pituitary adenoma. 25% of all patients with untreated macroprolactinoma suffered complications during pregnancy related to the pituitary tumour, whereas those with microprolactinomas had almost always uneventful pregnancies.

These observations are in agreement with the findings by Griffith et al. [29] who reported the course of 116 completed pregnancies in patients with prolactinomas. 8 patients developed visual field disturbances and in 9 pregnancies severe headaches were encountered.

Rjosk et al. [25] reported the outcome of 82 pregnancies in 62 of his own patients with hyperprolactinaemic anovulation. Thirty-four pregnancies occurred in patients with hyperprolactinaemia and a normal sella turcica and 25 pregnancies in patients with intrasellar prolactinomas. Though all patients were treated with bromocriptine only, no complications related to the sella turcica were observed. Thus, patients with intrasellar adenomas and no evidence of suprasellar extension before pregnancy do not experience adverse symptoms during pregnancy if hyperprolactinaemic sterility is treated with DA-agonists or GnRH only. The PRL-levels during pregnancy may differ widely in individual patients [25]. However, even though steep increases in PRL-levels during pregnancy may signal enhanced oestrogen sensitivity, the fact that PRL-levels 3 months after pregnancy are within the same range as before pregnancy excludes persistent adenoma growth [25].

In contrast, resolution of hyperprolactinaemia after pregnancy can be observed. In 6 out of 62 patients a sudden decrease in the PRL-levels was observed after an initial increase in PRL-secretion after bromocriptine withdrawal in the first trimester of pregnancy [25]. Resumption of ovulatory cycles after termination of pregnancy in these patients documents that the anterior pituitary lobe has not been affected and hyperprolactinaemia has selectively disappeared (tab. 2).

Table 2 Therapy of prolactinomas

	Normal sella	Microadenoma or small adenoma	Large (invasive adenoma
Medical therapy	+++	+++	+++
Transsphenoidal surgery	∅	++	+++ (before pregnancy) ++ (after medical therapy)
Radiotherapy	∅	∅	++ (no response to DA-therapy)
Observation only	++ (no clinical symptoms)	++ (no clinical symptoms)	∅

In patients with macroprolactinomas extending into the sphenoid sinus and into the suprasellar area surgery before pregnancy is necessary in order to prevent complications during pregnancy [1, 5, 25]. Since operative results are less satisfying in larger adenomas, persisting hyperprolactinaemia has to be treated postoperatively with DA-agonists. Occasionally large doses of bromocriptine have to be given over a long period of time to normalize high postoperative PRL-levels [1, 5]. However, also in these patients radical neurosurgical intervention is not advisable, since gonadotrophic function may deteriorate after surgery even though PRL-levels have become normal.

References

[1] Flückinger, F., E. del Pozo, K. von Werder: Prolactin physiology, pharmacology and clinical findings. In: Monographs in Endocrinology, Vol. 23. Springer, Berlin–Heidelberg–New York 1982.
[2] Jung, R. T., M. C. White, N. B. Bowley, et al.: CT abnormalities of the pituitary in hyperprolactinemic women with normal or equivocal sellae radiologically. Brit. Med. J. **285** (1982) 1078–1081.
[3] Editiorial: Hyperprolactinemia: Pituitary tumor or not? Lancet **2** (1980) 517–519.
[4] Robert, F.: Morphology of human prolactinomas: A study of invasive prolactin secreting adenomas. In: Prolactin and Prolactinomas (G. Tollis, C. Stefanis; T. Mountokalakis, F. Labrie, eds.), pp. 339–349. Raven Press, New York 1983.
[5] von Werder, K., T. Eversmann, R. Fahlbusch and H. K. Rjosk: Treatment of hyperprolactinemia. In: Frontiers in Neuroendocrinology (W. F. Ganong, L. Martini, eds.), pp. 123–159. Raven Press, New York 1982.

[6] Connell, J. M. C., P. L. Padfield, E. A. Bunting, et al.: Inhibition of prolactin secretion by low-dose dopamine infusion in patients with hyperprolactinemia. Clin. Endocrinol. **18** (1983) 527–532.
[7] Völker, W., W. G. Gehring, R. Berning, et al.: Impaired pituitary response to bromocriptine suppression: Reversal after bromocriptine + tamoxifen. Acta endocr. **101** (1982) 491–500.
[8] Chiodini, P. G., A. Liuzzi, R. Cozzi, et al.: Size reduction of macroprolactinomas by bromocriptine or lisuride treatment. J. Clin. Endocr. **53** (1981) 737–743.
[9] Wass, J. A. H., J. Williams, M. Charlesworth, et al.: Bromocriptine in management of large pituitary tumors. Brit. Med. J. **284** (1982) 1908–1911.
[10] Wollesen, F., T. Andersen, A. Karle: Size reduction of extrasellar pituitary tumors during bromocriptine treatment. Ann. Intern. Med. **96** (1982) 281–286.
[11] del Pozo, E., L. Gerber, S. Hunziker: Response to bromocriptine therapy in 115 prolactinoma cases. In: Prolactin and Prolactinomas (G. Tollis, C. Stefanis, T. Mountokalakis, F. Labrie, eds.), pp. 403–414. Raven Press, New York 1983.
[12] Thorner, M. O., R. L. Perryman, A. D. Rogol, et al.: Rapid changes of prolactinoma volume after withdrawal and reinstitution of bromocriptine. J. Clin. Endocrinol. **53** (1981) 480–483.
[13] Tindall, G. T., K. Kovacs, E. Horvath, et al.: Human prolactin producing adenomas and bromocriptine: A histological immunocytochemical, ultrastructural and morphometric study. J. Clin. Endocrinol. Metab. **55** (1982) 1178–1183.
[14] Basetti, M., A. Spada, G. Pezzo, et al.: Bromocriptine treatment reduces the cell size in human macroprolactinomas: A morphometric study. J. Clin. Endocrinol. Metab. **58** (1984) 268–273.
[15] Nissim, M., B. Ambrosi, V. Bernasconi, et al.: Bromocriptine treatment of macroprolactinomas: Studies on the time course of tumor shrinkage and morphology. J. Endocrinol. Invest. **5** (1982) 409–415.
[16] Eversmann, T., R. Fahlbusch, H. K. Rjosk: Persisting suppression of prolactin secretion after longterm treatment with bromocriptine in patients with prolactinomas. Acta Endocrinol. **92** (1979) 413–427.
[17] Winkelmann, W., Allolio, B., D. Heesen, et al.: TRH-stimulated prolactin release in patients with prolactinoma during longterm treatment with bromocriptine or lisuride. Acta Endocrinol. (Khb) **102** (1983) Suppl. 253, 37–38.
[18] von Werder, K.: Prolactinomas. An overview. In: Proceedings of the 3rd Europ. Workshop on Pituitary Adenomas, Amsterdam 1983. Blackwel Publications, Oxford 1984 (in press).
[19] Landolt, A. M., P. J. Keller, E. R. Frösch, et al.: Bromocriptine: Does it jeopardise the result of later surgery for prolactinomas? Lancet **2** (1982) 657–658.
[20] Faglia, G., P. Moriondo, P. Travaglini, et al.: Influence of previous bromocriptine therapy on surgery for microprolactinoma. Lancet **1** (1983) 133–134.
[21] Dallabonzana, D., B. Spelta, G. Oppizzi, et al.: Reenlargement of macroprolactinomas during bromocriptine treatment: Report of two cases. J. Endocrinol. Invest. **6** (1983) 47–50.
[22] Martin, N. A., M. Males, C. B. Wilson: Cerebellar metastasis from a prolactinoma during treatment with bromocriptine. J. Neurosurg. **55** (1981) 615–619.
[23] Cohen, D. L., J. V. Dienghdoh, D. G. T. Thomas, et al.: An intracranial metastasis from a PRL secreting pituitary tumour. Clin. Endocrinol. **18** (1983) 259–264.
[24] Serri, O., E. Rasio, H. Beauregard, et al.: Recurrence of Hyperprolactinemia after selective transsphenoidal adenomectomy in women with prolactinoma. N. Engl. J. Med. **309** (1983) 280–283.

[25] Rjosk, H. K., R. Fahlbusch, K. von Werder: Influence of pregnancies on prolactinomas. Acta Endocrinol. **100** (1982) 337–346.

[26] Berg, D., H. K. Rjosk, F. Jänicke, et al.: Behandlung der hyperprolaktinämischen Amenorrhoe durch pulsatile Gabe von gonadotropin Releasing Hormonen. Geburtsh. and Frauenheilk. **43** (1983) 686–688.

[27] Magyar, D. M., J. R. Marshall: Pituitary tumors and pregnancy. Am. J. Obstet. Gynaecol. **132** (1978) 739–775.

[28] Gemzell, C., C. F. Wang: Outcome of pregnancy in women with pituitary adenoma. Fertil. Steril. **31** (1979) 363–372.

[29] Griffith, R. W., I. Turkalj, P. Braun: Pituitary tumors during pregnancy in mothers treated with bromocriptine. Br. J. Clin. Pharmac. **7** (1979) 393–396.

Conservative management of prolactinoma

H. S. Jacobs

Introduction

The endocrinologist's present approach to the management of patients with prolactinomas has been influenced by three important advances. The first two – the wide spread availability of measurements of prolactin in serum and the introduction of an efficacious medical treatment – are well known and as they have been the subject of many reviews [14, 7] they will not be dealt with here in any detail.

Diagnosis

The development of high resolution CT scanning of the pituitary consitutes the third important advance. Earlier radiological methods, such as conventional lateral and anterio posterior radiographs, coned views and hypocycloidal polytomography of the fossa all suffer from the inherent disadvantage that they image not the pituitary gland, but the bones that encase it. The principle upon which they rely is, therefore, that lesions of soft tissue can be implied from changes detected in hard tissues. Uncertainty concerning the specificity of such changes has been voiced for several years. Very large fossas for instance, even when occurring in patients with endocrine symptomatology, can be largely empty (fig. 1). Less striking radiological changes, traditionally considered indicative of prolactinomas by most endocrinologists, have recently been the subject of careful review [4, 19] and results representative of one such study are shown in table 1. These data, taken from the paper by Burrow's group and based on post mortem material, show a very poor correlation of radiological diagnosis with the diagnosis established histologically. In common with most endocrine units, therefore, we have abandoned tomography of the sella turcica for the diagnosis of patients with hyperprolactinaemia.

Imaging the pituitary by CT scanning has the great advantage that the pituitary itself can be seen; with the newer techniques of reformating the images in any of several planes, available on 4th generation machines, the precision of diagnosis increases enormously [15]. We find axial scans, reformated in the sagittal plane, very helpful in the diagnosis of supra sellar extension and when reformated in the coronal plane the degree of symmetry can be easily seen, as can any tendency of the

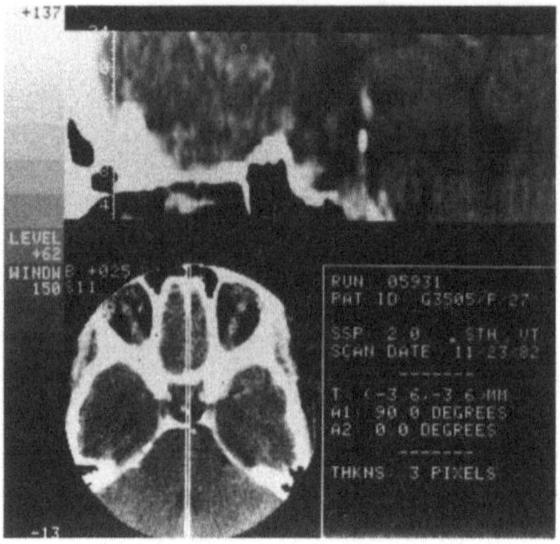

Fig. 1 a

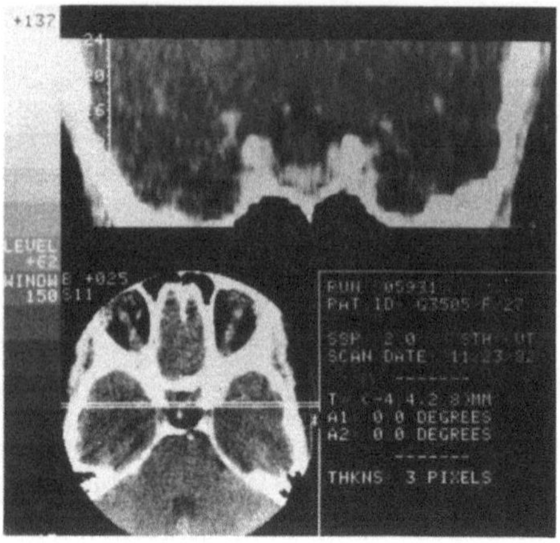

Fig. 1 b

Figs. 1 a and b Saggital (a) and coronal (b) reconstruction of CT-scan before treatment in a young qoman with amenorrhoea, galactorrhoea and a very high serum prolactin concentration (for details, see text).

Table 1 Correlation of pituitary tomogram appearance and histological findings in a post mortem study of 120 patients (Burrow et al. [4])

Tomogram +	27 cases	tumour	– 21
			+ 6
Tomogramm –	93 cases	tumour	– 67
			+ 26

tumour to invade the cavernous sinuses (fig. 2). Direct coronal scans are most helpful for the diagnosis of small intra pituitary lesions. They have the added advantage of markedly reducing the dose of irradiation sustained by the eyes [9].

Whilst CT has made air encephalography completely outdated and offers tremendous advantages to the patient and doctor alike, it is of course itself not without problems. Studies of CT results, parallel to those of polytomography mentioned above, have not yet been published, but it is inevitable that the specificity of any purely radiological diagnosis must have limitations. It is for instance well known that up to 20 per cent of women have incidental pituitary nodules found at autopsy [5] and that many of these nodules do contain prolactin, as assessed by immunocytochemical methods [1]. However, rather than lamenting the lack of 100 per cent specificity of a single diagnostic modality, the practical physician recognises that clinical diagnosis characteristically depends upon the coincidence of several lines of enquiry. We therefore base a diagnosis of micro prolactinoma on finding the association of a raised serum prolactin concentration with certain characteristic CT

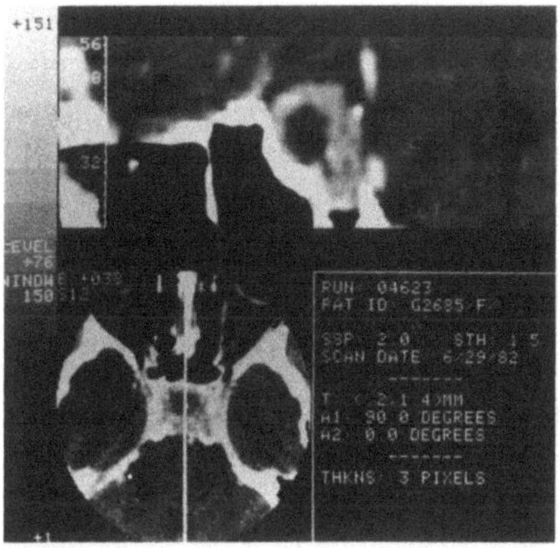

Fig. 2 a

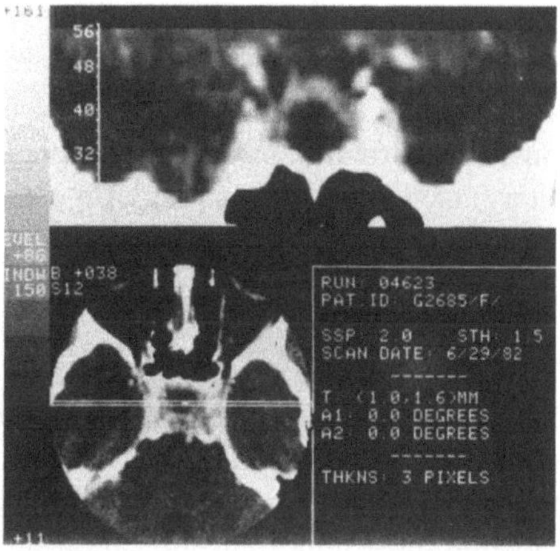

Fig. 2 b

Figs. 2 a and b Saggital (a) and coronal (b) reconstructions of CT-scans in the same patient as in figure 1 after 5 months treatment with bromocriptine.

changes, such as expansion of the pituitary (often giving its upper surface a convex upward surface) with distortion of its anatomy (often deviating the pituitary stalk to one side) with a radiological hetero-density (usually a discrete radiolucent area) in the substance of the expanded pituitary [15, 9]. We do not find dynamic tests of prolactin secretion helpful, although the probability of finding a prolactinoma is, of course, directly related to the height of the basal serum prolactin concentration. Few patients with prolactin concentrations exceeding 100 µg/l (4000 miu/l) do not have a radiologically demonstrable prolactinoma.

Clinical presentation

The presentation of patients with hyperprolactinaemia to the clinician is characteristic and is in most cases because of endocrine symptomatology – that is, with disturbances of reproduction associated, on occasion, with galactorrhoea [12]. Clinically the important point to make is that the endocrine deficiency reflects the associated gonadal inactivity, so symptoms of oestrogen deficiency in women [12] or of testosterone deficiency in men [8] dominate the picture. These gonadal steroid deficiences produce respectively dyspareunia and impotence. Quite apart from the immediate distress of these symptoms it behoves us to consider the longer term consequences of prolonged oestrogen deficiency because there are now data that indicate that chronic osteopoenia may be a feature of young women with hyperprolactinaemia. I consider oestrogen deficiency itself a sufficient reason on its own to constitute an important indication for treatment of hyperprolactinaemia. A few patients present for the first time with neurosurgical problems: the indication to treat such patients is obvious and is dealt with extensively elsewhere in this volume.

In my opinion most patients with prolactinomas, either macro- or micro-prolactinomas, need treatment, either for immediate local problems (expansion of the pituitary) or because of the longterm consequences of gonadal failure or because of infertility.

Treatment

The merits of surgical treatment of prolactinoma are discussed elsewhere in this volume and I will therefore concentrate on describing the possibilities of medical therapy. The conclusion is reached that, in the opinion of this endocrinologist at least, the most important indication for surgical extirpation of a prolactinoma is failure of medical treatment.

The principal of medical therapy is the now familiar observation that both normal and pathological secretion of prolactin is under dopaminergic control. In the physiological state this inhibitory control is supplied by dopamine released from hypothalamic neurones into the pituitary portal circulation [7]. In patients with prolactinoma, though the hypersecretion of prolactin clearly escapes from endogeneous dopamine inhibition, treatment with exogenous dopamine or with one of its longer acting agonists suppresses prolactin secretion to normal. Suppression of prolactin secretion to normal permits resumption of normal gonadotrophin secretion, with the evolution of ovulatory menstrual cycles and fertility in women and of testosterone secretion and return of potency and libido in men. Using the cumulative conception rate in women with hyperprolactinaemia as an index of successful treatment, most studies have shown that treatment with bromocriptine produces a normal rate of conception and of delivery [2].

There are in this area four relatively new pieces of information which are helpful to the clinician in deciding on whether to offer the patient with hyperprolactinaemia treatment with medical therapy.

Drugs available

2 alpha bromergocriptine (bromocriptine, Parlodel, Sandoz) is the long acting dopamine agonist that was first introduced into clinical practice and for which therefore there is greatest experience, both of its efficacy and of its safety. Efficacy is attested to by its ability to suppress serum prolactin concentrations, by the rate at which women on treatment resume ovulatory cycles and by their rate of return of fertility, which is normal [10]. Bromocriptine does however have side effects, both immediate and longterm. The immediate ones include nausea and vomiting and postural hypotension; they can usually be avoided by initiating treatment in small

doses and giving the drug at night time. Typically one starts with 1.25 mg at night with food and the dose of treatment is gradually raised to between 5 and 10 mg a day (in divided doses), although sometimes higher and occasionally lower. Once the prolactin concentration is suppressed into the normal range and ovulatory cycles have resumed, it is frequently possible to lower the dose and in our experience maintenance doses are 50–75 per cent of those needed for resumption of normal reproductive function. Longer term adverse reactions include nasal stuffiness and constipation, both of which can usually be dealt with symptomatically but both of which have on occasion been reasons for stopping the therapy. In patients on long-term therapy, we usually ask the patient to discontinue treatment at the beginning of a period every twelve months and to come up to hospital three weeks later for measurement of serum prolactin and progesterone concentrations. Decisions about further treatment are then determined by whether the patient retains ovulatory cycles (based on the serum progesterone concentration) and on whether the serum prolactin concentration remains in the normal range (based on a measurement on the same sample).

Since treatment with bromocriptine is very often given to women to permit them to conceive, it behoves us to consider whether the ensuing pregnancies are in fact safe. To date, follow-up studies indicate that even when treatment is carried over into the first few weeks of pregnancy no adverse effects can be detected on the pregnancy (as measured by the rate of abortion and of premature labour), on the newborn (as measured by the rate of congenital abnormalities, by the distribution of birth weights etc) or on growth and development, so far studied in a few cases up to the age of five years [16].

While these studies are most encouraging and provide no indication not to use bromocriptine to induce ovulation and therefore pregnancy, they do not in my opinion suggest that treatment with this drug should be carried on throughout pregnancy, unless there is some very specific indication to do so (see below). The reason is that bromocriptine, or some active metabolite thereof, certainly does cross at least the term placenta [3] and of course teratogenesis can in the longterm only be detected by very prolonged follow up. Thus the effects of diethylstilboestrol on the unborn child were only detected when the exposed fetuses were assessed at around the time of puberty.

Several other dopaminergic agonist drugs have been introduced in the last few years [18]. While there is no doubt that these compounds can suppress prolactin concentrations [6] no direct comparisons of their efficacy and safety are yet available. I personally have no experience of these drugs but anticipate a small role for them in patients intolerant of bromocriptine but tolerant of the other agonists. I suspect such cases are rare.

Shrinkage of prolactinomas on medical treatment

By obtaining CT scans before and at various stages of treatment with bromocriptine, it is now possible to observe considerable shrinkage of prolactinomas after remarkably short periods of time. Figure 2 indicates such a course of events: this young woman with amenorrhoea and galactorrhoea due to severe hyperprolactinaemia (40,000 mu/l [normal range <700 mu/l]) had an enlarged pituitary fossa containing a large prolactinoma showing extension both upwards and laterally. Treatment with bromocriptine led to normalisation of prolactin concentrations and a return of ovulatory menstrual cycles. After six months' treatment a repeat CT scan showed a marked decrease in the size of the prolactinoma (fig. 3). After a

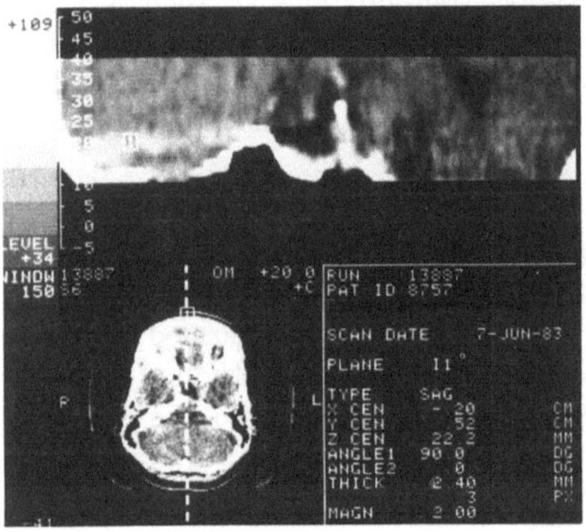

Fig. 3 a

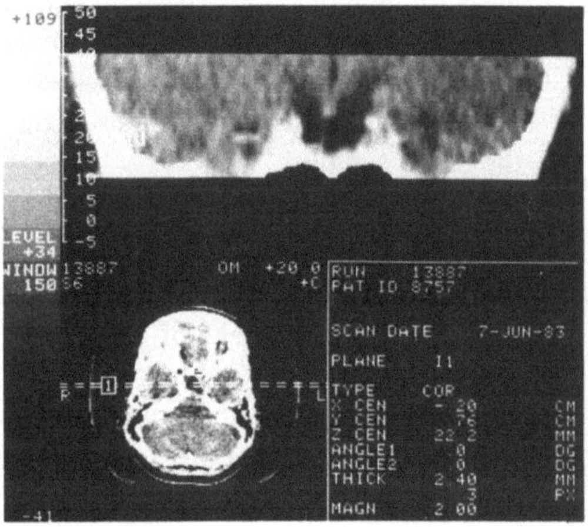

Fig. 3 b

Figs. 3 a and b Saggital (a) and coronal (b) reconstructions of CT-scans after treatment with bromocriptine for one year. The pituitary tumours has now disappeared, the sella is largely empty and the posterior long defect is beginning to heal.

further six months' treatment the enlarged fossa was almost empty and contained only a small amount of pituitary tissue (fig. 4). It is not possible to say whether there was any residual tumour at this stage, but quite fascinatingly an X-ray of the fossa taken after 12 months' treatment, ie at the same time as the CT shown in figure 4, showed radiological features indistinguishable from the pre treatment X-ray.

In our experience most prolactinomas shrink on medical treatment [7]. While there is debate amongst neuro-surgeons about whether medical treatment adversely affects subsequent surgical outcome, the fact that such shrinkage does occur becomes a significant factor in reaching a decision about optimal treatment. Thus in our practice, patients with prolactinomas presenting with visual field symptoms are usually treated with bromocriptine first and decisions about definitive surgical treatment can then be made at leisure.

Prolactinomas in pregnancy

While it is inappropriate in this review to consider the management of prolactinomas in pregnancy in any detail, it is pertinent to indicate here that the excellent prognosis of medically treated prolactinomas in pregnancy is due in large part to the pre pregnancy shrinkage of the prolactinoma on treatment with bromocriptine. In the rare situation in which such tumours do indeed enlarge in pregnancy, treatment with bromocriptine is safe and efficacious [20].

Longterm follow-up

Now that treatment with bromocriptine has been available for a decade, data on longterm follow-up are becoming available. Our early studies were first reported in 1981 and we found that after two to four years' treatment, a significant proportion of our patients were able to discontinue treatment with bromocriptine and yet retain normal ovulatory function and normal serum prolactin concentrations [13]. Patients with the most favourable prognosis for cure were those with pre-treatment prolactin concentrations of less than 40 μg/l (1600 miu/l). We are presently analysing the current neuro endocrine status of such patients. Further follow-up will be required to determine whether these patients, like many of those in remission after surgical treatment [17], relapse into hyperprolactinaemia after several years' remission.

Conclusion

A significant change in favour of longterm medical management of patients with prolactinomas has occurred in the last few years, due in large part to our ability to monitor the effects of treatment with CT scans. On reflection we should not really have been surprised by the remarkable changes in pituitary tumours revealed by CT, given the very effective suppression of hypersecretion of prolactin with which all endocrinologists are familiar. It has after all been known for many years that in patients with prolactinoma the serum prolactin concentration is an extremely accurate tumour marker.

References

[1] Asa, S. L., K. Koracs: Histological classification of pituitary disease. Clinics in Endocrinology and Metabolism **12** (1983) 567.

[2] Bergh, T., S. J. Nillius: Prolactinomas: follow up of medical treatment. In: A Clinical Problem: Microprolactinoma (G. M. Molinatti, ed.), p. 115. Excerpta Medica, Oxford 1982.
[3] Bigazzi, M., R. Ronga, I. Lancranjan, et al.: A pregnancy in an acromegalic woman during bromocryptine treatment: Effects on growth hormone and prolactin in the maternal, fetal and amniotic compartments. Journal of Clinical Endocrinology and Metabolism **48** (1979) 9.
[4] Burrow, G. N., G. Wortzman, N. B. Rewcastle, et al.: Microadenomas of the pituitary and abnormal sellar tomograms in an unselected autopsy series. N. Engl. J. Med. **304** (1981) 156.
[5] Costello, R. T.: Subclinical adenoma of the pituitary gland. Am. J. Pathol. **12** (1936) 205.
[6] Franks, S., P. M. Horrocks, S. S. Lynch, et al.: Effectiveness of pergolide mesylate in long term treatment of hyperprolactinaemia. British Medical Journal **286** (1983) 1177.
[7] Franks, S., H. S. Jacobs: Hyperprolactinaemia. Clinics in Endocrinology and Metabolism **12** (1983) 641.
[8] Franks, S., H. S. Jacobs, N. Martin, et al.: Hyperprolactinaemia and impotence. Clinical Endocrinology **8** (1978) 277.
[9] Hall, K.: Neuroradiology of prolactinomas. In: Prolactinomas and Pregnancy (H. S. Jacobs, ed.). Proceedings of 11th World Congress on Fertility and Sterility, Dublin, June 1983, Symposium. MTP Press, Lancaster–Boston–The Hague–Dordrecht 1983.
[10] Hull, M. G. R., P. A. Savage, H. S. Jacobs: Investigation and treatment of amenorrhoea resulting in normal fertility. British Medical Journal **1** (1979) 1257.
[11] Jacobs, H. S.: Prolactin and amenorrhoea. N. Eng. J. Med. **295** (1976) 954.
[12] Jacobs, H. S., S. Franks, M. A. F. Murray, et al.: Clinical and endocrine features of hyperprolactinaemia. Clinical Endocrinology **5** (1976) 439.
[13] Jacobs, H. S., S. U. Thobani: Long term follow-up of medically treated hyperprolactinaemia (including prolactinoma) – evidence for cure. In: Advances in Diagnosis and Treatment of Infertility (V. Insler, G. Bettendorf, eds.), p. 263. Elsevier North Holland, New York 1981.
[14] Jeffcoate, S. L.: Diagnosis of hyperprolactinaemia. Lancet **ii** (1978) 1245.
[15] Kendall, B.: Current approaches to hypothalamic pituitary radiology. Clinics in Endocrinology and Metabolism **12** (1983) 535.
[16] Krupp, P., I. Turkalj: Surveillance of Parlodel (bromocriptine) in pregnancy and offspring. In: Prolactinomas and Pregnancy (H. S. Jacobs, ed.). Proceedings of 11th World Congress on Fertility and Sterility, Dublin, June 1983 Symposium. MTP Press, Lancaster–Boston–The Hague–Dordrecht 1984.
[17] Serri, O., E. Rasio, H. Beauregard, et al.: Recurrence of hyperprolactinaemia after selective transsphenoidal adenomectomy in women with prolactinoma. N. Engl. J. Med. **309** (1983) 280.
[18] Thomas, J. P., R. Hall: Medical management of pituitary disease. Clinics in Endocrinology and Metabolism **12** (1983) 771.
[19] Turski, P. A., T. H. Newton, B. H. Horten: Sellar contour: anatomic-polytomographic correlation. Am. J. Radiol. **137** (1981) 213.
[20] van der Spuy, Z. M., H. S. Jacobs: Management of endocrine disorders in pregnancy. Part II – pituitary, ovarian and adrenal disease. Postgraduate Medical Journal **60** (1984) 312.

Effect of bromocriptine therapy on large prolactinomas

G. Galvan, T. Irnberger

Introduction

Although dopamine agonists are effective in the treatment of prolactinomas, leading to suppression of prolactin as well as to diminution of adenoma size, it seems not quite certain whether surgery or medication of dopamine agonists is the preferential treatment [1].

Patients and methods

We have been studying 4 patients with large prolactinomas and 2 patients with large recurrent tumours after surgery for macroprolactinomas. All patients have been treated with bromocriptine (BR) for 1 to 5 years in a wide dose range from 3.75 to 30 mg BR daily, varying also in the case of the same patient, depending on PRL levels and side effects. CT was done at the beginning and repeated in the course of the treatment.

Patient 1

In a 66 year old women an inoperable, invasive 4.6 × 3.3 × 3.5 cm prolactinoma with suprasellar and retrosellar extension was diagnosed in 1979 (fig. 1). There was no visual field defect. PRL was increased to 862 ng/ml. HGH, LH and FSH were low and could not be stimulated. T4 and cortisol were normal. BC-therapy was started initially with 2.5 mg daily. 4 weeks later PRL was reduced to 220 ng/ml. As a liquorrhoea appeared, probably because of the shrinking of the tumour, radiation therapy in a dose of 1600 rad was additionally carried out. BC was increased to 3 ×10 mg. Subsequently the PRL level was reduced to 4–30 ng/ml. A temporary reduction of the dose to 3 × 5 mg in 1981 was followed by an increase in PRL to 46 ng/ml within 4 weeks. The patient has been kept under 3 × 10 mg BC daily up to now for 62 months, PRL levels being about 15 ng/ml. An extensive shrinkage of the tumour occurred within the first 8 months. The intrasellar tumour remnant showed an almost complete cystic regression in the course of the 62 months treatment (fig. 2).

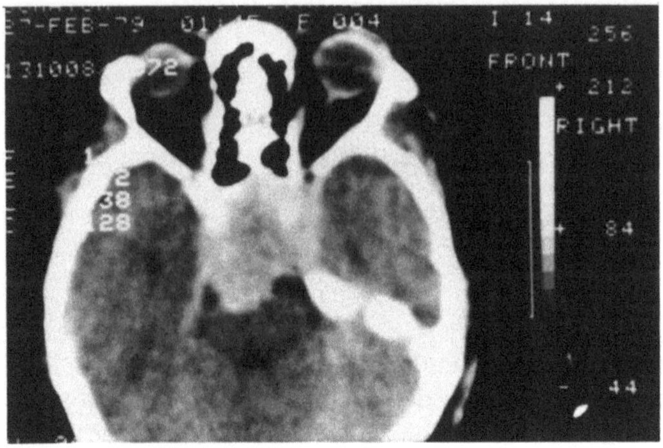

Fig. 1 Effect of long-time bromocriptine therapy on macroprolactinomas of patient 1. CT of the prolactinoma before treatment.

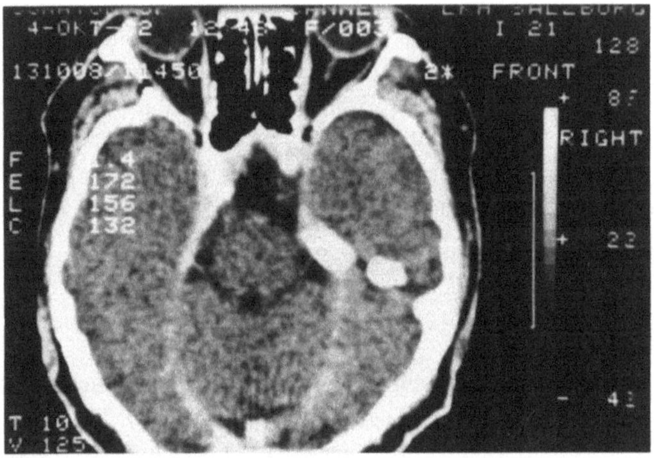

Fig. 2 CT of the prolactinoma after treatment.

LH and FSH increased to subnormal values in the last 3 months. Possible side effects of the BC-therapy were an enlargement of the liver without any notable increase in the enzymes, an infiltration of the lung with haemoptysis and oedema of the legs in the 10th month of treatment.

Patient 2

A craniotomy was carried out in 1973 on a 39 year old man with a 2 cm basophilic adenoma of the pituitary with suprasellar extension and a visual field defect. In

1974 an intrasellar recurrent tumour was twice removed through the transsphenoidal route. In 1978 a 2 cm recurrent tumour was diagnosed near the fissura orbitalis superior (fig. 3). There was no visual field defect. PRL was increased to 615 ng/ml, all other hormones were normal. BC-therapy was started with 3 × 1.25 mg daily. Three days later PRL was reduced to 247 ng/ml and 21 days later to 17 ng/ml. This dose has been maintained now for 66 months, PRL now being stabilized at about 2–5 ng/ml without response after stimulation with TRH. 5 months after starting the therapy the tumour showed a marked cystic regression. 53 months later no residual tumour could be documented (fig. 4). A possible side effect was an extremely increased libido throughout the whole period.

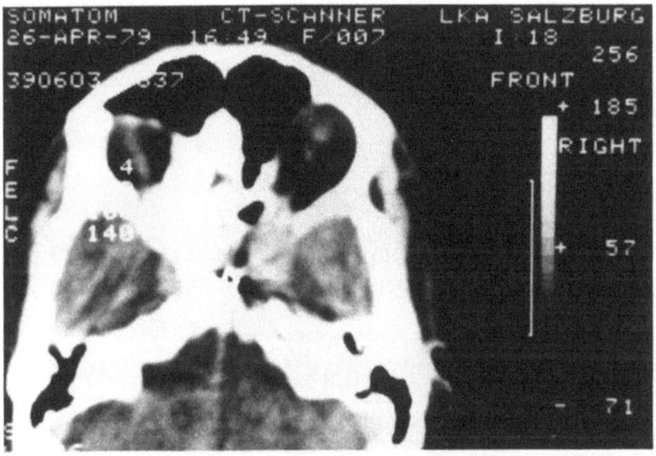

Fig. 3 Effect of long-time bromocriptine therapy on macroprolactinomas of patient 2. CT of the prolactinoma before treatment.

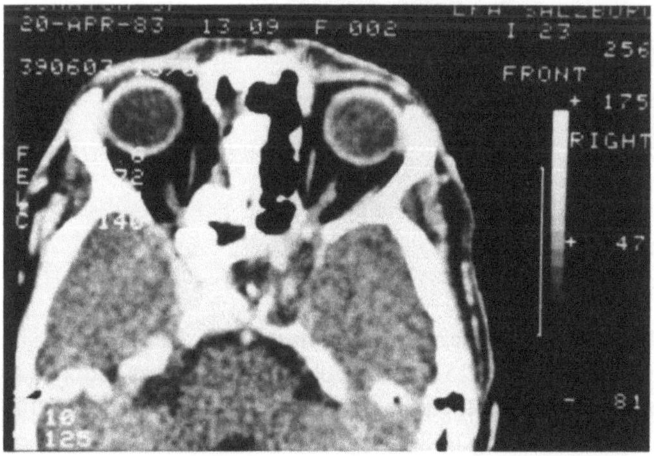

Fig. 4 CT of the prolactinoma after treatment.

Patient 3

In a 55 year old man an intrasellar cystic prolactinoma of 1.8 cm was diagnosed in 1978 (fig. 5). There was no visual field defect. PRL was increased to 88 ng/ml.

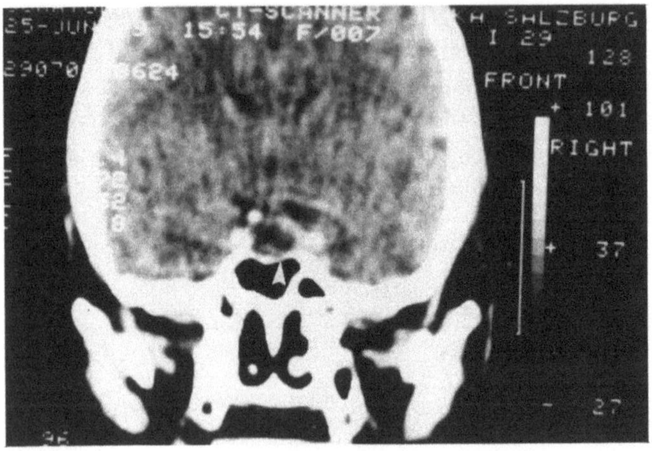

Fig. 5 Effect of long-time bromocriptine therapy on macroprolactinomas of patient 3. CT of the prolactinoma before treatment.

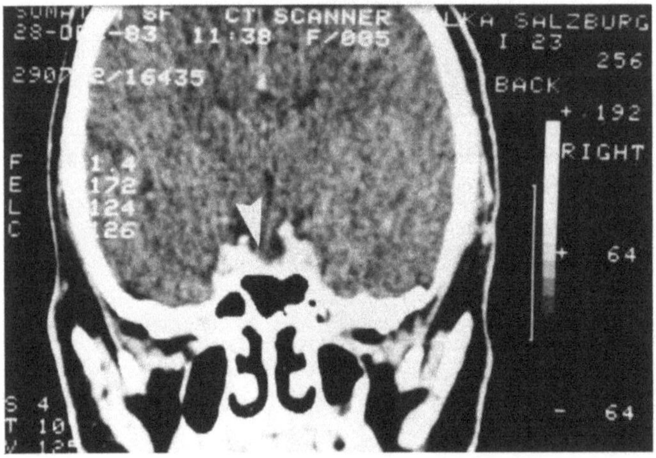

Fig. 6 CT of the prolactinoma after treatment.

Stimulation tests showed a decreased reserve of the pituitary for HGH and FSH. BC-therapy was commenced with 3 × 1.25 mg. 4 weeks later PRL was reduced to 9.7 ng/ml. As PRL did not sink to undetectable values, the dose was increased to 3 × 2.5 mg 10 months later, PRL falling to 2–5 ng/ml. This dose was maintained for 26 months and then reduced to 2.5 mg daily up to now.

PRL has stabilized at about 2 ng/ml after a total of 68 months. In the CT the tumour became gradually cystic, shrinking from 1.8 to 0.9 cm. Now, 68 months after the beginning of therapy the entire tumour is cystic (fig. 6). HGH, LH and FSH are now normalized. A possible side effect was unconsciousness for 3 minutes 7 weeks after the beginning of the therapy.

Patient 4

In a 50 year old man a 3.7 cm partly calcified prolactinoma with suprasellar extension was diagnosed in 1981 (fig. 7). There was no visual field defect. PRL was in-

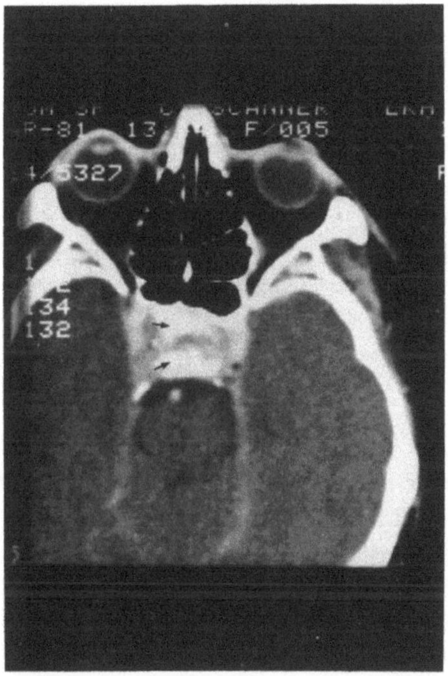

Fig. 7 Effect of long-time bromocriptine therapy on macroprolactinomas of patient 4. CT of the prolactinoma before treatment.

creased to 5500 ng/ml. There was a secondary hypogonadism, hypothyreoidism and adrenal insufficiency. BC-therapy was started with 3 × 1.75 mg, PRL was reduced to 1750 ng/ml within 2 months and to 288 ng/ml after 5 more months. Then PRL rose to 1000 ng/ml in spite of maintaining the dose. The dose was increased to 3 × 10 mg daily and PRL was gradually reduced to 48 ng/ml after a total of 36 months. The tumour was reduced to 2.2 × 1.8 cm after 7 months. As the PRL increased the tumour grew. After increasing the dose there was a considerable decrease in the size of the tumour 34 months after the beginning of the therapy (fig. 8). Testosteron, Cortisol, T4, LH and FSH were normalized. No side effects were observed.

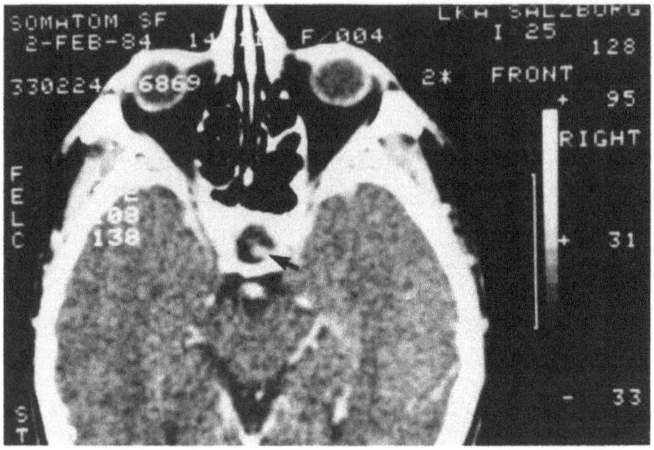

Fig. 8 CT of the prolactinoma after treatment.

Patient 5

In a 40 year old woman a transsphenoidal hypophysectomy was performed in 1972. In 1982 a recurrent invasive prolactinoma of 4.5 × 5 cm with suprasellar and retrosellar extension was diagnosed (fig. 9). A homonymous incomplete visual field defect was confirmed. PRL was increased to 3500 ng/ml. HGH was increased to 12 ng/ml, but could be suppressed to 2 ng/ml by glucose (mixed adenoma?). T4 was low, LH and FSH were in the upper borderline range and could not be stimulated, the patient being amenorrhoeal. BC-therapy was started with 3 × 1.25 mg. 4 weeks later PRL had fallen to 1540 ng/ml, then increased to 4600 ng/ml in spite of unchanged BC-therapy. The dose was increased to 3 × 10 mg and PRL decreased to 790 ng/ml up to now within a total period of 19 months. There is a shrinkage of the tumour to 2.8 × 2.5 cm with a regression of the suprasellar and retrosellar part of the tumour (fig. 10). The visual field defect has normalized completely. HGH is low, T4 and T3 are in the lower range. No side effects were observed.

Patient 6

In a 61 year old woman a 3 × 3 cm invasive prolactinoma with a large suprasellar extension was diagnosed (fig. 11). There was a large visual field defect of the right

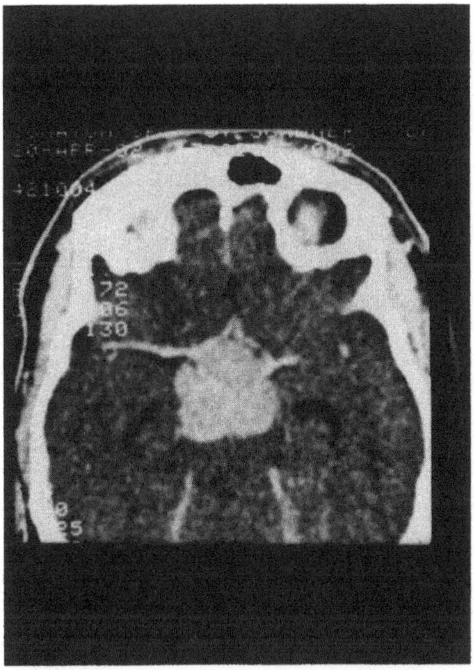

Fig. 9 Effect of long-time bromocriptine therapy on macroprolactinomas of patient 5.
CT of the prolactinoma before treatment.

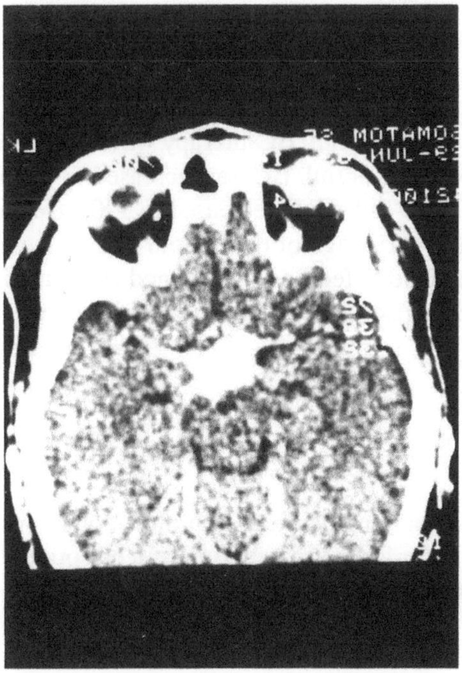

Fig. 10 CT of the prolactinoma after treatment.

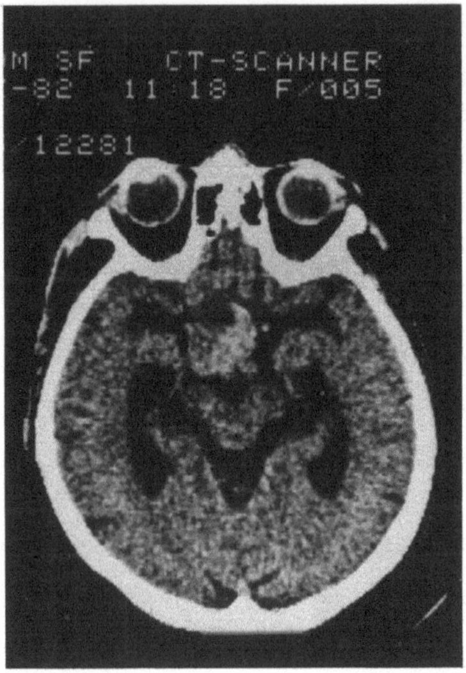

Fig. 11 Effect of long-time bromocriptine therapy on macroprolactinomas of patient 6. CT of the prolactinoma before treatment.

eye and a complete amaurosis of the left. PRL was increased to 3818 ng/ml. HGH, LH, FSH, TSH, T4 and cortisol were subnormal. BC-therapy was started with 3 × 2.5 mg daily. 4 months later PRL was 712 ng/ml. BC was increased to 15 mg daily and the tumour was irradiated with 4680 rad. PRL decreased to 390 ng/ml after 13 months of the BC-therapy. There is a shrinkage of the tumour to 2 × 2 cm with a cystic regression (fig. 12). The visual field defects are unchanged without any deterioration. HGG, LH, FSH, T4 and cortisol have remained unchanged up to now. No side effects were observed.

Summary

As a result of our observations in 6 patients with large prolactinomas we prefer BC-therapy as an effective treatment for large prolactinomas. In our opinion this is also true for patients with visual field defects.

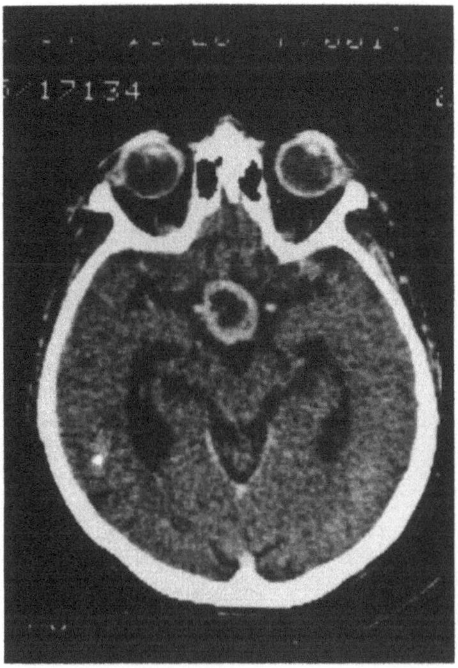

Fig. 12 CT of the prolactinoma after treatment.

References

[1] Von Werder, K., R. Fahlbusch, H. K. Rjosk: Macroprolactinomas: Clinical and Therapeutic Aspects. In: Prolactin and Prolactinomas (G. Tolis, C. Stefanis, T. Mountokalakis, F. Labrie, eds.), pp. 415. 427. Raven Press, New York 1983.

Macroprolactinomas in male patients: efficiency of treatment with a new dopaminergic drug (CU 32-085-Sandoz), tumour calcification and relative significance of preoperative tumour volume regression as estimated by CT-scan

J. Mockel, J. D'Haens, D. Désir, J. P. Denayer, R. Dayeh, M. L'Hermite, D. Balériaux, J. Flament-Durand, J. Brotchi

The case reports described concern three male patients presenting with macroprolactinomas. The particular points of interest of these cases were

1. the efficiency of the new dopaminergic drug CU 32-085 in normalizing prolactin (PRL) levels,

2. the occurrence of massive homogeneous calcifications of the tumour in 2 of the cases,

3. the *non*-shrinkage of the 3 tumours despite adequate medical treatment and the surgically confirmed diagnosis of prolactinoma.

All CT-scans were performed with a last generation high resolution machine allowing 2 mm thickness contiguous enhanced sections in the coronal and axial planes, with reformated images in the coronal and sagittal planes. Endocrine evaluation included basal measurement of all the hormones in the plasma and 24h-urine samples, 2 hourly samples for ACTH, cortisol, GH and prolactin for 24 hours, a TRH 200 μg – LHRH 100 μg IV test measuring TSH-PRL-LH and FSH, an insulin induced hypoglycaemia with appreciation of the ACTH-cortisol-GH and PRL responses, and a CRF 100 μg IV test performed at 23.00 H when judged necessary. Histological examination of the surgical samples included standard microscopy with conventional stains, electron microscopy and immunocytochemistry by the peroxidase technique as well as with antibodies labelled by colloidal gold for EM.

Case 1: This 38 year old patient was completely impotent in the last 3 years, was shaving more and more rarely in the last 2 years and was almost blind at presentation. Visual function was deteriorating progressively since 15 months and for the last 3 months the patient was unable to drive his car and recognize his neighbours. He also complained of increased weight and muscle cramps. Except moderate gynecomastia and paucity of axillary and pubic hair examination was unremark-

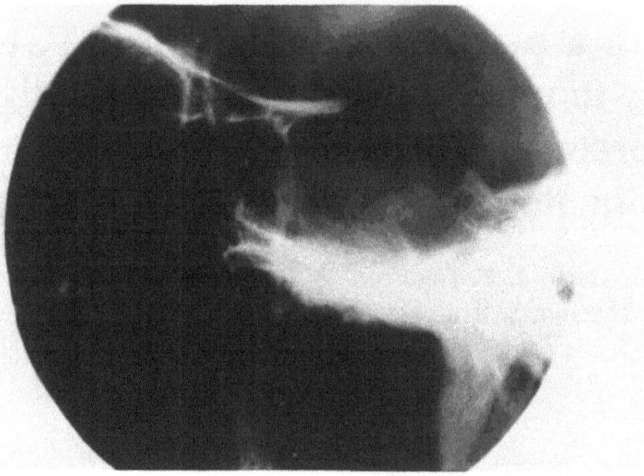

Fig. 1a Sellar X-ray: complete destruction of the bony sella (case 1).

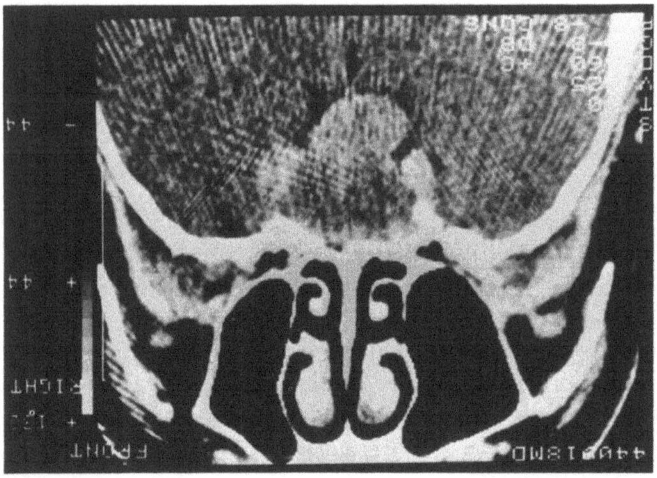

Fig. 1b CT-scan at diagnosis. Macroadenoma with irregular hypodensities (case 1).

able. Standard X-ray of the sella and CT-scan showed complete destruction of the sella and a macroadenoma extending into the third ventricle (figs. 1 a–b). Visual acuity was 2/10 for the right eye, the left one being nearly blind with severe bitem-

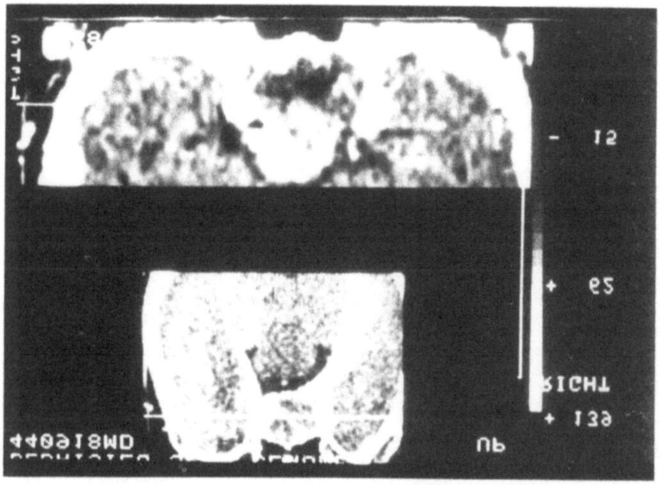

Fig. 1c CT-scan after one month of bromocriptine treatment (case 1).

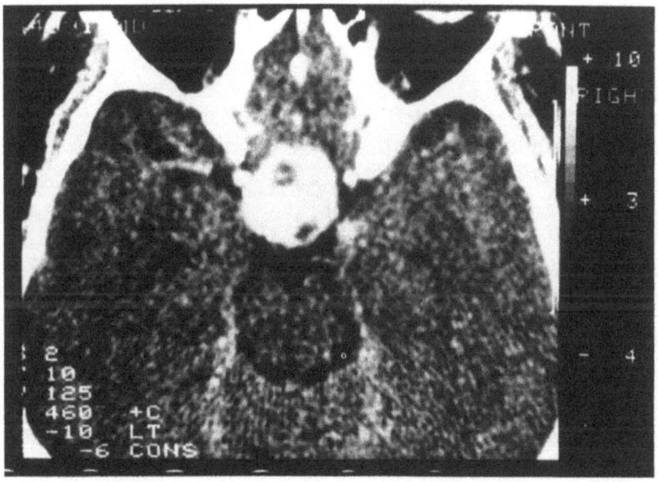

Fig. 1d CT-scan after six month of bromocriptine treatment: note no regression of tumour volume.

poral hemianopsia (fig. 2a). Endocrine evaluation demonstrated PRL levels exceeding 100 × the upper normal limit, not responsive to TRH, and a complete pituitary insufficiency.

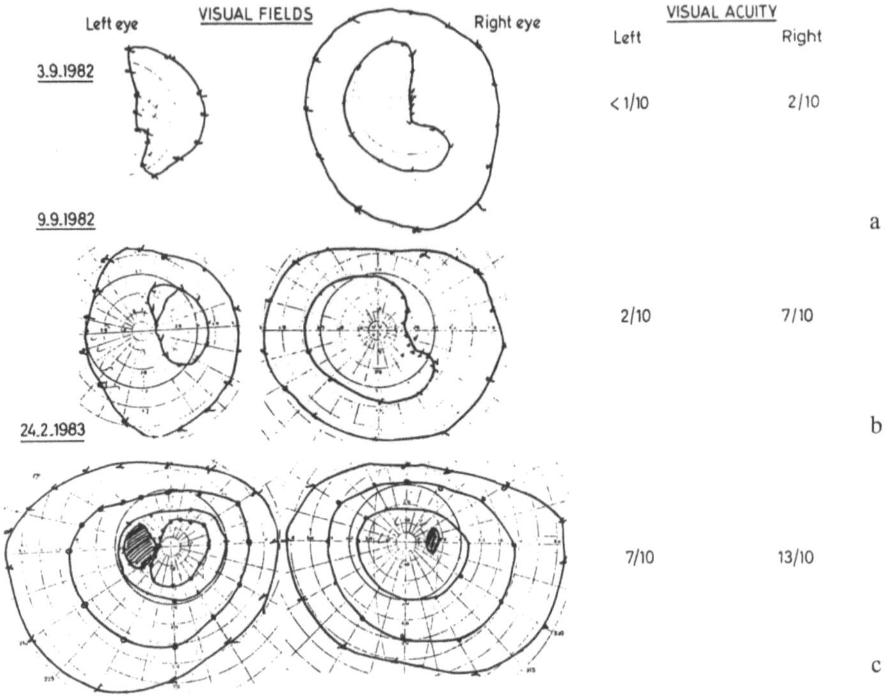

Fig. 2 Visual fields and visual acuity (case 1).
a) at diagnosis, bitemporal hemianopsia left macular amputation;
b) after six days of bromocriptine treatment;
c) after six month of bromocriptine treatment.

The patient was treated with cortisone acetate, L-thyroxine and bromocryptine 7.5 mg/daily. Within 6 days, erections had reappeared and visual acuity and fields were greatly improved (fig. 2b), with PRL reduced to 10× the upper normal limit. The bromocryptine dosage was rapidly raised to 15 mg daily to normalize PRL levels. After six months, sexual function was normal despite persistently low testosterone, LH and FSH, PRL was normal (tab. 1), visual fields and visual acuity were nearly normal. Despite this complete biological and clinical cure of the disease, the CT-scan performed *1* and *6* months after the start of bromocryptine therapy did *not* show any tumour shrinkage. A transsphenoidal adenomectomy was then performed, histology confirming the diagnosis of macroprolactinoma.

Case 2: This 43 year old patient's major complaints consisted of frontal headaches, increasing during the last 3 years, and of complete impotency since 2 years. Sella X-ray and CT-scan demonstrated an enlarged sella with a completely calcified intra- and suprasellar tumour (figs. 3a–b). The ocular fundus, visual acuity and visual fields were normal. Endocrine evaluation showed euthyroidism, eucortisolism, a

Table 1 Case 1: Endocrine evaluation

	Normal values	Patient's values	Maximum values after TRH-LHRH
T_4 c*	6.3–12 μg/dl	1.7	–
T_3 c*	85–195 ng/dl	48	–
TSH	<5 μU/ml	4	17.1
Cortisol	8–9 a. m. 90–220 ng/ml	*1 × 2 h/24 h*	
Plasma	20–23 p. m. 20–90 ng/ml	25–60	–
Free cortisol/24 h urines	25–100 μg	15	–
Testosterone	400–1200 ng/dl	100	–
Free testosterone	8–32 ng/dl	3.9	–
LH	1.2–2.2 ng/ml	0.7	0.7
FSH	1.3–3.3 ng/ml	<0.5	<0.5
Prolactin	<250 μU/ml	*1 × 2/24 h* 25000–35000	unchanged
Time after bromocryptine administration	10 days	1800–3500	
15 mg	6 months	240–530	

* c = corrected for TBG values of the patient.

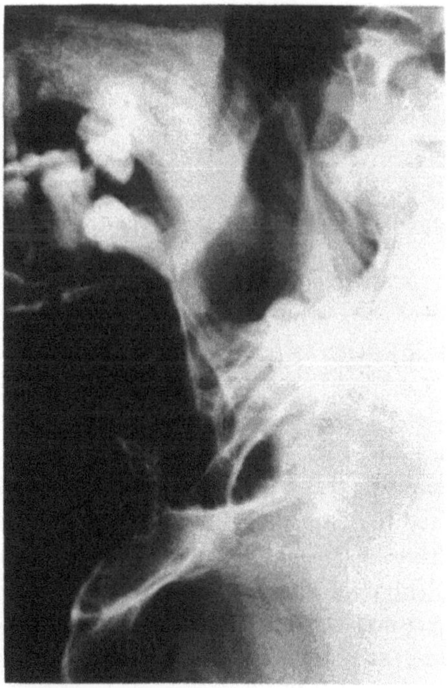

Fig. 3a Sellar X-ray: enlarged sella with calcified content (case 2).

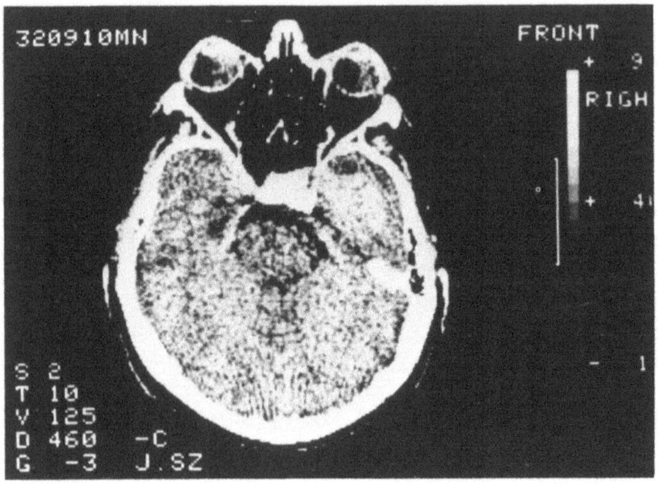

Fig. 3b CT-scan at diagnosis: calcified macroadenoma with suprasellar extemsion (case 2).

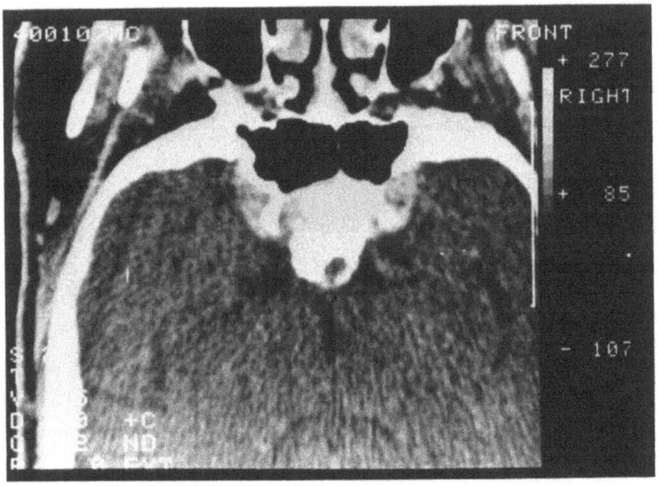

Fig. 3c CT-scan after six weeks of treatment CU 32-085 (case 2).

slight secondary gonadal insufficiency and PRL levels nearly reaching 100× the upper normal limit (tab. 2). The patient was treated with a new dopaminergic drug CU 32-085 (Sandoz, Basle), 0.5 raised to 2 mg/daily. Within 2 weeks, the headaches disappeared while normal erections were again present. PRL was nearly normalized after 6 weeks, while no change of the CT-appearance was observed (fig. 3c). A transsphenoidal adenomectomy was then performed. The tumour was surprisingly soft and easy to extrude, as shown by the postoperative CT-scan (fig. 3d). PRL was still elevated (60–80 ng/ml) this being normalized by resuming

Table 2 Case 2: Endocrine evaluation

– Euthyroidism		
– Eucortisolism		
– Testosterone	3.5–4.2 ng/ml	(N.: ≥5)
– FSH	1.0 ng/ml	→1.0
	after	
– LH	1.4 ng/ml LHRH	→2.3
	– 1×2 h – 1720 – 1950 ng/ml (N.: ≤20)	
– *Prolactin*	– After TRH – unchanged	
	– After 6 weeks	
	of CU 32-085 – 2 mg/daily	35–47 ng/ml

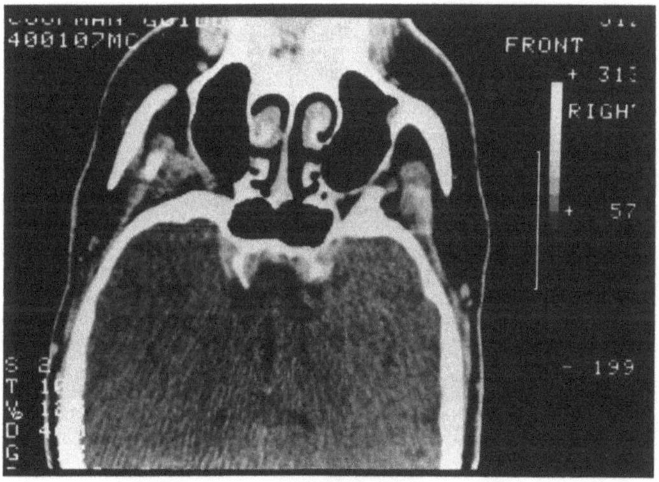

Fig. 3d Postoperative CT-scan (case 2).

treatment with CU 32-085–1 mg daily. Histology confirmed the diagnosis of a calcified macroprolactinoma.

Case 3: This 50 year old man was suffering from headaches since 1 year, since 3 months a progressive blurring of the right eye's vision and a left hemiparesis were slowly developing. The patient was admitted as an emergency case because of confusion and left Bravais-Jacksonian epileptic fits occurring in the last 2 days. Standard X-ray showed a dense intrasellar calcification and the CT-scan a calcified intrasellar lesion extending into a large right temporal tumour (figs. 4a–b).

Ophthalmological examination disclosed a right papilloedema with a left temporal hemianopsia. Except the above mentioned neurological signs, the physical examination was normal and did not evoke such a diagnosis as acromegaly, hypercorti-

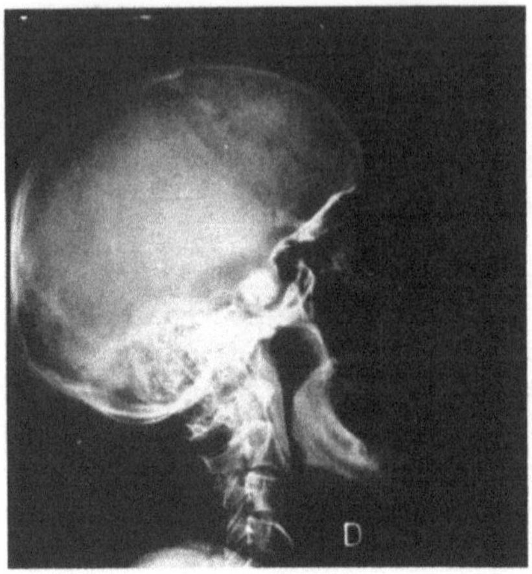

Fig. 4a X-ray – enlarged sella with cacified content (case 3).

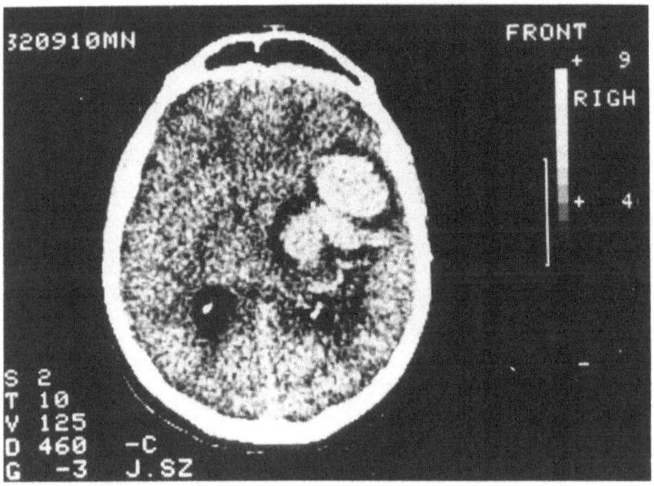

Fig. 4b CT-scan at diagnosis: calcified tumour, intrasellar extending into right temporal mass (case 3).

cism or pituitary insufficiency. An emergency excision of the right temporal mass was performed, and 6000 rads administered postoperatively to the right temporal field. The clinical status returned to normal within 2 months. Histology showed a calcified tumour, with numerous mitoses, densely granulated cells containing ACTH and prolactin. Endocrine evaluation was done 6 months after surgery and 4 months after the end of radiotherapy. Prolactin levels exceeded 100× the upper normal limit, but were still weakly responsive to TRH. All other pituitary function were entirely normal, including ACTH and the cortisol response to 100 μg CRF

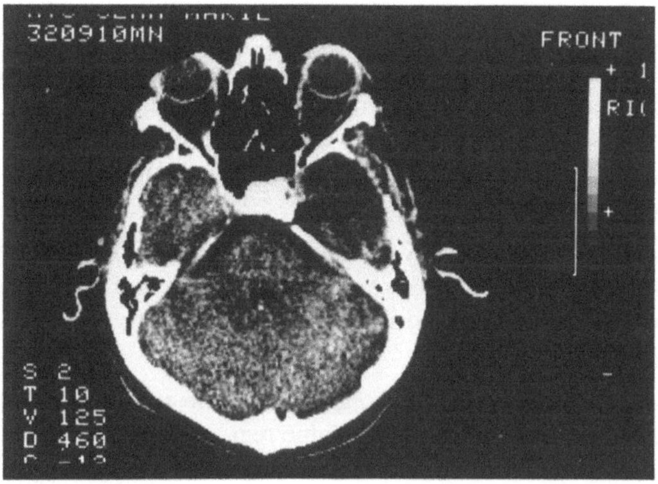

Fig. 4c Postoperative (temporal mass) CT-scan after six month of CU 32-085 treatment: unchanged sellar calcification (case 3).

IV. Treatment was then started with CU 32-085 0.5 → 2 mg daily, PRL being almost normal with that dose (tab. 3). After 6 months of treatment, the radiological appearance of the calcified tumour was unchanged. A transsphenoidal adenomectomy was then performed, removing a calcified tumour whose histology was identical to the temporal tumour removed one year before. A residue from the tumour infiltrating the right cavernous sinus could not be extirpated. Postoperative PRL reached 2500–4000 μU/ml, while all other pituitary functions remained normal. Treatment with CU 32-085 1.5 mg daily was resumed with normalization of PRL.

Table 3 Case 3: Endocrine evaluation

– Euthyroidism	
– Eugonadism	
– Cortisol ng/ml	9 – 12 – 16 – 20 – 23 – 08 h 181 152 71 74 44 155
– Cortisol after at 23.00 pm	100 μg I.V. CRF 40 ng/ml → peak 185 ng/ml
– Free cortisol/24 h urine samples: 60 μg (N.: 25–100)	
– *Prolactin*:	– 1 × 2 h/24 h – 26700–42000 μU/ml (N.: ≤250) – peak after TRH – 73600 μU/ml – after 6 months of CU 32-085 – 2 mg/daily – 260–450 μU/ml

Discussion

1. These case reports demonstrate the efficiency of CU 32-085 in the treatment of major hyperprolactinaemias encountered in macroadenomas. This drug has been used since 2–3 years and seems to have an efficiency comparable to that of bromocryptine with perhaps fewer side effects. In the two high dose treatments applied in our 2 cases, tolerance was excellent.

2. Calcifications are seen in 3–5% of pituitary tumours, most often in prolactinomas, but are usually curvilinear, adjacent to the capsule [1]. Massive nodular homogeneous calcifications such as those observed in cases 2 and 3 seem to be exceptional.

3. It has been reported that up to 90 percent of prolactinomas efficiently treated by dopaminergic agents showed evidence of tumour volume regression by sequential radiological and ophthalmological examination [2]. The suggestion has even been made that the "non-responders" may in fact all have secondary hyperprolactinaemia associated with large non-pituitary tumours like meningiomas or craniopharyngiomas [3]. If such cases evidently exist, they cannot explain all non-responders", as clearly demonstrated by case 1, in which complete clinical and biological cure of the disease was not accompanied by any tumour shrinkage of a non calcified tumour confirmed to be a prolactinoma at surgery. In cases 2 and 3, the calcifications easily explain the same phenomenon of "non-shrinkage" despite efficient medical treatment. The evolution of case 1 also demonstrates surprinsingly that severe hemianopsia can evolve to near normalization without regression of tumour volume, and that repeated visual fields cannot thus be a direct indicator of tumour volume evolution.

References

[1] Kendall, B.: Current approaches to hypothalamic pituitary radiology. Clin. Endoc. Metab. **12** (1983) 535–566.

[2] Bergh, T., S. J. Nillius: Prolactinomas: follow-up of medical treatment. In: A clinical problem: microprolactinoma (Molinatti, ed.), pp. 115–130. Excerpta Medica, Oxford 1982.

[3] Franks, S., H. S. Jacobs: Hyperprolactinemia. Clin. Endoc. Metab. **12** (1983) 641–668.

Evidence for spontaneous tumour shrinkage in a 45-year-old patient with a 20-year history of untreated microprolactinoma

E. Jungmann, P.-H. Althoff, H. Hacker, K. Schöffling

Introduction

Our knowledge of the natural history of prolactin-secreting pituitary microadenomas is still rudimentary [9]. It is commonly accepted and is considered to justify primary surgery of microprolactinoma that, in some of the prolactinoma patients, small adenomas may grow into large tumours [7]. Because nearly all patients with microprolactinoma are usually treated with transsphenoidal operation and/or dopaminergic agonists, only few data are available on the spontaneous outcome of patients harbouring untreated microprolactinoma. So far there are case reports on 29 patients observed for 2 up to 13 years. In 2 patients there was a tumour progression and in 27 patients no change in tumour size or prolactin levels was found. In none of the patients was a spontaneous remission documented [3, 12, 14]. In a further report on the spontaneous development of hyperprolactinaemia describing spontaneous normalization of prolactin levels in three patients unfortunately no detailed information about CT results were given. In 2 out of 43 patients of this study tumour progression became evident [10]. Therefore, the question awaits to be answered, whether spontaneous tumour shrinkage does occur in microprolactinoma.

A second question remains unanswered: Does long-term prolactin excess and, thus, missing gonadotrophin stimulation induce a complete and, therefore, irreversible secondary atrophy of the gonadotroph cells as previously postulated [15]?

Case report

Our now 45-year-old female patient first noticed galactorrhoea, amenorrhoea and complete loss of libido in 1962. Therefore, in 1964 a gynaecological examination was done. In laparoscopy, inactive ovaries were seen, an abrasion revealed an atrophic endometrium. An X-ray of the sella was misinterpreted as being normal (fig. 1). 17-ketosteroids were found normal. Argonz-Del-Castillo-syndrome was presumed and no treatment started. Galactorrhoea disappeared spontaneously lat-

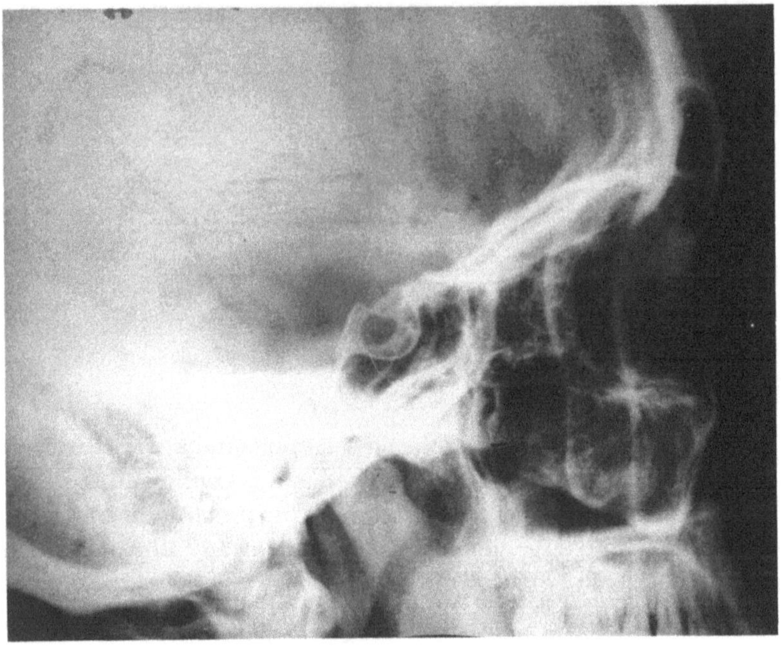

Fig. 1 X-ray of the sella of the patient of our case report misinterpreted in 1964 as being normal.

er in 1964. Amenorrhoea persisted until 1981 when endocrinological reexamination was performed. Prolactin levels were clearly increased above the normal range: the basal prolactin value was 87 ng/ml, the peak value 20′ after TRH 200 μg i.v. was 102 ng/ml. Adrenal and thyroid function as well as visus were normal (fig. 2). The plain X-ray of the sella was more or less identical with that from 1964 except for a different projection (fig. 3). Sella tomography demonstrated left-sided (fig. 4) and ventrocaudal (fig. 5) excavation of the sella floor as an indicator of pituitary microadenoma. In computerized tomography, no tumour tissue could be visualized but the pituitary stalk was found to be shifted to the right. The third ventricle was seen in the entrance of the sella (fig. 6). These findings were interpreted as evidence for a left-sided pituitary microadenoma which had undergone spontaneous tumour shrinkage and given way to a partly empty sella. Because of still elevated prolactin levels and persisting secondary amenorrhoea, bromocriptine treatment was started which promptly normalized the prolactin concentration (fig. 2). The first menstruation was induced after 3-weeks of bromocriptine treatment. After reduction of the bromocriptine dose to 1.25 mg b.i.d. because of migraine, the prolactin increased up to 39 ng/ml and amenorrhoea recurred. Whereas LH levels were unchanged (7 mU/ml vs. 6 mU/ml), FSH rose from 12 mU/ml to

17 mU/ml. Oestradiol was increased from 38 pg/ml to 95 pg/ml. Testosterone (35 ng/ml vs. 36 ng/ml) and DHEAS (873 ng/ml vs. 921 ng/ml) were unchanged.

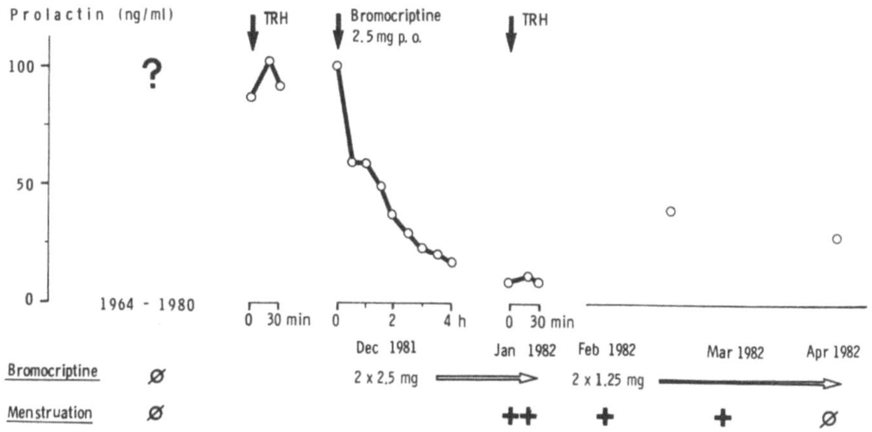

Fig. 2 Prolactin levels in our 45-year-old patient with microprolactinoma before and during bromocriptine treatment in 1981/1982.

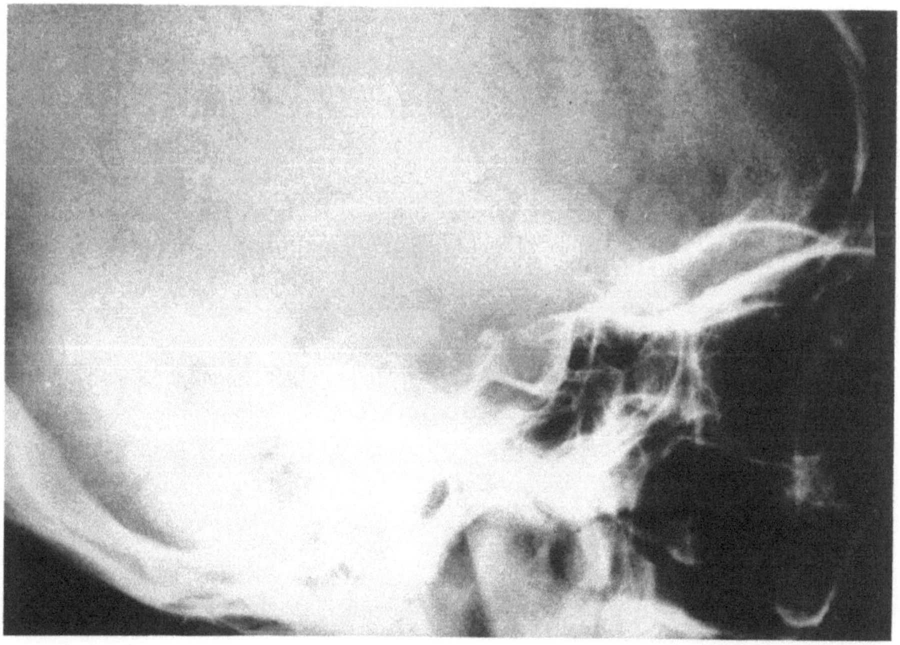

Fig. 3 X-ray of the sella of the patient of our case report in 1981.

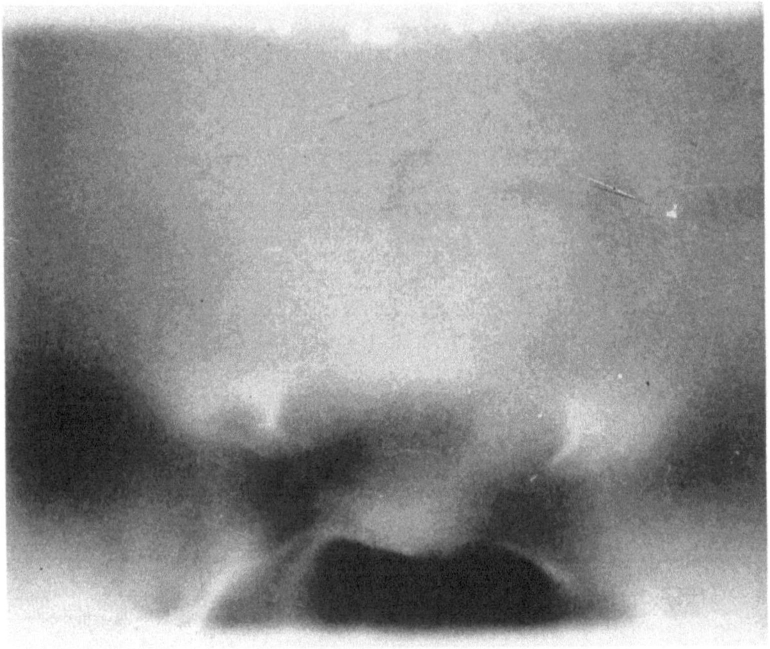

Fig. 4 Sella tomography (a.-p.) of the patient of our case report in 1981.

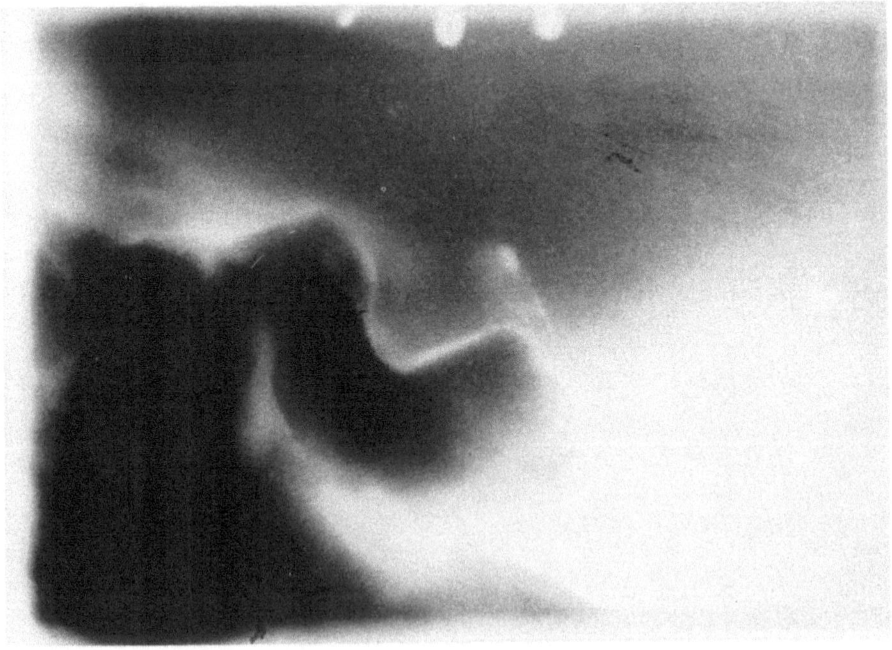

Fig. 5 Sella tomography (lateral) of the patients of our case report in 1981.

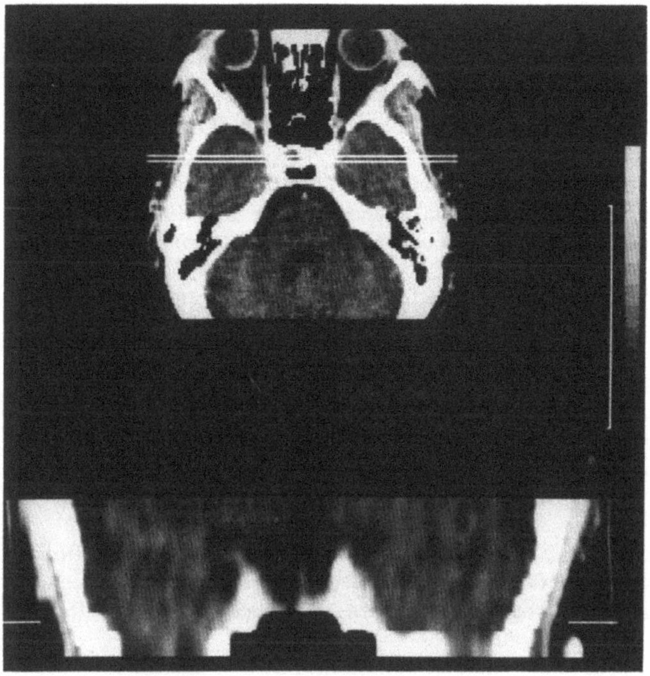

Fig. 6 CT scan (reconstruction) of the sella of the patient of our case report in 1981.

Discussion

There was good evidence for the possibility of a spontaneous remission of microprolactinoma, since in patients with pituitary microadenoma a partial or complete empty sella syndrome is frequently found [2, 4, 6, 8, 11, 13]. It is a widely accepted hypothesis for the pathogenesis of an empty sella syndrome that it takes place after spontaneous disappearance of pituitary tumour tissue. As demonstrated by our case report, spontaneous tumour shrinkage does indeed occur in microprolactinoma which should be considered when tumour shrinkage as result of treatment, particularly bromocriptine treatment, is discussed [1, 5]. Moreover, we could demonstrate that in hyperprolactinaemic states in contrast to previous suggestions [15] no complete atrophy of gonadotroph cells is present, and that successful bromocriptine treatment restores normal menstrual cycles even after a 20-year history of prolactin excess due to untreated microprolactinoma.

References

[1] Bergh, T., S. J. Nillius: Prolactinomas: follow up of medical treatment. In: A clinical problem: microprolactinoma (G. M. Molinatti, ed.). Excerpta Medica, Oxford 1982.

[2] Bertrand, G., G. Tolis: Surgical treatment of prolactinomas. In: clinical neuroendocrinology and treatment (G. Tolis, F. Labrie, J. B. Martin, F. Naftolin, eds.). Raven Press, New York 1979.
[3] Fahlbusch, R.: Surgical failures in prolactinomas. In: Pituitary adenomas: biology, physiopathology and treatment (P. J. Derome, C. P. Jedynak, F. Peillon, eds.). Asclepios France, Paris 1980.
[4] Fahlbusch, R., M. Giovanelli, P. G. Crosignani, et al.: Differentiated therapy of microprolactinomas: significance of transsphenoidal adenomectomy. In: Pituitary microadenomas (G. Faglia, R. M. McLeod, M. A. Giovanelli, eds.). Academic Press London 1980.
[5] Frantz, A. G.: Personal communication. Cited in: Franks, S., H. S. Jacobs: Hyperprolactinemia. Clinics in Endocrinology and Metabolism **12** (1983) 641–668.
[6] Giovanelli, M. A., R. Fahlbusch, S. M. Gaini, et al.: Surgical treatment of growth hormone-secreting microadenomas. In: Pituitary microadenomas (G. Faglia, R. M. McLeod, M. A. Giovanelli, eds.). Academic Press London 1980.
[7] Hardy, J., H. Beauregard, F. Robert: Prolactin-secreting pituitary adenomas: transsphenoidal microsurgical treatment. In: Progress in prolactin physiology and pathology (C. Robyn, M. Harter, eds.). Elsevier/North Holland Biomedical Press, Amsterdam 1978.
[8] Klijn, J. G. M., S. W. K. Lamberts, F. H. de Jong, et al.: Relationship between pituitary tumour size, hormonal parameters and extrasellar extension in patients with prolactinomas. In: Pituitary microadenomas (G. Faglia, M. A. Giovanelli, R. M. McLeod, eds.). Academic Press, London 1980.
[9] Landolt, A. M.: Biology of pituitary microadenomas. In: Pituitary microadenomas (G. Faglia, A. M. Giovanelli, R. M. McLeod, eds.). Academic Press, London 1980.
[10] March, C. M., O. A. Kletzky, V. Davajan, et al.: Longitudinal evaluation of patients with untreated prolactin-secreting pituitary adenomas. Am. J. Obstet. Gynecol. **139** (1981) 835–844.
[11] Melancon, D., F. Bedard, G. Belanger, et al.: Radiological assessment of the pituitary fossa. In: Clinical neuroendocrinology (G. Tolis, F. Labrie, J. B. Martin, F. Naftolin, eds.). Raven Press, New York 1979.
[12] Nabarro, J. D. N.: Pituitary prolactinomas. Clinical Endocrinology **17** (1982) 129–155.
[13] Newton, T. H., I. Richmond: Radiologic evaluation of pituitary microadenomas. In: Pituitary microadenomas (G. Faglia, A. M. Giovanelli, R. M. McLeod, eds.). Academic Press, London 1980.
[14] Rjosk, H.-K., K. v. Werder, R. Fahlbusch: Spontaneous development of hyperprolactinemia. Acta endocrinol. **100** (1982) 333–336.
[15] Rjosk, H.-K., K. v. Werder, R. Fahlbusch: Hyperprolactinämische Sterilität. Arch. Gynäk. **228** (1979) 518–530.

The influence of various forms of treatment on serum levels of prolactin, growth hormone and insulin-like growth factors I and II in patients with hyperprolactinaemia and acromegaly

H. Stracke, J. Zierski, J. Zapf, H. Schatz

Hyperprolactinaemia caused by a demonstrable pituitary tumour can often be normalized by adenomectomy if the basal prolactin level is about 200 ng/ml (fig. 1). Surgical therapy of tumours with higher prolactin values usually leads only to a partial reduction in the levels. Dopamine agonists are therefore indicated not only for the therapy of hyperprolactinaemia with no definite proof of "tumour" but also, at least when the prolactin levels have failed to return to normal, following surgery.

Not all patients, however, tolerate bromocriptine (BC) because of side effects related to its dopaminergic activity (nausea, emesis, orthostatic hypotension). As an alternative treatment we used lisuride (L), another semi-synthetic ergot derivative with a very high affinity for dopamine receptors at the pituitary level [2]. Both BC and L directly stimulate dopamine receptors, thereby inhibiting prolactin release and synthesis in normal pituitary cells as well as in prolactinomas [6].

We started a comparative study in hyperprolactinaemic patients whose condition was mostly caused by micro- and macroprolactinomas as demonstrated by surgery and/or radiological investigation. Treatment with BC was stopped for one month and treatment with L started thereafter. Another smaller group was first treated with L and then with BC after L had been stopped in a similar way. 27 hyperprolactinaemic patients were treated with both dopamine agonists. 20 patients had undergone transsphenoidal or transfrontal surgery for pituitary tumours, but the elevated prolactin levels had not fully returned to normal. The general effect of L and BC on prolactin levels can be seen from figures 2 and 3. During treatment with L the prolactin levels fell by an average of 83%. Side effects occurred in a total of 11 patients and consisted of hypotension (7), vomiting (5) and nausea (10). 14 patients tolerated L without side effects. During treatment with BC the prolactin levels fell by an average of 87%. Side effects occurred in 13 patients: hypotension (8), vomiting (4) and nausea (11). 13 patients experienced no side effects. If one compares the two forms of treatment, 11 patients were normalized by both BC and L. 10 patients could not be normalized by either L or BC. In 4 patients normalization

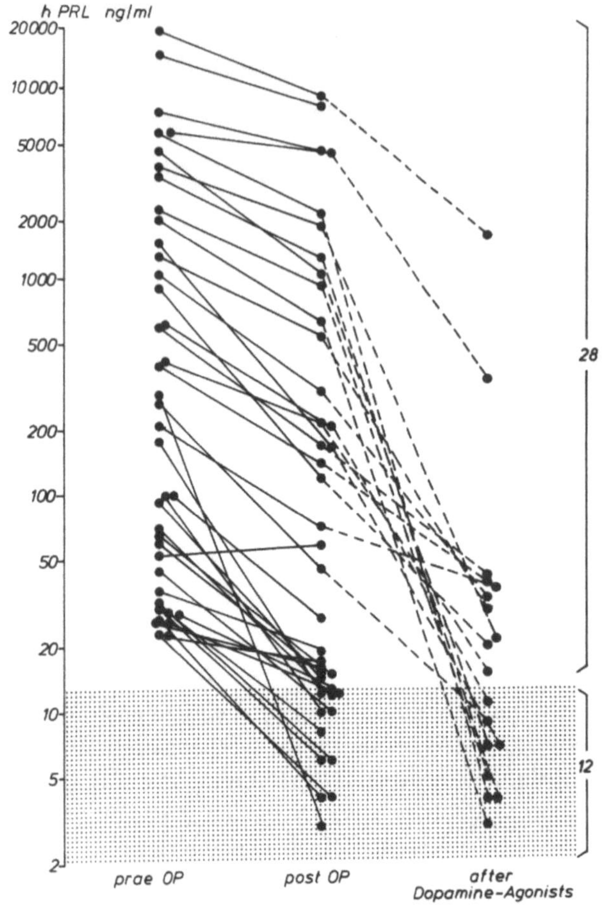

Fig. 1 Prolactin plasma levels before and after pituitary surgery in 40 hyperprolactinaemic patients and after treatment with dopamine agonists (dashed line).

was achieved only by BC, and in 2 only by treatment with L. Thus, BC and L were both equally effective in reducing serum prolactin levels. With regard to side effects, there seem to be no major differences between the two drugs. Since it was found, however, that some patients tolerated L better and others BC, L can be considered as an enrichment in the established therapy of hyperprolactinaemia.

In acromegaly due to growth hormone cell adenomas or to mixed cell adenomas with hypersecretion of growth hormone and prolactin, dopamine agonists were only partly effective in reducing growth hormone levels, in contrast to prolactin.

The effect of growth hormone (GH) on peripheral tissue is partially mediated by somatomedins or "insulin-like growth factors" (IGF) [3, 7] which exist in two forms, IGF I and IGF II. The diagnostic value of IGF I determination as a parame-

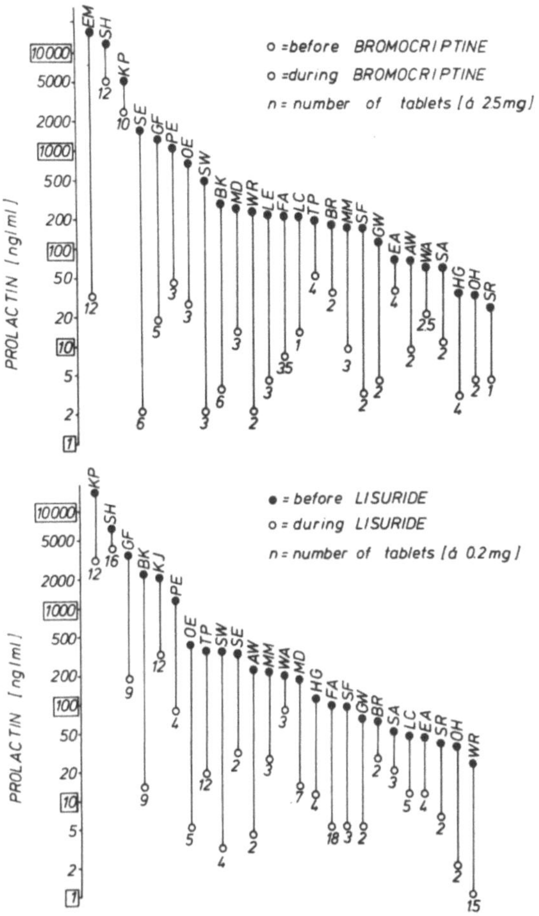

Fig. 2 Influence of bromocriptine and lisuride on prolactin plasma levels in hyperprolactinaemic patients. The dosage (number of tablets) is indicated below the individual results.

ter for the activity of acromegaly is controversial. Whereas Stonesifer [5] is sceptical about IGF determination, Clemmons [1] and Rieu [4] consider it to be of great value in appraising the activity degree of acromegaly. It was the objective of our study to determine the clinical importance of IGF I determination in comparison to GH measurement before and after glucose loading. An attempt was made to establish new criteria for a normal or normalized suppressibility of the GH level after glucose administration.

To test the clinical value of IGF measurement as compared to that of GH, IGF I and IGF II were determined radio-immunologically in 24 acromegalic patients. In 10 of these patients IGF was measured for several months to years after surgery, drug therapy or radiotherapy. In cases of untreated acromegaly the IGF I levels

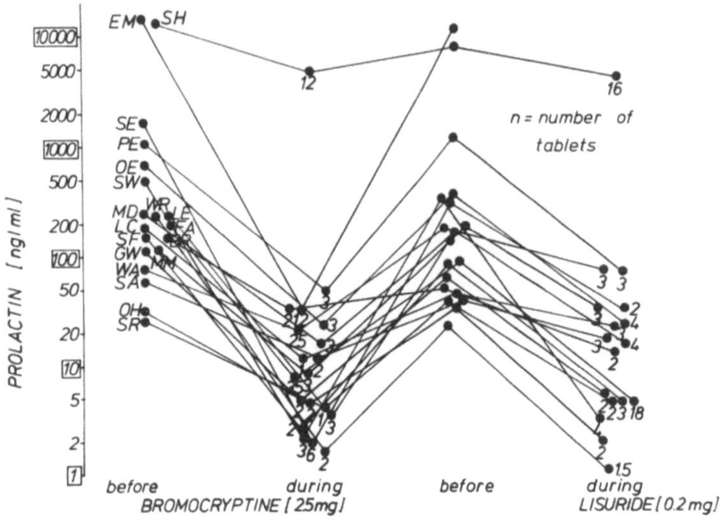

Fig. 3 a

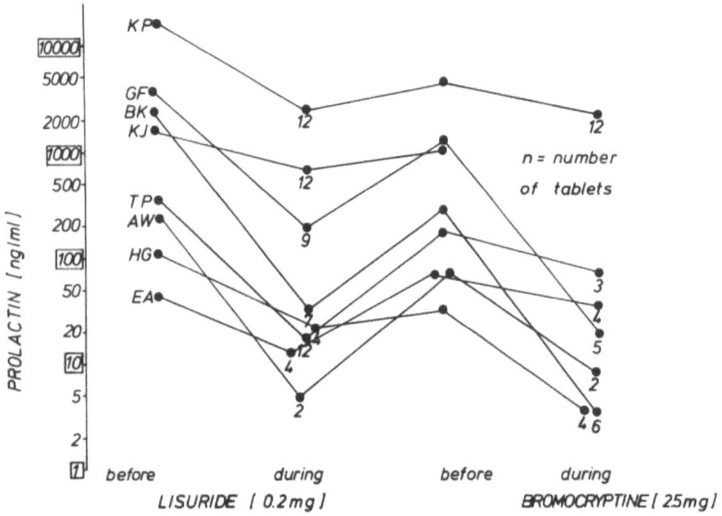

Fig. 3 b

Fig. 3 Prolactin levels of patients first treated with bromocriptine (3a, n = 18) or lisuride (3b, n = 8) before and during treatment with both compounds.

were always found to be elevated (553 ± 75 ng/ml). The corresponding IGF II levels were within the normal to subnormal range (553 ± 38 ng/ml). After surgery or after radiotherapy and/or administration of dopamine agonists, the IGF I levels dropped with a delay in time averaging 6–8 weeks in comparison to the GH levels (figs. 4 and 5). Table 1 summarizes the results after surgery. It can be seen that no patient whose GH level could be suppressed below 1 ng/ml after oral glucose displayed an elevated IGF I level. When the GH value after glucose administration was over 5 ng/ml, IGF I was always elevated (over 300 ng/ml). The following criteria are therefore suggested for evaluating somatotropic function under oral glucose:

A normal or no longer elevated somatotropic function can be diagnosed when a GH value under 1 ng/ml is measured after glucose administration. This value is normally reached after 1 h, in some cases even later, so that in addition to the 1 h value at least also the 2 h value should be determined.

2. If the GH level is not suppressed below 5 ng/ml after oral glucose, then hypersomatotropism or a residual acromegalic activity is present with certainty.

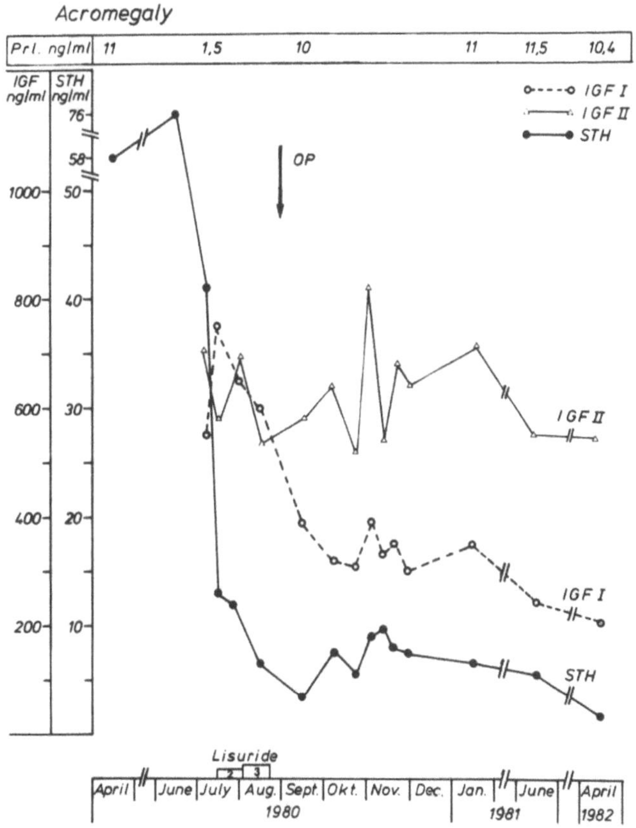

Fig. 4 Course of IGF I, IGF II and GH levels in an acromegalic patient under dopamine agonist (lisuride) therapy and after operation. Prl = prolactin level.

Table 1 Basal and maximally suppressed growth hormone level, IGF I and IGF II after glucose administration (fasting blood sugar as well as some of the blood sugar values (0 h, 1 h and 2 h) during oral glucose loading (100 g) in patients after surgical treatment of an acromegaly

Patient	GH (ng/ml) basal	GH (ng/ml) after glucose	IGF I (ng/ml)	IGF II (ng/ml)	Fasting blood sugar (mg/dl)	Σ 0+1+2 h
A. W.	2.45	→ 0.2	47	391	82	314
B. H.	0.37	→ 0.29	22	236	75	222
C. M.	2.94	→ 0.45	56	642	59	218
Z. H.	1.6	→ 0.54	95	586	65	328
B. I.	3.79	→ 0.60	204	545	64	222
T. M.	12.2	→ 0.98	113	444	70	260
J. F.	2.91	→ 1.76	323	697	97	625
M. H.	2.52	→ 1.88	122	610	77	239
S. E.	3.47	→ 1.94	183	325	116	725
M. K.	3.62	→ 1.99	404	539	98	358
B. G.	2.7	→ 2.9	268	467	90	343
F. E.	3.22	→ 4.87	523	607	88	364
W. K.	8.5	→ 5.6	502	709	88	364
H. R.	7.8	→ 5.7	510	469	103	646
S. H.	7.1	→ 5.98	319	481	103	515
K. W.	5.7	→ 6.3	410	500	89	376
L. H.	4.6	→ 6.3	478	720	77	323
S. I.	7.7	→ 6.7	335	594	72	458
D. A.	18.3	→10.5	411	398	74	433
K. J.	17.0	→19.0	438	260	86	325
B. G.	36.2	→26.1	364	187	106	496
G. B.	33.6	→28.4	898	314	102	524
L. H.	18.1	→30.1	1066	317	84	365
B. I.	41.2	→57.4	576	702	76	334

3. GH values between 1 and 5 ng/ml after oral glucose characterize the initial range in which IGF I determination for evaluation of activity is particularly helpful and important.

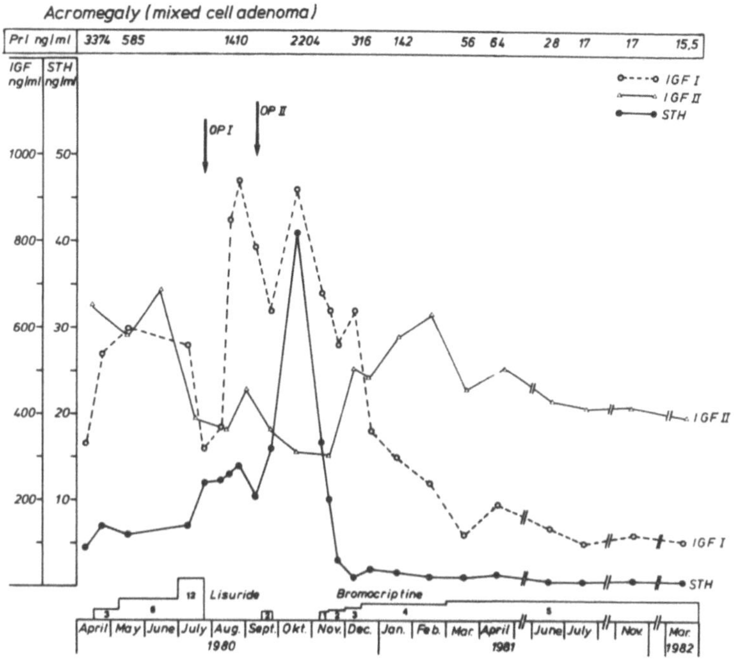

Fig. 5 Course of IGF I, IGF II and GH as well as prolactin levels (Prl) in an acromegalic patient with mixed cell adenoma under therapy with dopamine agonists (lisuride or bromocriptine) and two pituitary operations.

References

[1] Clemmons, D. R., J. J. van Wyk, E. G. Ridgway, et al.: Evaluation of acromegaly by radioimmunoassay of somatomedin C. New Engl. J. Med. **301** (1979) 1138.

[2] Cronin, M. J., C. A. Valdenegro, S. N. Perkins, et al.: The 7315a pituitary tumor is refractory to dopaminergic inhibition of prolactin release but contains dopamine receptors. Endocrinology **109** (1981) 2160.

[3] Daughaday, W. H., K. Hall, M. S. Raben, et al.: Somatomedin: a proposed designation for the sulfation factor. Nature **235** (1972) 107.

[4] Rieu, N., F. Girard, H. Bricaire, et al.: The importance of insulin-like growth factor (somatomedin) measurements in the diagnosis and surveillance of acromegaly. J. Clin. Endocrinol. Metab. **50** (1982) 322.

[5] Stonesifer, L. D., R. M. Jordan, P. O. Kohler: Somatomedin C in treated acromegalic: poor correlation with growth hormone and clinical response. J. Clin. Endocrinol. Metab. **53** (1981) 931.

[6] Thorner, M. O., J. A. Burdman, M. T. Calabrese, et al.: Dopamine agonists and prolactinomas: clinical and basic considerations of the mechanism of action. In: Lisuride and other dopamine agonists. (D. B. Cahne, R. Horowski, R. J. McDonald, W. Wuttke, eds.), p. 213. Raven Press, New York 1983.

[7] van Wyk, J. J., Underwood, L. E.: The somatomedins and their actions. In: Biochemical actions of hormones (G. Litwack, ed.), p. 101. Academic Press, New York 1978.

Persisting partial suppression of growth hormone excess in acromegaly after long term treatment with bromocriptine

E. Leicht, G. Biro

During the last ten years conservative management of acromegaly with bromocriptine has been extensively studied. It was found that growth hormone (GH) levels are depressed by bromocriptine in about 60–75% of the patients. In only about 15–20% of the patients, however, GH concentrations were found to decrease into the range below 5 ng/ml [9, 12], which is considered to indicate successful therapy. After longterm treatment of acromegaly with bromocriptine GH rapidly rises in most cases to initial values, when the administration of the drug is stopped [6]. For these reasons we have had all our patients with acromegaly operated on in the last years, except those who refused surgical treatment.

We now report on a patient who refused surgery and was followed during six years of bromocriptine therapy.

In 1977, when the diagnosis of acromegaly was established, the patient was 56 years of age. She had observed an increase in shoe size since 1974. The sella turcica was found to be enlarged and GH values were fluctuating between 20 and 110 ng/ml. GH was suppressible to 13 ng/ml in the oral glucose tolerance test, rose to 153 ng/ml after 400 μg thyrotropin releasing hormone (TRH) and dropped for about 8 hours to 13–15 ng/ml after a single oral dose of 2,5 mg bromocriptine. The excretion of hydroxyproline in the urine was elevated to 31 mg/24 hrs/m^2 body surface (normal 6.5–21 mg/24 hrs/m^2).

Bromocriptine therapy, initiated in November 1977, was well tolerated. When 30 mg/day, divided into four equal doses, were administered, GH values were found between 11 and 14 ng/ml (control intervals 1–3 months). After 7,5 months the drug was discontinued for one day. 36 hours after the last dose, GH concentration was elevated to 135 ng/ml and suppressed to 121 ng/ml in the oral glucose tolerance test. Hydroxyproline excretion had returned to normal and during the following years gradually fell to the low normal range. GH concentrations were found between 4,0 and 35 ng/ml in the years 1978–1980, and 6.0–17 ng/ml when the daily dose of bromocriptine was reduced to 15 mg from June 1980 to February 1981. Subsequently, the dose was increased to 25 mg/day and GH values gradually fell to the range of 4–7 ng/ml. Without interruption of therapy a TRH-test was performed in August 1983 (400 μg TRH i.v.) and a rise in GH to 8 ng/ml was found.

In September 1983 bromocriptine therapy was discontinued. The following two tests were performed in Erlangen. We thank Prof. Fahlbusch for the results.

Ten days after cessation of therapy GH concentration was 2.5 ng/ml and did not rise after TRH. In the oral glucose tolerance test, suppression to 1.9 ng/ml was observed. Five weeks after termination of therapy, when the glucose tolerance test was repeated, GH concentration was 6 ng/ml and suppressed to 4.9 ng/ml. Nine weeks after the end of therapy, however, GH concentration was elevated to 11 ng/ml and the patient complained of swelling of the hands and feet. In December 1983 bromocriptine therapy was reinstituted. Three weeks later GH concentration was 5 ng/ml, in April 1984 4 ng/ml and at this time, 36 hours after a short interruption of treatment 4,5 ng/ml. No rebound effect [8] was observed as in 1978. Daily fluctuations of growth hormone values and their progressive fall are demonstrated in figure 1.

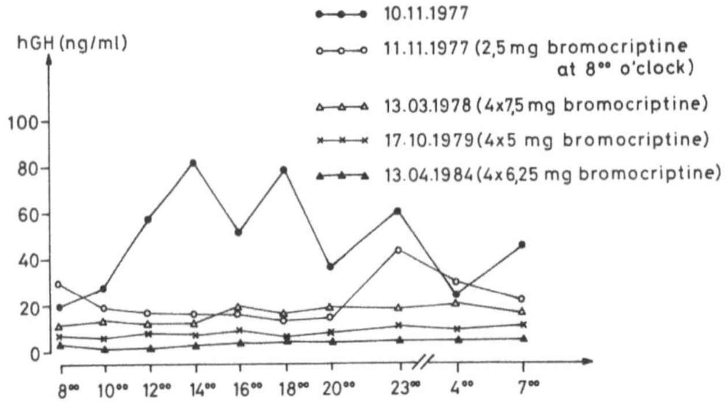

Fig. 1 Growth hormone day profiles before and during therapy with indicated doses of bromocriptine.

In summary, GH values gradually fell to the range of about 5 ng/ml in six years of bromocriptine therapy. The patient was free of symptoms during this time and no side effects of the drug were noticed. Headaches or other symptoms indicating pituitary necrosis [15] were not complained of before, during or after therapy, nor was there a sudden fall in GH values. We therefore believe, that this course of events was due to bromocriptine therapy, the effects of which outlasted the end of treatment for several weeks. It remains to be expected if further administration of bromocriptine will lead to additional improvement of the disease.

Unfortunately we have not measured prolactin concentrations before therapy. After termination of bromocriptine treatment prolactin rose to 20 ng/ml and did not rise further after intravenous TRH. The patient may well be suffering from a GH and prolactin producing adenoma [4].

Reduction of tumour size [5, 7, 10, 11] and persisting suppression of prolactin secretion [2, 13] have been repeatedly reported in patients with prolactinoma. In contrast, GH producing adenomas have much less tendency to shrink during dopamin agonist therapy [6, 10, 14]. GH concentrations generally return to pretreatment levels within 24–48 hours after termination of therapy, even if it has been used for years [6]. In our patient a persisting partial suppression of GH values was found after a very long time of uninterrupted bromocriptine treatment. Recently Happ and coworkers [3] and earlier Althoff and coworkers [1] reported that in some of their patients with acromegaly GH concentrations did not rise to pretreatment values after termination of long-term bromocriptine therapy. Further observations are necessary to answer the question if there exists a subpopulation of acromegalics in whom a similar development of the disease during long-term dopamin agonist therapy may be expected.

References

[1] Althoff, P. H., M. Neubauer, B. Böttger, et al.: Zur Langzeitbehandlung der Akromegalie mit Bromokryptin – Ergebnisse und Erfahrungen nach 3 Jahren Therapie. Verh. Dtsch. Ges. Inn. Med. **84** (1978) 1441–1446.

[2] Eversmann, T., R. Fahlbusch, H. K. Rjosk, et al.: Persisting suppression of prolactin secretion after long-term treatment with bromocriptine in patients with prolactinomas. Acta endocrinol. (Kbh.) **92** (1979) 413–427.

[3] Happ, J., O. Hey, S. Klien, et al.: Bromocriptine therapy in acromegalic patients. Third European workshop on pituitary adenomas, September 7–10, 1983 (Amsterdam), abstract p. 31.

[4] Lamberts, S. W. J., J. G. M. Klijn, C. C. J. van Vroonhoven, et al.: The role of prolactin in the inhibitory action of bromocriptine on growth hormone secretion in acromegaly. Acta endocrinol. (Kbh.) **103** (1983) 446–456.

[5] Landolt, A. M., R. Wüthrich, H. Fellmann: Regression of pituitary prolactinoma after treatment with bromocriptine. Lancet **1** (1979) 1082–1083.

[6] Liuzzi, A., P. G. Chiodini, G. Opizzi, et al.: Medical treatment of pituitary adenomas: effects on hormonal secretion and tumor size. In: Lisuride and other dopamin agonists (D. B. Calne, R. Horowski, R. J. McDonald, W. Wuttke, eds.), pp. 231–238. Raven Press, New York 1983.

[7] McGregor, A. M., M. F. Scanlon, K. Hall, et al.: Reduction in size of a pituitary tumour by bromocriptine therapy. N. Engl. J. Med. **300** (1979) 291–293.

[8] Nortier, J. W. R., R. J. M. Croughs, J. H. H. Thijssen, et al.: Plasma growth hormone (GH) suppressive effect of bromocriptine in acromegaly. Evaluation by plasma GH day profiles and plasma GH concentrations during oral glucose tolerance tests. Third European workshop on pituitary adenomas, September 7–10, 1983 (Amsterdam), abstract p. 29.

[9] Quabbe, H. J.: Treatment of acromegaly by trans-sphenoidal operation, 90 Yttrium implantation and bromocriptine. Results in 230 patients. Clin. Endocrinol. **16** (1982) 16.

[10] Spark, R. F., R. Baker, D. C. Bienfang, et al.: Bromocriptine reduces pituitary tumor size and hypersecretion. Requiem for pituitary surgery? J.A.M.A. **247** (1982) 311–316.

[11] Thorner, M. O., W. H. Martin, A. D. Rogol, et al.: Rapid regression of pituitary prolactinomas during bromocriptine treatment. J. Clin. Endocrinol. Metab. **51** (1980) 438–445.
[12] Wass, J. A. H., M. O. Thorner, D. V. Morris, et al.: Long-term treatment of acromegaly with bromocriptine. Br. Med. J. **1** (1977) 875–878.
[13] Winkelmann, W., B. Allolio, U. Deuß, et al.: Medikamentöse Langzeittherapie bei Patienten mit prolactinproduzierenden Hypophysentumoren. Akt. Endokr. Stoffw. **4** (1983) 163–169.
[14] Wollesen, F., T. Andersen, A. Karle: Size reduction of extrasellar pituitary tumors during bromocriptine treatment. Ann. intern. Med. **96** (1982) 281–286.
[15] Yamaji, T., M. Ishibashi, K. Kosaka: Pituitary apoplexy in acromegaly during bromocriptine therapy. Acta endocrinol. (Kbh.) **98** (1981) 171–177.

Medical and surgical treatment of micro and macroprolactinomas: seven years follow-up of 65 cases

C. Cecotto, M. Leonardi, G. Fabris, C. Taboga, F. Bertolissi, F. De Nardi

Introduction

Since Cushing's era the treatment of pituitary's adenomas has been surgical, by a superior or inferior approach, with subsequent radiological treatment. Since a few years the introduction of bromocriptine has offered new therapeutical possibilities: prolactin secreting adenomas are sensitive to this drug, which results in normal serum prolactin levels and frequently also a reduction in the mass volume.

The diagnosis of a prolactin secreting adenoma needs a complete evaluation, endocrinological and neuroradiological, before the beginning of the treatment, with careful follow-up. In many cases in fact hyperprolactinaemia is possible without evidence of an adenoma. Cases of this kind as clynoid meningiomas, arachnoid cysts and cases with normal CT findings have been excluded from the series reported in this paper.

Material and methods

The group of 62 patients in this paper is composed of 59 females and 3 males, aged from 18 to 54 years.

The neuroradiological examinations were accomplished by means of a G.E. CT/T 8.800, computerized tomograph, and a LU/D F 3000, digital angiograph.

The patients were divided into three subgroups, on the basis of their neuroradiological findings:

1st subgroup: 45 patients, ♀, aged from 18 to 40 years, with CT evidence of a pituitary's microadenoma, clinical syndrome of amenorrhoea-galactorrhoea (serum prolactin levels between 40 and 350 ng/ml).

2nd subgroup: 5 patients: 3 ♂; 15, 30 and 50 years old; 2 ♀, 28 and 37 years old. In these cases there was CT evidence of a sellar mass with extension into the suprasellar cysterns (Serum prolactin levels between 800 and 16000 ng/ml).

3rd subgroup: 11 patients, ♀ aged from 26 to 54 years, with CT evidence of an intrasellar mass (serum prolactin levels between 180 and 1100 ng/ml).

All patients underwent a complete endocrinological evaluation. Their prolactin reserve was investigated under basal conditions and after 200 μg TRH i.v. and also after administration of 10 mg of metoclopramide. All the patients of the 1st and 3rd subgroups were treated with bromocriptine, from 2.5 to 12.5 mg pro die. The medical treatment was chosen also for 4 patients of the 2nd subgroup after a surgical approach, which did not result in the normalization of the prolactin levels.

CT of the pituitary was accomplished before the beginning of the treatment with a follow-up at one month, six months and every year.

Results

1st subgroup: these patients, with CT evidence of microadenoma, received as medical treatment a dose of 2.5–7.5 mg pro die of bromocriptine. As a result the serum levels of prolactin were normalized within 15–60 days, with normal menstruations and ovulations. In 40 patients, the CT follow-up investigation showed modification of the microadenoma in a lucent zone.

2nd subgroup: 4 patients underwent surgery by the transsphenoidal/subfrontal approach for the suprasellar extension of the mass causing a visual deficit. In no case was surgery followed by normalization of the prolactin serum levels. The bromocriptine medical treatment was chosen, 12.5 mg pro die, with endocrinological normalization. One case was submitted to the medical treatment only, with the same dose resulting in normalization of the prolactine serum levels, from 16000 ng/ml, and also with a great reduction in the sellar and extrasellar mass (figs. 1 and 2).

3rd subgroup: all these patients were treated with 2.5–7.5 mg pro die of bromocriptine. The normalization of the serum levels of prolactin was associated with a reduction in the sellar mass and frequently with cystic evolution of the CT images (fig. 3). In two cases the interruption of the treatment was followed by new hyperprolactinaemia and sellar mass growth.

Conclusion

From our experience, which is in accordance with the extensive literature on the subject, we think that the treatment of choice in cases of prolactin secreting pituitary mass lesions should be with bromocriptine. In fact the administration of this drug offers satisfactory results even in those cases unsatisfactorily treated by the surgical approach.

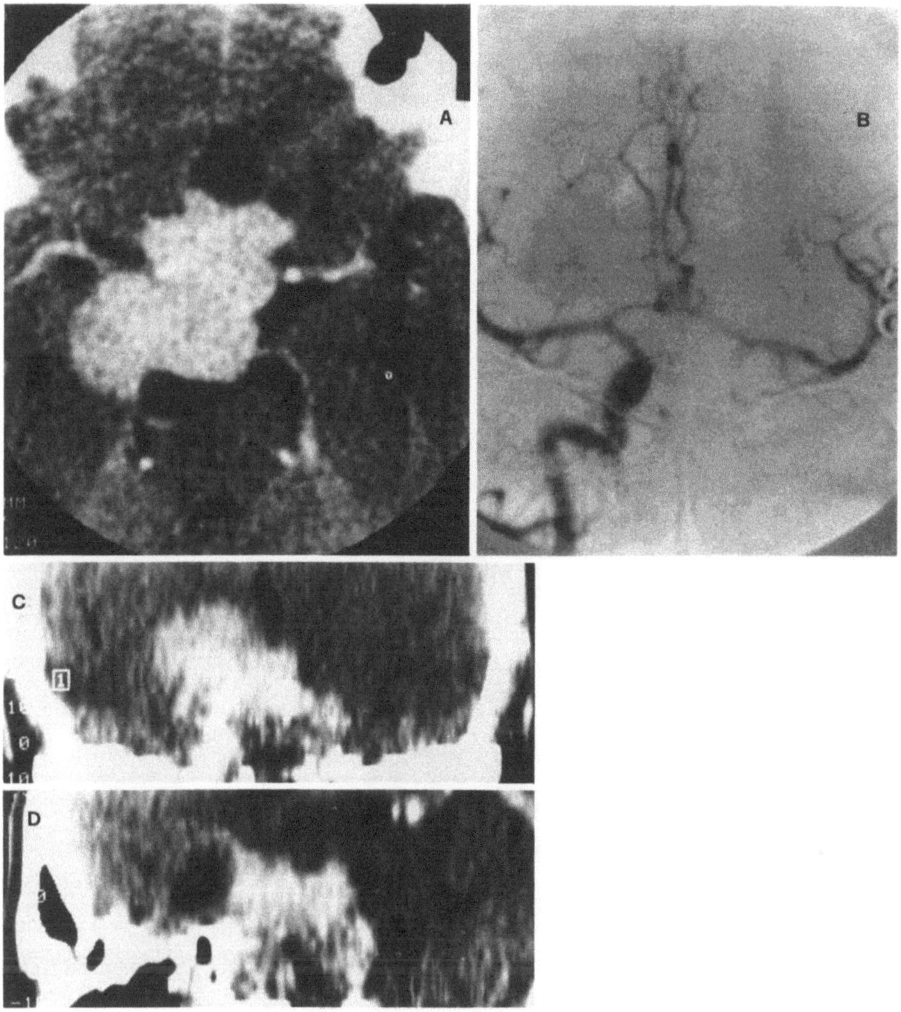

Fig. 1 Fifth case from the second subgroup: very large prolactin-secreting adenoma, examinations before medical treatment.
(A) axial view, (B) angiography, (C) coronal reconstruction, (D) sagittal reconstruction. The total extention of the mass is clearly evaluated.

In our cases we have positive results in 93%, with various CT appearances: normalization of CT findings, CT lucency (cystic evolution? necrosis?), reduction in the mass volume.

The surgical approach is now confined to the patients who do not respond positively to the bromocriptine treatment and, moreover, in all cases with a visual deficit due to the mass effect on the optic chiasma.

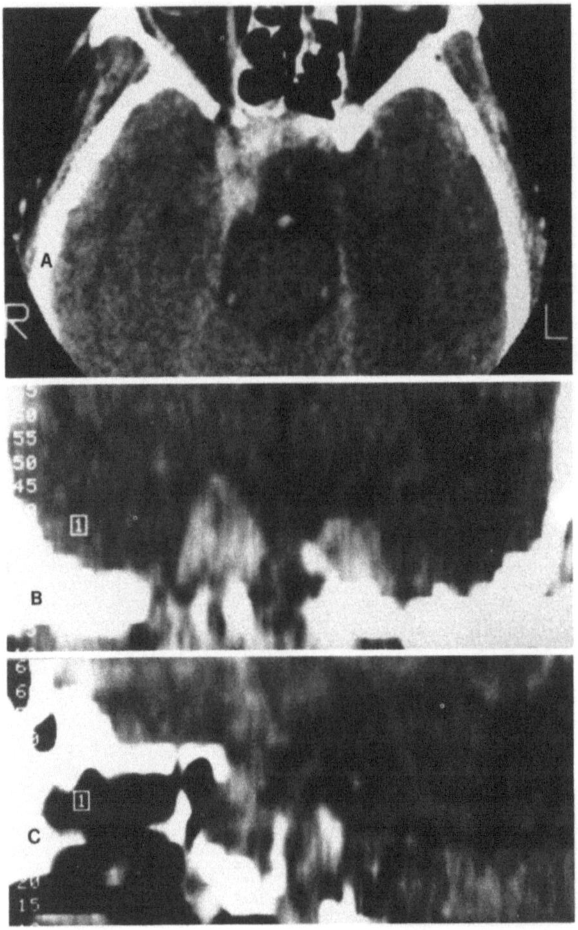

Fig. 2 Same case as figure 1 examinations after six month of bromocriptine medical treatment, at a dose of 12.5 mg pro die.
(A) axial view, (B) coronal reconstruction, (C) sagittal reconstruction.
Enormous reduction in mass volume. Normalization of prolactin serum levels, from the starting point of 16000 ng/ml.

Summary

Forty-six female patients (aged 18 to 40) with high serum prolactin levels (40 ng/ml–350 ng/ml) and with CT evidence of microprolactinoma were studied during long term bromocriptine treatment (2.5–7.5 mg pro die). In forty patients the effects of bromocriptine on the changes in the microadenoma in the CT scans were shown as a region of hypodensity. Four patients showed a complete remission of the microadenoma and two cases showed no change in their CT scans. The normal-

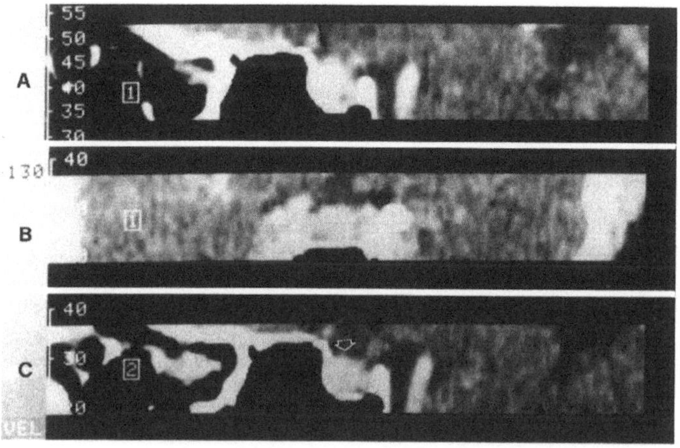

Fig. 3 Young patient from the third subgroup.
(A) sagittal computer reformatted image, clear evidence of an intrasellar mass. arrow. The patient underwent bromocriptine medical treatment, (B) and (C) examination after four months' of treatment (coronal and sagittal reconstructions): evidence of mass reduction, open arrow; normalization of serum prolactin levels from the starting point of 300 ng/ml.

ization of serum prolactin levels after bromocriptine treatment in all patients occurred before the CT changes.

Four patients with macroprolactinoma underwent surgery; none of these patients had a normalization of serum levels of PRL postoperatively. One patient with an extrasellar macroprolactinoma (16000 ng/ml) showed a normalization of the prolactin level and a rapid regression of the tumour mass at CT after two months of bromocriptine treatment (12.5 mg/day). Twelve patients with intrasellar prolactinomas were successfully treated with bromocriptine and showed a size reduction in the tumour and in two patients the withdrawal of the drug was followed by reenlarging of the tumour mass.

References

[1] Landolt, A. M., R. Wütherich, H. Fellmann: Regression of pituitary prolactinoma after treatment with bromocriptine. Lancet **1** (1979) 1082–1083.

[2] Leonardi, M., F. Bertolissi, G. Fabris, et al.: CT evidence of functioning microadenomas of the pituitary. In: Pituitary Microadenomas, pp. 329–335. Academic Press, London 1980.

[3] Leonardi, M., F. Bertolissi, G. Fabris, et al.: CT checking of a series of endocrinological patients under medical treatment. Congress of the European Society of Neuroradiology, Milan 1981.

[4] Niwa, J., O. Sato, S. Tanabe: Effects of bromocriptine for prolactin-secreting adenomas: analysis by CT scan. Computerized Radiol. **7** (1983) 237–241.

VI Aspects of gynecology and obstetrics

Management of prolactinomas in pregnancy

S. J. Nillius, A. Rojanasakul, T. Bergh

Introduction

During the seventies, the management of infertile women with symptoms and signs of a prolactinoma was a most controversial issue in clinical reproductive medicine. Most authorities were of the opinion that the risk of rapid pituitary enlargement during pregnancy was considerable. Treatment with either surgery nor radiotherapy or both was therefore normally advocated for such patients before they were allowed to attempt to conceive [24]. Experiences gained during the last five years have shown that neither surgery nor radiotherapy provides a definitive cure for most infertile women with prolactinomas [25]. Transsphenoidal operations on the pituitary can have disastrous results in inexpert hands and, even when performed by experienced surgeons, hypopituitarism may follow [23]. Long-term follow-up results after pituitary surgery of prolactinomas are still limited but suggest a surprisingly high recurrence rate [32].

Medical therapy with bromocriptine was suggested by Bergh et al. [1] to be the most suitable primary treatment for many infertile women with prolactinomas. This therapeutic alternative has been backed up by the clinical experience gained during recent years. Induction of ovulation has been shown to be remarkably safe in most infertile women with prolactinomas.

This paper on prolactinomas and pregnancy is an up-dated review of the literature published after 1979.

Patients and methods

Incidence of prolactinoma complications during pregnancy

The first reports on the incidence of pituitary tumour complications during pregnancy consisted of patients, most of whom had been treated with other ovulation-inducing agents than bromocriptine [14, 22]. In many of these women with amenorrhoea and sometimes also galactorrhoea, there was no biochemical evidence of hyperprolactinaemia. During recent years, 13 series of a total of 430 hyperprolactinaemic women, who had been given primary dopamine agonist therapy to induce ovulation and pregnancy, have appeared (tab. 1). Sixty-six per cent of these women had radiological signs consistent with a pituitary tumour. The information on clinical details in the 13 papers usually does not permit a separation of the patients with presumptive prolactinomas into sub-groups of micro- and macroadenomas. Unfortunately, there is not yet any uniformly accepted classification of patients with prolactinomas treated primarily with medical therapy. The introduction of a new generation of high resolution computerized tomography (CT) scanners may make a better delineation of particularly the small prolactinomas possible in the future.

It is evident from table 1 that the incidence of severe pituitary tumour complications during pregnancy is low in prolactinoma patients treated primarily with dopamine agonists, mostly bromocriptine. Only 2 per cent of the hyperprolactinaemic women developed reversible visual complications due to rapid prolactinoma enlargement during dopamine agonist-induced pregnancy. In the last few years it has been clearly documented that dopamine agonist treatment causes a regression of prolactin-secreting pituitary tumours [12]. This may, at least in part, explain the rare occurrence of prolactinoma complications during pregnancy.

The risk of pregnancy-induced pituitary expansion is small also in bromocriptine-treated women with large prolactinomas. Bergh et al. [3] described the outcome of 19 pregnancies induced by bromocriptine in 14 women with large prolactinomas. Only one patient had clinical symptoms of marked tumour enlargement with visual field defects during pregnancy. Post-partum X-ray of the sella turcica showed signs of tumour expansion in another woman who had a clinically uneventful pregnancy. The other 12 patients experienced 17 pregnancies with no complications caused by their prolactinomas. One of them was a 36-year-old infertile woman with 10 years of amenorrhoea-galactorrhoea and the highest pretreatment serum prolactin concentration (1470 μg/l; normal <15 μg/l). Her pretreatment sellar X-ray is shown in figure 1. Since we described the outcome of her first pregnancy, she has experienced a second bromocriptine-induced uneventful term pregnancy. Her serum prolactin level 2 months after this pregnancy was only 98 μg/l [25].

Thus, even in patients with large prolactinomas serious pituitary complications seldom develop during bromocriptine-induced pregnancies. It is therefore warranted to treat most infertile women with prolactinomas primarily with dopamine agonists.

Monitoring of pregnancies in women with prolactinomas

As soon as pregnancy is suspected in a dopamine agonist-treated woman with hyperprolactinaemia, the drug should be discontinued. The low incidence of pituitary tumour complications during pregnancy does not justify prophylactic treat-

Table 1 Incidence of pituitary tumour complications during 488 term pregnancies in 430 hyperprolactinaemic women given primary dopamine agonist therapy

Reference	Patients	Patients with presumtive prolactinoma	Pregnancies	Visual complication	Diabetes insipidus	Progression of sella X-ray change after pregnancy
	n	n	n	n	n	n
Present study	61	44	71	2	0	6
Corenblum & Taylor (1983)	37	30	52	1	0	0
Crosignani et al. (1981)	28	13	29	1	0	4
Divers & Yen (1983)	48*	48*	48	4	0	0
Hammond et al. (1983)	13*	13*	16	0	1	0
Jewelewicz & Vande Wiele (1980)	25*	25*	25	0	0	0
Kletzky et al. (1983)	20	14*	20	0	0	0
Nyboe-Anderson et al. (1983)	15	8*	17	0	0	1
Pepperell (1981)	61	8	79	1	0	0
Randall et al. (1982)	30	5	40	0	0	1
Rjosk et al. (1982)	48*	48*	47	0	0	0
Shewchuk et al. (1980)	27	19*	27	1	0	6
Weinstein et al. (1981)	17	10	17	0	0	0
Total	430	285	488	10 (2%)	1 (0.2%)	18 (3.7%)

* Only patients with microadenoma treated

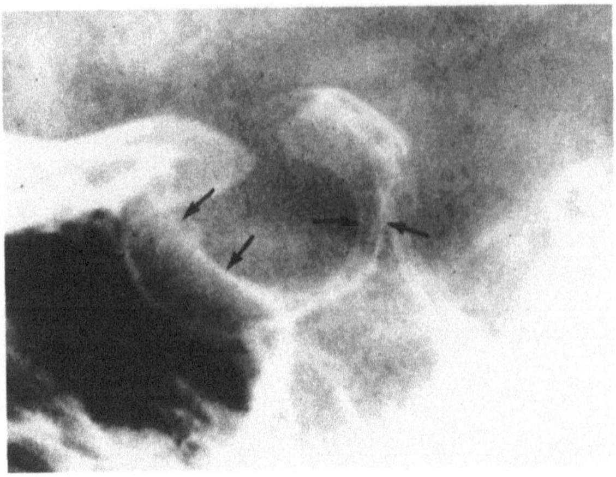

Fig. 1 Pretreatment X-ray of the sella turcica in a 36 year old hyperprolactinaemic woman. The pituitary fossa is markedly asymmetric. She was successfully treated with bromocriptine and experienced two uneventful term pregnancies. (From Bergh et al. [3] with permission).

ment throughout pregnancy. Already before the ovulation-inducing treatment is instituted the patient should have been carefully informed about symptoms and signs of possible rapid pituitary enlargement during pregnancy. This information is brought up again and forwarded to the antenatal clinic, where frequent clinical examinations are performed throughout pregnancy.

Visual field examinations should be performed regularly during the pregnancy. This monitoring should be initiated already in the first trimester, since prolactinoma complications may develop early in pregnancy (fig. 2). Our practice is to perform these examinations every 1–2 months for earliest possible detection of visual impairment. Every woman with hyperprolactinaemia before pregnancy, regardless

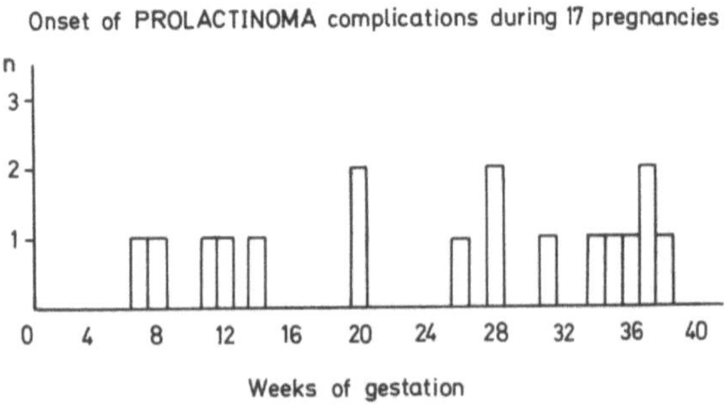

Fig. 2 Onset of prolactinoma complications during 17 pregnancies described in detail in table 2.

of the presence of radiological signs of a prolactinoma or not, should really be monitored in this way. Severe visual complications have been described in bromocriptine-treated pregnant women with normal pretreatment radiology of the sella turcica (see table 2 and case report below).

Repeated serum prolactin determinations at monthly intervals throughout pregnancy have been advocated by some authorities [14]. In our opinion this is of limited value for the management of the pregnant prolactinoma patient. Indication for treatment of a prolactinoma during pregnancy should not be based solely on a biochemical test but rather on clinical symptoms or signs of a pituitary tumour complication. There are few data on the clinical value of repeated prolactin measurements during pregnancy in patients with prolactinomas. The general opinion seems to be that maternal prolactin levels are not predictive of any complications [10, 26, 30]. A case report by Nabarro [23] may be one exception. This patient had a dramatic increase of her serum prolactin level at 20 weeks of gestation but had no visual field abnormalities. After pregnancy, she was found to have an invasive prolactinoma, which was difficult to treat. However, in most instances, the finding of a markedly raised serum prolactin level in a pregnant asymptomatic prolactinoma patient only raises questions and is of little help for the clinical management.

Radiological check-ups during pregnancy are not indicated unless the patient has clinical symptoms or signs of a prolactinoma complication.

Management of prolactinoma complications during pregnancy

Should symptoms or signs of a pituitary tumour complication (severe headache, visual impairment, cranial nerve palsies, diabetes insipidus, etc.) occur during pregnancy in a patient with a prolactinoma, there are several therapeutic alternatives available. If the symptoms are mild and not rapidly progressive, conservative treatment under close surveillance may be warranted. However, in most other instances, reinstitution of bromocriptine treatment during pregnancy should be the primary therapy [1]. If the pregnancy is close to term, labour should be induced. After interruption of pregnancy, even severe symptoms of pituitary tumour complications rapidly improve [24].

Dopamine agonist therapy for pregnancy-induced prolactinoma complications may well be used in combination with corticosteroid treatment, which formerly was the medical therapy of choice in such situations [16]. Bromocriptine with its tumour-regressing effect has been successfully used for treatment of prolactinoma complications during pregnancy (tab. 2). This is also illustrated by the following case report.

A 21-year-old woman with one year of amenorrhoea-galactorrhoea was evaluated elsewhere and found to have a serum prolactin level of 160 μg/l. A plain sellar X-

Table 2 Cases of symptomatic pituitary tumour complications during pregnancy and their management in women with hyperprolactinaemia

References	Sella turcica X-ray before pregnancy*	Serum prolactin before treatment	Complication	Onset (week)	Management
Bergh et al. (1984)	normal plain X-ray	160 μg/l	bitemporal hemianopsia	31	Bromocriptine
Corenblum and Taylor (1983)	macroadenoma		visual field defect	12	Bromocriptine
Crosignani et al. (1981)	macroadenoma	36 ng/ml	visual field defect	36	Surgery
Dommerholt et al. (1981)	slight asymmetry	100 μg/l	bitemporal hemianopsia	20	Surgery
Divers and Yen (1983)	microadenoma		bitemporal hemianopsia	37	Induction of labour
	microadenoma		bitemporal hemianopsia	38	Induction of labour
Furuhjelm et al. (1980)	normal plain X-ray	>200 μg/l	visual field defect	26	Bromocriptine Induction of labour
Hammond et al. (1983)	microadenoma		severe headache	28	Bromocriptine
	macroadenoma		diabetes insipidus	37	Bromocriptine
Konopka et al. (1983)	macroadenoma	54 ng/ml	bitemporal hemianopsia	20	Bromocriptine
	macroadenoma	115 ng/ml	bitemporal hemianopsia	28	Bromocriptine
Maeda et al. (1983)	macroadenoma		ptosis, diplopia, oculomotor nerve paralysis	14	Bromocriptine
Pepperell (1981)	microadenoma		temporal visual field abnormality	last trimester	Bromocriptine
Rjosk et al. (1980)	double contour	2700 μu/ml	visual field defect	34	Bromocriptine, surgery
Shewchuk et al. (1980)	microadenoma	98 ng/ml	diplopia, third nerve palsy	7	Surgery
van der Spuy & Jacobs (1984)	macroadenoma	22000 mu/l	severe headache regrowth of tumour	11	Bromocriptine
van Roon et al. (1981)	normal plain X-ray	150 ng/ml	bitemporal hemianopsia severe galactorrhoea	8	Bromocriptine

* as judged by the authors

ray was judged to be normal (fig. 3). Bromocriptine treatment (3.75 mg/day) restored ovulatory function and she conceived after 5 months of therapy. In the third trimester of pregnancy she was found to have progressing visual field defects and decreased visual acuity. CT scan at admittance to our department showed suprasellar extension (SSE) of a pituitary tumour. Bromocriptine treatment (7.5 mg/day) was reinstituted in pregnancy week 31. The visual impairment rapidly improved and was normalized after 3 weeks of therapy. A repeat CT scan showed regression of the SSE. The pregnancy continued uneventfully and a healthy girl was delivered at term. Bromocriptine was discontinued 2 days post-partum and the patient breast-fed normally for 8 months. Post-partum CT-scan showed no SSE [4]. After weaning, amenorrhoea persisted. The serum prolactin level was 52 µg/l. Bromocriptine was reinstituted and ovulation returned with conception after 4 months of treatment. Bromocriptine was then discontinued. The second pregnancy was clinically uneventful with normal visual fields.

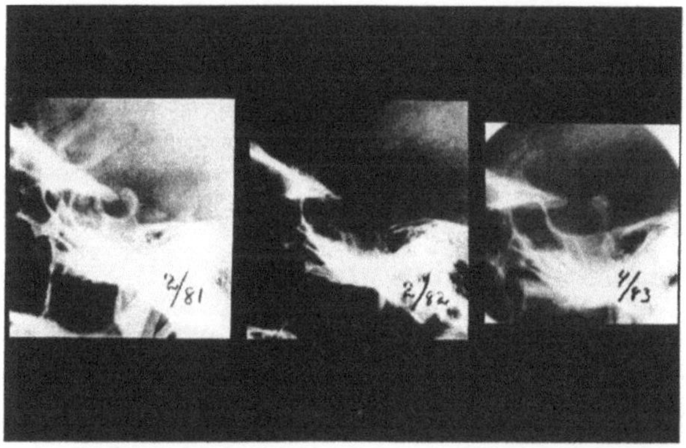

Fig. 3 Plain sellar X-ray of a 21 year old hyperprolactinaemic woman with a prolactinoma complication during pregnancy. Before bromocriptine therapy, the X-ray was interpreted as normal (left). A marked expansion of the sella turcica was noted in the 31st week of pregnancy when pronounced visual impairments occurred (middle). After delivery and lactation a remodelling of the pituitary fossa with recalcification occurred (right).

This case report illustrates that severe visual impairment can occur during pregnancy also in hyperprolactinaemic patients with no evident radiological changes of the sella turcica. Rapid tumour enlargement with visual complications does not necessarily occur during a second bromocriptine-induced pregnancy in prolactinoma patients who have had SSE of their tumour during the first pregnancy. It also illustrates that lactation does not exert any untoward effects on a prolactinoma.

Should medical therapy with dopamine agonists alone or in combination with corticosteroids fail to improve the prolactinoma complication there is yet another therapeutic alternative, namely surgery. There are several reports in the literature on pituitary surgery during pregnancy with a successful outcome both for mother and child [24].

Safety of bromocriptine treatment during pregnancy

Recent data on the outcome of bromocriptine-induced pregnancies indicate that there is no special risk for the foetus inherent in the dopamine agonist therapy. Turkalj et al. [34] obtained information from 1410 pregnancies in 1335 women treated with bromocriptine before and after conception. Eighty-two foetuses were exposed to bromocriptine for more than 8 weeks. Nine patients were treated throughout pregnancy and all of them delivered healthy children with no abnormalities. A second survey of bromocriptine in pregnancy is ongoing [20]. Intense monitoring of 563 pregnancies in bromocriptine-treated women confirms the reassuring results of the first study published. There was no increased incidence of spontaneous abortion nor of congenital malformations in the babies born. Neither was there any specific pattern of abnormal postnatal development in 212 Caucasian and 134 Japanese infants born to bromocriptine-treated mothers.

Prophylactic bromocriptine therapy during pregnancy

Continuation of bromocriptine treatment during pregnancy to prevent tumour complications was described by Yuen [38], who treated two women with microprolactinomas to the third trimester of pregnancy. Bromocriptine was then discontinued for fear of development of respiratory distress syndrome in the infants due to subnormal cord prolactin levels. Prophylactic use of bromocriptine during pregnancy in women with prolactinomas has been used by clinical investigators but few reports on the results of this practice have appeared in the literature.

Four patients with macroprolactinomas were treated by Canales et al. [5] with bromocriptine (5–20 mg/day) throughout the entire pregnancy and puerperium. In two other women with macroprolactinomas, bromocriptine was discontinued after conception. None of their patients had any pituitary tumour complication. Recently, Konopka et al. [19] reported on continuous bromocriptine therapy for the prevention of neurological complications in 10 pregnant women with prolactinomas. The bromocriptine dosage (5–20 mg/day) was modified to reduce the serum prolactin level to below 20 ng/ml. Eight patients continued without interruption throughout pregnancy and had no serious complications. Two other patients, who were not treated from the start of pregnancy, developed bitemporal hemianopsia at 5 and 7 months of pregnancy, respectively. In both, reinstitution of bromocriptine rapidly normalized their visual fields.

Prophylactic bromocriptine treatment during the second and third trimester of pregnancy was used by de Wit et al. [9] in 13 women with macroprolactinomas. One of their patients had signs of tumour enlargement during the first trimester but the others had uncomplicated term pregnancies with delivery of healthy normally-developing infants. The authors stated in their conclusion that they are no longer in favour of prophylactic bromocriptine therapy during pregnancy because of the low incidence of pregnancy-induced prolactinoma complications. This is in accordance with our policy. Instead we, like them, favour close surveillance during pregnancy and reinstitute bromocriptine therapy only if symptoms or signs of severe prolactinoma complications occur.

Postpartum management of patients with prolactinomas

During the first months of normal lactation, suckling has a marked stimulatory effect on the prolactin secretion. Some authors have therefore advised against breast-feeding in patients with prolactinomas in order to decrease this stimulatory effect on the pituitary lactotrophs [31, 33]. However, all our patients with prolactinomas have been permitted to breast-feed without any untoward effects being observed. The patient described above, with visual field defects developing during pregnancy, breast-fed normally when bromocriptine was discontinued two days after delivery. Further tumour regression was verified by CT scan during the period of lactation. In our opinion, there is therefore no reason to withhold the women with prolactinomas from the advantages of breast-feeding.

Repeat radiological investigations of the sella turcica should be with-held until after delivery unless serious neurological complications occur. Subtle radiological changes in the bony structure of the pituitary fossa have been observed by many investigators at postpartum X-ray (tab. 1). These findings have been interpreted as asymptomatic prolactinoma enlargement during pregnancy.

Prolactin determinations in serum are usually performed only after weaning. If hyperprolactinaemia and anovulation persist, bromocriptine treatment is indicated to restore normal gonadal function.

Influence of pregnancy on prolactinomas

Resolution of hyperprolactinaemia after bromocriptine-induced pregnancy has been described but is a rather infrequent finding [2, 8, 30]. On the other hand, it is very uncommon that pregnancy makes the hyperprolactinaemic condition worse. In 19 women with presumptive prolactinomas, the mean serum prolactin concentration after pregnancy and lactation was similar to that before bromocriptine-induced pregnancy (fig. 4). This was confirmed by Rjosk et al. [30], who studied the outcome of 38 uncomplicated term pregnancies in 33 patients with prolactinomas.

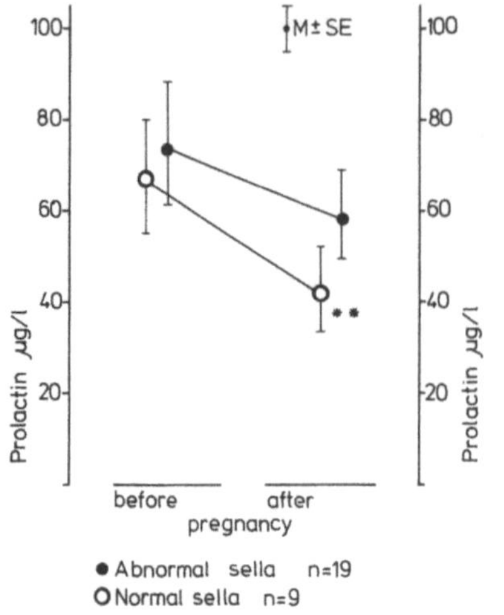

Fig. 4 Mean serum prolactin levels before bromocriptine therapy and after pregnancy and lactation in 28 hyperprolactinaemic women. (Data from Bergh et al. [2]).

They also observed that even several pregnancies following each other do not lead to persistent enlargement of prolactinomas.

The development of a severe prolactinoma complication during a previous pregnancy does not necessarily contraindicate medical induction of ovulation and pregnancy [1 and case report above]. Should a complication recur during the next pregnancy, reinstitution of bromocriptine therapy has proved to improve the symptoms rapidly [6].

Summary

The management of infertile women with prolactinomas is much less controversial today than it used to be. Most authorities now agree that primary medical therapy with dopamine agonists is the treatment of choice for most of these patients. Induction of ovulation by dopamine agonists is highly effective in prolactinoma patients. The incidence of complications caused by rapid pituitary tumour enlargement is remarkably low not only in women with micro- but also macroprolactinomas without evident suprasellar extension.

Before pregnancy, the patient should be carefully evaluated by modern neuroradiological techniques. She should be informed about the low risk of rapid pituitary enlargement during dopamine agonist-induced pregnancy and the symptoms and signs of such a complication. The dopamine agonist therapy should be discontinued as soon as pregnancy is suspected. The low risk of tumour complications does not justify prophylactic treatment.

During the pregnancy, the patient should be monitored by regular antenatal visits and repeated visual field determinations should be carried out. Should a prolactinoma complication occur during pregnancy, reinstitution of bromocriptine is the primary treatment. Bromocriptine has no teratogenic effects or any other untoward effects on the pregnancy. It should be discontinued after delivery to permit normal lactation which has not been shown to have any adverse effect on prolactinomas. Nor does pregnancy make the hyperprolactinaemic condition worse. If bromocriptine treatment fails to markedly improve the prolactinoma complication, there are other therapeutic alternatives which have been used to treat pregnancy-induced prolactinoma complications with successful outcome for both the mother and child.

A properly evaluated, well informed and carefully supervised infertile woman with a prolactinoma can be effectively treated with dopamine agonists. The rare prolactinoma complications during pregnancy can be safely managed. The risk of irreversible sequelae after a pituitary tumour complication during dopamine agonist-induced pregnancy is remote in infertile patients with prolactinomas under close surveillance.

References

[1] Bergh, T., S. J. Nillius, L. Wide: Clinical course and outcome of pregnancies in amenorrhoeic women with hyperprolactinaemia and pituitary tumours. Br. Med. J. **1** (1978) 875–880.

[2] Bergh, T., S. J. Nillius, S.-G. Larsson, et al.: Effects of bromocriptine-induced pregnancy on prolactin-secreting pituitary tumours. Acta endocrinol. **98** (1981) 333–338.

[3] Bergh, T., S. J. Nillius, P. Enoksson, et al.: Bromocriptine-induced pregnancies in women with large prolactinomas. Clin. Endocrinol. **17** (1982) 625–631.

[4] Bergh, T., S. J. Nillius, P. Enoksson, et al.: Bromocriptine-induced regression of a suprasellar extending prolactinoma during pregnancy. J. Endocrinol. Invest. **7** (1984) 133–136.

[5] Canales, E. S., I. C. García, J. E. Ruíz, et al.: Bromocriptine as prophylactic therapy in prolactinoma during pregnancy. Fertil. Steril. **36** (1981) 524–526.

[6] Corenblum, B., P. J. Taylor: Long-term follow-up of hyperprolactinemic women treated with bromocriptine. Fertil. Steril. **40** (1983) 596–599.

[7] Crosignani, P. G., C. Ferrari, C. Scarduelli, et al.: Spontaneous and Induced Pregnancies in Hyperprolactinaemic Women. Obstet. Gynecol. **58** (1981) 708–713.

[8] Daya, W., A. B. Shewchuk, N. Bryceland: The effect of multiparity on intrasellar prolactinomas. Am. J. Obstet. Gynecol. **148** (1984) 512–515.

[9] de Wit, W., H. J. T. Coelingh Bennink, L. J. Gerards: Prophylactic bromocriptine treatment during pregnancy of women with macroprolactinomas: report of 13 pregnancies. International Symposium on Prolactinomas, Graz, April 29-May 2, 1984. Abstract 54, p. 135.

[10] Divers, W. A. Jr., S. S. C. Yen: Prolactin-Producing Microadenomas in Pregnancy. Obstet. Gynecol. **61** (1983) 425–429.
[11] Dommerholt, H. B. R., J. Assies, A. J. M. van der Werf: Growth of a prolactinoma during pregnancy. Case report and review. Br. J. Obstet. Gynaecol. **88** (1981) 62–70.
[12] Franks, S., H. S. Jacobs: Hyperprolactinaemia. Clin. Endocrinol. Metabol. **12** (1983) 641–668.
[13] Furuhjelm, M., T. Rydner, K. Carlström: Hyperprolactinemia in cases of infertility and amenorrhea. Acta Obstet. Gynecol. Scand. **59** (1980) 137–141.
[14] Gemzell, C., C. F. Wang: Outcome of pregnancy in women with pituitary adenoma. Fertil. Steril. **4** (1979) 363–372.
[15] Hammond, C. B., A. F. Haney, M. R. Land, et al.: The outcome of pregnancy in patients with treated and untreated prolactin-secreting pituitary tumors. Am. J. Obstet. Gynecol. **147** (1983) 148–157.
[16] Jewelewicz, R., E. A. Zimmerman, P. W. Carmel: Conservative management of a pituitary tumor during pregnancy following induction of ovulation with gonadotropins. Fertil. Steril. **28** (1977) 35–40.
[17] Jewelewicz, R., R. L. Van de Wiele: Clinical course and outcome of pregnancy in twenty-five patients with pituitary microadenomas. Am. J. Obstet. Gynecol. **136** (1980) 339–343.
[18] Kletzky, O. A., R. P. Marss, V. Davajan: Management of patients with hyperprolactinemia and normal or abnormal tomograms. Am. J. Obstet. Gynecol. **147** (1983) 528–532.
[19] Konopka, P., J. P. Raymond, R. E. Merceron, et al.: Continuous administration of bromocriptine in the prevention of neurological complications in pregnant women with prolactinomas. Am. J. Obstet. Gynecol. **146** (1983) 935–938.
[20] Krupp, P., I. Turkalj: Surveillance of Parlodel (bromocriptine) in pregnancy and offspring. In: Prolactinomas and Pregnancy (H. S. Jacobs, ed.), pp. 45–50. MTP Press Ltd., Lancaster 1984.
[21] Maeda, T., T. Ushiroyama, K. Okuda, et al.: Effective bromocriptine treatment of a pituitary macroadenoma during pregnancy. Obstet. Gynecol. **61** (1983) 117–121.
[22] Magyar, D. M., J. R. Marshall: Pituitary tumours and pregnancy. Am. J. Obstet. Gynecol. **132** (1978) 739–751.
[23] Nabarro, J. D. N.: Pituitary Prolactinomas. Clin. Endocrinol. **17** (1982) 129–155.
[24] Nillius, S. J., T. Bergh, S.-G. Larsson: Pituitary tumours and pregnancy. In: Pituitary Adenomas. Biology, Physiopathology and Treatment (J. P. Derome, C. P. Jedynak, F. Peillon, eds.), pp. 103–111. Asclepios France, Paris 1980.
[25] Nillius, S. J., T. Bergh: Prolactinomas and Pregnancy. In: Proceedings from the 3rd European Workshop in Pituitary Adenomas (S. W. J. Lamberts, J. Assies, F. J. H. Tilders, E. A. van der Veen, eds.). Blackwell, London 1984 (in press).
[26] Nyboe Andersen, A., J. Starup, A. Tabor, et al.: The possible prognostic value of serum prolactin increment during pregnancy in hyperprolactinaemic patients. Acta Endocrinol. **102** (1983) 1–5.
[27] Pepperell, R. J.: Prolactin and reproduction. Fertil. Steril. **35** (1981) 267–274.
[28] Randall, S., I. Laing, A. J. Chapman, et al.: Pregnancies in women with hyperprolactinaemia: obstetric and endocrinological management of 50 pregnancies in 37 women. Br. J. Obstet. Gynaecol. **89** (1982) 20–23.
[29] Rjosk, H. K., R. Fahlbusch, J. H. Greite, et al.: Prevention and therapy of visual complications during pregnancy in patients with prolactinomas. In: Pituitary Adenomas. Biology, Physiopathology and Treatment (P. J. Derome, D. P. Jedynak, F. Peillon, eds.), p. 340. Asclepios France, Paris 1980.

[30] Rjosk, H.-K., R. Fahlbusch, K. von Werder: Influence of pregnancies on prolactinomas. Acta Endocrinol. **100** (1982) 337–346.

[31] Shewchuk, A. B., G. D. Adamson, P. Lessard, et al.: The effect of pregnancy on suspected pituitary adenomas after conservative management of ovulation defects associated with galactorrhea. Am. J. Obstet. Gynecol. **136** (1980) 659–666.

[32] Serri, O., E. Rasio, H. Beauregard, et al.: Recurrence of hyperprolactinemia after selective transsphenoidal adenomectomy in women with prolactinoma. N. Engl. J. Med. **309** (1983) 280–283.

[33] Thorner, M. O., G. M. Besser, A. Jones, et al.: Bromocriptine treatment of female infertility: report of 13 pregnancies. Br. Med. J. **4** (1975) 694–697.

[34] Turkalj, I., P. Braun, P. Krupp: Surveillance of bromocriptine in pregnancy. Jama **247** (1982) 1589–1591.

[35] van der Spuy, Z. M., H. S. Jacobs: Management of endocrine disorders in pregnancy. Part II – pituitary, ovarian and adrenal disease. Postgrad. Med. J. **60** (1984) 312–320.

[36] van Roon, E., J. C. M. van der Vijver, G. Gerretsen, et al.: Rapid regression of a suprasellar extending prolactinoma after bromocriptine treatment during pregnancy. Fertil. Steril. **36** (1981) 173–177.

[37] Weinstein, D., S. Yarkoni, J. G. Schenker, et al.: Conservative management of suspected prolactin secreting pituitary adenoma during pregnancy. Europ. J. Obstet. Gynec. Reprod. Biol. **11** (1981) 305–312.

[38] Yuen, B. H.: Bromocriptine, pituitary tumours, and pregnancy. The Lancet **II** (1978) 1314.

Long-term follow-up of hyperprolactinaemia in women

R. J. Pepperell

Introduction

In order to gather information about the natural history of hyperprolactinaemia, irrespective of its cause, all patients found to have elevated serum PRL levels at the Royal Women's Hospital, Melbourne were reviewed. This review took place during 1984 and all patients included in this report have been followed for at least 12 months since the discovery of the elevated PRL level.

Materials and methods

The prolactin (PRL) level in at least 3 separate blood samples had to be elevated above the normal range before the patient was deemed to have sustained hyperprolactinaemia and to be suitable for follow-up. Patients taking medications which were known to elevate PRL levels were excluded, but patients with primary hypothyroidism with hyperprolactinaemia were not.

All patients with elevated PRL levels had previously had coned lateral and postero-anterior views of the pituitary fossa in addition to a Town's view. Some patients had had hyper-cycloidal pituitary polytomography performed, however this procedure was discontinued in 1981 when its accuracy was seriously questioned [1, 7]. Very few patients seen prior to 1980 had computerized axial tomography (CAT scan) performed due to the lack of suitable equipment in this city, however during the last 2 years this procedure has been performed more frequently.

Most hyperprolactinaemic patients had presented to the Royal Women's Hospital since 1975, however, some had been seen many years previously when a prolactin assay was not available. These latter patients were still included for follow-up when hyperprolactinaemia was found, as it was assumed the PRL levels had been elevated previously. At the time of latest review the clinical condition of each patient was documented and compared with that at the time of the initial presentation, and the PRL and thyroid hormone levels were measured again. Note was made of any treatment given during the intervening period, the incidence of spontaneous or drug induced pregnancies and complications during such pregnancies. Radiographic evaluation was repeated with coned views of the pituitary fossa being performed in almost all instances. CAT scans were not performed routinely on all hyperprolactinaemic patients although they were done frequently where the coned views were abnormal or the PRL level was very high.

The PRL level, measured in duplicate by double antibody RIA, for each patient was noted as:

$1 = 1.1 - 1.4 \times N$;	$4 = 3.5 - 4.4 \times N$;	$7 = \geq 6.5$ N.
$2 = 1.5 - 2.4 \times N$;	$5 = 4.5 - 5.4 \times N$;	
$3 = 2.5 - 3.4 \times N$;	$6 = 5.5 - 6.4 \times N$;	

This method of handling the data permitted comparisons between different assay systems used in the same hospital over a period of many years.

Results

One hundred and twenty women with elevated PRL at the time of initial presentation were reviewed during 1983, all being followed-up for at least 12 months. One of these patients had primary hypothyroidism, however, the remaining 119 had normal thyroid function and are those who will be analysed further.

Most patients had mild or moderate elevation of their PRL levels with 82% of subjects having a PRL level less than 4 times the upper limit of normal. The overall incidence of galactorrhoea was 52%, this incidence being similar at all levels of PRL and not being more common in the patients with abnormal coned views of the pituitary fossa.

The duration of follow-up (mean ± SEM) of the 119 patients was 66.3 ± 3.9 months. No significant difference in duration of follow-up was found between the varying degrees of hyperprolactinaemia, or between the different menstrual pattern groups at presentation.

Menstrual pattern

Where the PRL level was >4 times normal, the menstrual pattern at presentation was always amenorrhoea, however oligomenorrhoea or even regular cycles were seen in patients with lesser degrees of hyperprolactinaemia (tab. 1). A spontaneous return of regular menses, in patients with secondary amenorrhoea or oligomenorrhoea, was seen in almost one third of patients with PRL levels less than 4 times normal but was not seen at all where the initial PRL level was >4 times normal. The return of regular menses was almost always associated with a concurrent return of PRL levels to normal and was much more likely where bromocriptine had been administered in the interim, even where it had only been given for a short time to produce a pregnancy (tab. 2).

Pregnancy rate

Pregnancies occurred in 67 of the 78 patients (86%) in patients who wished to conceive and were treated with bromocriptine, irrespective of the presence or absence of a pituitary tumour or the degree of elevation of the PRL level; 10% of these patients required clomiphene citrate administration in addition to bromocriptine.

Spontaneous pregnancies occurred in 11 patients, 10 of these having had bromocriptine induced pregnancies in the interim. In all instances the PRL level had returned to normal whilst not taking bromocriptine.

Incidence of pituitary tumours at the time of presentation (table 1)

Nine of the 98 patients (9%) with PRL levels <4 times normal and 4 of the 21 (19%) with higher PRL levels had abnormalities discovered on their coned view assessment. All were seen prior to 1981, when the phase 3 or 4 CAT scan facilities were not available, and only 4 have had a CAT scan performed during the last 18 months – in 3 instances an intrasellar tumour (with no suprasellar extension) was diagnosed, but the CAT scan was normal in the fourth subject.

None of the tumours produced any visual field abnormality, 11 being grade I in type and the remainder grade II [11]. Four of these patients received prolonged treatment with bromocriptine given in a dose usually sufficient to suppress the PRL levels to normal – none became pregnant and none showed tumour progression during follow-up of 41, 41, 44 and 161 months respectively; the latter patient receiving bromocriptine only for the last 2 years of this follow-up period. Five patients were treated successfully with bromocriptine to induce pregnancy; in all instances the therapy was ceased at 6 weeks of gestation, the pregnancies were uncomplicated and there was no evidence of tumour progression following pregnancy or during follow-up for 40, 54, 64, 65 and 123 months respectively.

The remaining 4 patients did not receive bromocriptine therapy at all. One, whose initial PRL level was 30 times the upper limit of normal, showed a progressive increase in her PRL levels during a follow-up interval of 41 months during which time her plain X-rays showed tumour progression from grade I to grade II. Treatment with bromocriptine had been refused initially but has now been commenced. The other 3 patients who have currently been followed for 26, 60 and 224 months respectively, have shown no change in their pituitary fossae during this period.

Incidence of tumour development during follow-up (tables 1 and 2)

Radiographic evidence of tumour development during follow-up was seen in 16 of the 106 patients with normal coned views initially. In all instances the visual fields

Table 1 Analysis of hyperprolactinaemic women seen at the Royal Women's Hospital between 1/4/1975 and 31/12/1981

Serum PRL level at presentation or when first measured (xN)	Number of patients	Menstrual pattern at presentation				Coned view assessment at presentation		
		Regular cycles	Oligo-menor-rhoea	Second-ary amenor-rhoea	Prim-ary amenor-rhoea	Normal	gradeI tumour	grade II tumour
1.1–1.9	46	4	16	26	–	41	5	–
2.0–2.9	33	1	11	21	–	31	2	–
3.0–3.9	19	2	4	13	–	17	1	1
4.0–4.9	9	–	–	8	1	8	1	–
5.0–5.9	3	–	–	3	–	3	–	–
≥6	9	–	–	7	2	6	2	1
All elevated cycles	119	7	31	78	3	106	11	2

* Patients with regular cycles at presentation have been excluded from this assessment;
† Patients not receiving treatment with bromocriptine at time of measurement of PRL;
+ Coned view radiological assessment;
The figure underlined in tumour progression is duration of follow-up of patient who showed tumour progression.

remained normal. Tumour development was more common when the PRL level was greater than 4 times the upper limit of normal at the time of presentation chi-square = 8.46, $p<0.005$) but was still observed in 10% of patients where the PRL level was less than 4 times normal. Although 7 patients showed an increase in PRL levels, 5 patients showed a decrease in PRL levels and in 4 the levels actually returned to normal. The remaining 4 patients were being treated with bromocriptine when the PRL level was last measured, no assay being performed prior to commencing bromocriptine at the time of diagnosis of tumour development.

CAT scans were performed in 12 of these 16 patients following the discovery of the normal X-rays. One failed to reveal any evidence of a pituitary tumour but an empty sella was present. Tumours were confirmed in the remainder – 9 had intrasellar tumours with no suprasellar extension, 1 had an intrasellar tumour with <1 cm suprasellar extension and the other had a normal pituitary fossa but a suprasellar tumour.

Bromocriptine treatment (table 2)

Eight of the 16 patients had been treated with bromocriptine during the follow-up period. In all instances only short-term therapy was given in an attempt to achieve

Spontaneous return of regular menses*	Serum PRL at latest review		Evidence of tumour development since time of presentation+		Evidence of tumour progression since time of presentation+	
	Currently receiving bromocriptine	Normal PRL†	Incidence	Duration of follow-up of tumour patients (months)	Incidence	Duration of follow-up (months)
14/42 (33%)	4	15 (36%)	4/41 (10%)	48, 49, 129, 131	–/5	26, 44, 54, 60, 65
12/32 (38%)	2	11 (35%)	3/31 (10%)	59, 61, 78	–/2	64, 123
2/17 (12%)	1	1 (6%)	2/17 (12%)	37, 56	–/2	41, 224
–	1	–	4/8 (50%)	30, 38, 94, 152	–/1	40
–	–	–	–/3 (0%)	–	–	–
–	3	–	3/6 (50%)	15, 18, 120	1/3	*41*, 41, 161
28/112 (25%)	11	27 (25%)	16/106 (15%)	15–152 (Mean = 80.9)	1/13 (8%)	26–224 (Mean = 75.7)

a pregnancy. Six of these patients conceived, had uneventful pregnancies, and their visual fields which were assessed 3-monthly remained normal throughout.

Discussion

Because this series represents a follow-up of all hyperprolactinaemic patients seen at one institution during a 7 year period, it allows conclusions to be made concerning the long-term follow-up of such patients which were not possible for most previous reports. The likelihood of discovery of a pituitary tumour on coned view assessment of the pituitary fossa at the time of presentation was 10.9%, and 15% of patients with normal coned views initially developed evidence of a tumour during a mean follow-up in excess of 5 years. All of the tumours were small (grades I or II) although those associated with markedly elevated PRL levels (>6 normal) were more likely to show evidence of suprasellar extension. Administration of bromocriptine was associated with a reduction of tumour growth or a prevention of progression in all instances, this feature being reported previously by other workers [2, 5, 8, 9, 10].

It is well known that polytomography of the pituitary fossa enables more 'abnormalities' to be detected than when plain coned-views alone are used, however false

Table 2 Effect of treatment with bromocriptine on subsequent menstrual pattern, serum PRL levels and risk of tumour development or tumour progression

Treatment	Menstrual pattern at presentation	Number of patients Normal X-ray at presentation	Tumour evident at presentation
Bromocriptine	Primary amenorrhoea	1	1
	Secondary amenorrhoea	49	6
	Oligomenorrhoea	20	2
	Regular cycles	7	–
Not given bromocriptine	Primary amenorrhoea	1	–
	Secondary amenorrhoea	20	3
	Oligomenorrhoea	8	1
	Regular cycles	–	–
All patients	All patterns	106	13

* Only patients not currently receiving treatment with bromocriptine assessed;
† Coned view radiological assessment.

Statistics:

Return of regular cycles	Secondary amenorrhoea	treated: not treated	$X^2 = 1.78$, NS.
	Oligomenorrhoea	treated: not treated	$X^2 = 6.90$, $p<0.01$
	Both sec. a. + oligo.	treated: not treated	$X^2 = 8.31$, $p<0.005$

positive and false negative rates of 28% and 81% respectively have led most clinicians to abandon the use of polytomography in the assessment of hyperprolactinaemic subjects. The latest generation of CAT scan machines (phase III or phase IV) allows accurate definition of small microadenomas (>2 mm in diameter) as well as enabling recognition of the empty sella syndrome and accurate diagnosis of the extent or presence of suprasellar tumour. This examination has now become an integral part of the initial evaluation of all hyperprolactinaemic patients but at the time many of the patients in the current study were first seen, CAT scan facilities were not available. This has necessitated statements being made in regard to changes observed following coned view reassessment; although such statements are not as informative as those able to be made following CAT scan assessment the conclusions drawn would appear to be valid.

Treatment with bromocriptine not only controls tumour growth, but usually lowers PRL levels to normal and restores ovulatory cycles where these are absent. Pregnancy commonly occurs during such treatment whereas pregnancies are rare in untreated hyperprolactinaemic subjects. There is no evidence from this series that

Menstrual pattern at latest review				
Patients currently receiving treatment with bromocriptine	Regular cycles (not on bromocriptine)	Normal s. PRL at latest review*	Evidence of tumour development since time of presentation†	Evidence of tumour progression since time of presentation†
1	–/1 (0%)	–/1 (0%)	–/1 (0%)	–/1 (0%)
8	12/47 (26%)	13/47 (28%)	6/49 (12%)	–/6 (0%)
2	12/20 (60%)	11/20 (55%)	1/20 (5%)	–/2 (0%)
–	7/7 (100%)	2/7 (29%)	1/7 (14%)	–
–	–/1 (0%)	–/1 (0%)	1/1 (100%)	–
–	2/23 (9%)	1/23 (4%)	7/20 (35%)	1/3 (33%)
–	–/9 (0%)	–/9 (0%)	–/8 (0%)	–/1 (0%)
–	–	–	–	–
11	33/108 (31%)	27/108 (25%)	16/106 (15%)	1/13 (8%)

Return of PRL to normal	Secondary amenorrhoea	treated: not treated	$X^2 = 3.89, p<0.05$
	Oligomenorrhoea	treated: not treated	$X^2 = 5.81, p<0.02$
	Both sec. a. + oligo.	treated: not treated	$X^2 = 10.59, p<0.005$
Incidende of tumour development	Secondary amenorrhoea	treated: not treated	$X^2 = 3.44, 0.05<p<0.10$
	All patients	treated: not treated	$X^2 = 3.61, 0.05<p<0.10$

pregnancy increases the risk of tumour expansion where the pregnancy follows treatment with bromocriptine.

In addition to achieving pregnancy, treatment with bromocriptine may restore PRL levels to normal (and result in a resumption of spontaneous menstruation and fertility) after the treatment is ceased, these features being more likely when the PRL levels are only moderately elevated [3, 4]. For this reason, bromocriptine therapy may be indicated in patients with moderately elevated PRL levels even though a pregnancy is not desired. The required duration of such therapy is not known but few patients in the current series were treated for more than 6 months unless they were known to have a pituitary tumour.

There is no doubt that contraceptive advice is necessary for patients who do not wish to conceive but are receiving treatment with bromocriptine. In the past combined oestrogen/progestogen oral contraceptive preparations have usually been avoided because of the theoretical risk of tumour expansion during such therapy, however, such advice may no longer be necessary [6]. From the results presented here it is apparent that contraceptive advice should also be offered to patients whose PRL level is only moderately elevated (<4 times normal) even when they are not receiving treatment with bromocriptine. About 30% of such patients can be expected to resume normal menstruation, this phenomenon being more likely to follow short-term treatment with bromocriptine, usually given to induce pregnancy, than observations alone.

Abstract

One hundred and nineteen women with sustained hyperprolactinaemia were followed for a mean duration of 5.5 years. One-third of subjects whose initial PRL level was <4 × normal had a 'spontaneous' resolution of their hyperprolactinaemia and resumed cyclical menstrual activity and fertility after receiving short term treatment with bromocriptine, usually to induce a pregnancy. Subjects with higher PRL levels or those not treated with bromocriptine, did not show this beneficial effect. Pituitary or hypothalamic tumours were identified in 11% of subjects at the time of presentation and developed in a further 15.1% during follow-up. Most of these tumours were small, occurred more commonly when the PRL level was >4 × normal, and were less likely to develop when treatment with bromocriptine had been administered.

Acknowledgements

We thank the Consultant Medical Staff of the Royal Women's Hospital for referring patients to the Endocrine Clinic for investigation and management. Funds were provided by Sandoz Australia for establishment of the register of hyperprolactinaemic subjects.

References

[1] Burrow, G. N., G. Wortzman, N. B. Rewcastle, et al.: Microadenomas of the pituitary and abnormal sellar tomograms in an unselected autopsy series. New England Journal of Medicine **304** (1981) 156.

[2] Eversmann, T., R. Fahlbusch, H. K. Rjosk, et al.: Persisting suppression of prolactin secretion after long-term treatment with bromocriptine in patients with prolactinomas. Acta Endocrinologica (Kbh) **92** (1979) 413.

[3] Isaacs, A. J.: Resolution of hyperprolactinaemia after bromocriptine-induced pregnancy. Lancet **i** (1979) 784.

[4] Jacobs, H. S., S. U. Thobani: Long term follow-up of medically treated hyperprolactinaemia (including prolactinoma) – evidence for cure. In: Advances in Diagnosis and Treatment of Infertility (V. Insler, G. Bettendorf, eds.), p. 263. Elsevier North Holland, New York 1981.

[5] McGregor, A. M., M. F. Scanlon, R. Hall, et al.: Effects of bromocriptine on pituitary tumour size. British Medical Journal **2** (1979) 700.

[6] Moult, P. J. A., J. E. Dacie, L. H. Rees, et al.: Oral contraception in patients with hyperprolactinaemia. British Medical Journal **284** (1982) 868.
[7] Nachtigall, R. D., S. E. Monroe, C. B. Wilson, et al.: Prolactin-secreting pituitary adenomas in women: Absence of demonstrable adenomas in patients with altered menstrual function and abnormal sellar polytomography. American Journal of Obstetrics and Gynecology **140** (1981) 303.
[8] Sobrinho, L. G., M. C. P. Nunes, M. A. Santos, et al.: Radiological evidence of regression of prolactinoma after treatment with bromocriptine. Lancet **ii** (1978) 257.
[9] Thorner, M. O., W. H. Martin, A. D. Rogol, et al.: Rapid regression of pituitary prolactinomas during bromocriptine treatment. Journal of Clinical Endocrinology and Metabolism **51** (1980) 438.
[10] Thorner, M. O., R. L. Perryman, A. D. Rogol, et al.: Rapid changes of prolactinoma volume after withdrawal and reinstitution of bromocriptine. Journal of Clinical Endocrinology and Metabolism **53** (1981) 480.
[11] Vezina, J. L.: Prolactin secreting pituitary adenomas; radiologic diagnosis. In: Progress in Prolactin Physiology and Pathology (C. Robyn, M. Harter, eds.), p. 351. Elsevier North Holland, New York 1978.

Prophylactic bromocriptine treatment during pregnancy of women with macroprolactinomas: report of thirteen pregnancies*

W. de Wit, H. J. T. Coelingh Bennink, L. J. Gerards

Introduction

Since 1974 bromocriptine has been used at our institute for the induction of ovulation in hyperprolactinaemic women. We allowed our patients with prolactinomas to become pregnant without any pre-treatment, except bromocriptine. However, during the mid-seventies it was suggested that pregnancy in women with previously untreated prolactinomas might be extremely hazardous. Therefore it was recommended that before embarking on pregnancy such patients should undergo prophylactic irradiation or surgery of the pituitary gland.

We did not feel justified in exposing so many young women to the risks of these therapies for a nonmalignant disease. Especially since many patients who would not experience complications during pregnancy would also be treated. We felt that in patients with microprolactinomas the risk of complications during pregnancy was very low, justifying no prophylactic treatment before embarking on pregnancy. However, we felt that in patients with macroprolactinomas some form of prophylactic treatment was necessary when embarking on pregnancy.

Other's [14] and our own [5] experience with bromocriptine treatment during pregnancy for another indication indicated that bromocriptine is not teratogenic and does not interfere with the normal development of pregnancy. Also this dopamine-agonist had been shown to reduce mitotic activity and to inhibit oestrogen induced proliferation of the pituitary lactotrophs in experimental animals [9, 15] and to have a probable anti-tumour effect in men [6].

In view of the above we decided to treat our patients with a macroprolactinoma prophylactically with bromocriptine during pregnancy. As the greatest proliferation of the lactotrophs occurs during the third trimester of pregnancy [11] and most complications develop or become troublesome after the first trimester and in order to avoid bromocriptine treatment during embryogenesis prophylactic bromocriptine treatment was only given during the second and third trimester of pregnancy.

* A more extensive version has been accepted for publication by the British Journal of Obstetrics and Gynaecology.

Patients and methods

We treated ten women during thirteen pregnancies prophylactically with bromocriptine. The main characteristics these patients are shown in table 1. Patients A, C

Table 1 Main characteristics of the patients

Patient	Age[1]	Gynaecological, endocrinological and obstetrical history	Prolactin (IU/L) Basal	TRH-test[2]
A	32	R→O→A+G→Cl→Cl+Gon→BCT→P→A+G	5.8	5.8−6.3−5.7
B	27	A+G→OCA→A+G→TA→A+G	61	61−66−53
C	35	R→OCA→A+G→Cl→Gon→WR→BCT→P→A+G	1.8	not tested
D_1	24	O→A→Gon→LAb→A+G	8.0	8.0−8.0−8.0
D_2	26	→BCT→P→A+G		
E_1	22	R→A+G	7.3	7.3−>8−>8
E_2	23	→BCT→P→A+G		
F	32	R→R+G→IAb→R+G→OCA→A+G→BCT→P→A+G	2.0	1.8−2.1−1.8
G	39	R+G→A+G	7.8	7.8−12−8.4
H_1	28	R→A+G→Cl→Gon	3.5	3.5−3.7−3.6
H_2	31	→BCT→P→A+G		
I	27	R+G→OCA→A+G→Cl→Gon	8.8	8.8−10.4−9.2
J	28	R→OCA→A→BCT→P→A+G	1.1	1.2−1.6−1.7

[1] At conception.
[2] Response to 200 μg TRH at 0−20−60 min.
R = regular menstrual cycle; O = oligomenorrhoea; A = amenorrhoea; G = galactorrhoea; P = parturition; Cl = clomiphene; Gon = gonadotropins; BCT = bromocriptine; OCA = oral contraceptive agent; TA = transphenoidal adenectomy; WR = wedge resection; LAb = late abortion; IAb = induced abortion.

and F had their first pregnancy before we started with prophylactic bromocriptine treatment. Patient J was referred to us after her first pregnancy. Patient B was operated elsewhere because of suprasellar extension. However, postoperatively prolactin levels were only slightly decreased. Though this patient became euprolactinaemic with bromocriptine treatment amenorrhoea persisted. Only when gonadotropins were added did she became pregnant.

Bromocriptine was reinitiated at a dosage of 7.5 mg per day to all patients at 16 to 20 weeks gestation with the exception of patient B who recieved 15 mg per day in view of her extremely high prolactin levels. Patient E experienced nausea and dizziness caused by orthostatic hypotension before her pregnancies. As bromocriptine increased her complaints she did not take prophylactic bromocriptine medication consistently. During a routine visual field control towards the end of patient H's second pregnancy a small defect was noted, which did not progress and which persisted after delivery. There was no associated rise in prolactin levels and as there had been a change in the examining oculist, we think this was an old defect which previously had gone unnoticed. Patient I developed a severe headache almost immediatly after discontinuing bromocriptine treatment at seven weeks gestation. Additional complaints of nausea, vomiting and slight diplopia occurred at 9 weeks gestation. In a few days the headache decreased and nausea, vomiting and diplopia disappeared spontaneously. After this period the prolactin level fell spontaneously to approximately 40% of the original high levels registered during the period of nausea and vomiting. This history may be attributed to tumour enlargement and partial apoplexy of the tumour.

The prolactin levels of patient B rose to 110 IU/l during the first trimester. During prophylactic bromocriptine treatment they were suppressed to levels of approximately 25 IU/l. In most other pregnancies prolactin levels were suppressed to levels in the lower range of normal or even lower (fig. 1).

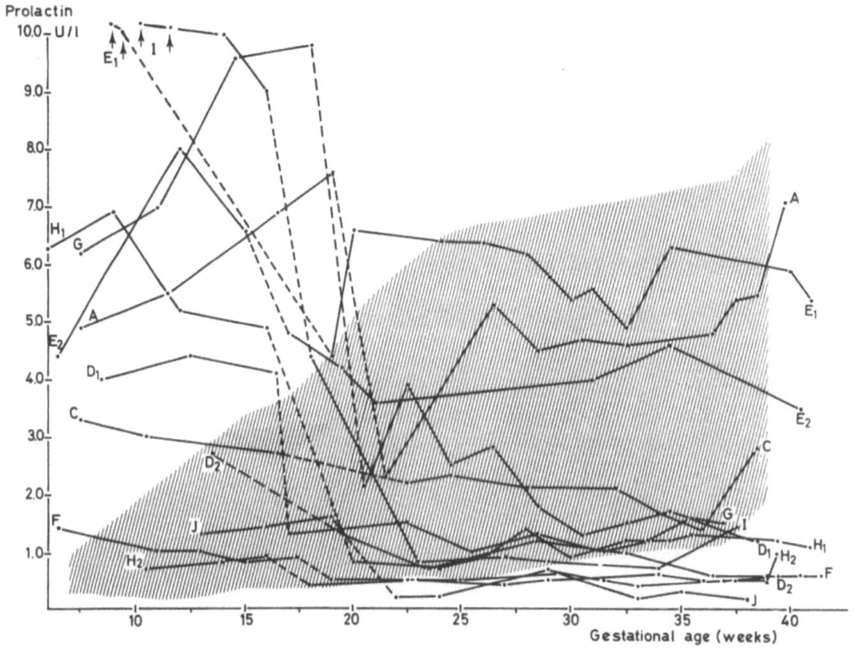

Fig. 1 Prolactin serum levels during 13 pregnancies in 10 women with microprolactinoma. Shaded area: normal prolactin levels during pregnancy. Interrupted: start of bromocriptine treatment in this period.

All pregnancies progressed to term. None of the children showed congenital abnormalities. The neonatal period was normal and during the follow-up period (at present $1^7/_{12}$ to $6^4/_{12}$ years) growth and psychomotoric development were normal in all the children (tab. 2).

Table 2 Main characteristics of the infants (February 1983)

Child	Sex	Gestation (weeks)	Birth weight (g)	Apgar scores (1 & 5 min)	Percentiles L	W	HC	Age[1] (years)
A	F	40 1/7	3710	9/10	50	50	75	2 5/12
B	F	40 1/7	2940	9/10	25	25	25	10/12
C	M	38 6/7	2700	10/10	50	10	50	3 7/12
D_1	M	38 5/7	3500	9/10	75	75	90	4 3/12
D_2	F	39 4/7	3080	9/10	75	50	50	2 8/12
E_1	F	40 6/7	3460	9/10	50	25	50	5 2/12
E_2	F	40 4/7	3180	9/10	25	25	50	3 6/12
F	F	41 5/7	3760	10/10	75	50	50	4 7/12
G	M	37 1/7	2540	8/10	75	50	75	3 7/12
H_1	F	41 1/7	4150	9/10	50	50	50	5 2/12
H_2	M	39 4/7	4380	9/10	75	90	50	2 3/12
I	F	37 2/7	2470	7/8	25	25	50	1 3/12
J	F	38	3410	10/10	75	50	75	7/12

[1] Age at latest follow-up visit.
L = length; W = weight; HC = head circumference.

Cord prolactin levels were suppressed, but in the amniotic fluid they were normal, supporting the view that amniotic fluid prolactin originates from the decidua and is not under dopaminergic control (fig. 2) [24].

Discussion

The question is whether bromocriptine treatment during pregnancy is safe. Bromocriptine treatment during pregnancy suppresses cord prolactin levels, therefore bromocriptine treatment might interfere with the possible physiological actions of prolactin in the foetus. A role for prolactin in foetal lung maturation, a stimulating action of foetal prolactin on the foetal adrenal cortex and an inhibiting action on testosterone-secretion in the male foetus have been postulated [1, 10, 12, 26]. However, work from other groups argues against these roles for fetal prolactin [13, 18, 20, 21].

Data collected from 1410 pregnancies in which bromocriptine had been given during early pregnancy showed a normal incidence of congenital malformations and a normal progress of pregnancy [25]. In addition to our thirteen pregnancies we are aware of thirty-nine other pregnancies in which bromocriptine had been used during the mid- and latefetal period for various indications. In none of the infants was a congenital malformation reported. In conclusion our results comfirm other reports that even if prolactin has a physiological role in the fetus, suppression of prolactin levels and bromocriptine treatment during pregnancy is not harmful to

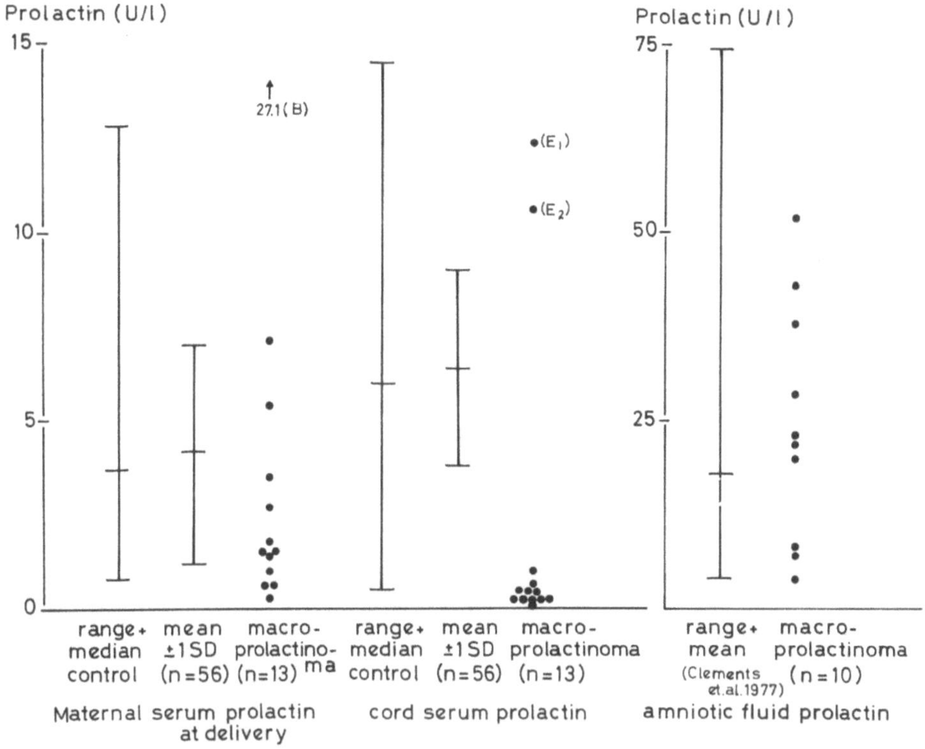

Fig. 2 Prolactin levels at delivery in maternal serum, cord serum and amniotic fluid.

the fetus and it does not interfere with the normal development of pregnancy and postnatal development seems to be normal. However, it should be realized that there is only limited information on long-term follow-up at present.

In our opinion obstetricians should be very careful with prescribing any medication during pregnancy, and weigh very careful the possible advantages to the mother against the possible risks to the foetus.

Recent reports show that the incidence of tumour complications during pregnancy is low and that the risk of permanent sequelae is very small in carefully supervised patients. Also it has been shown that reinstitution of bromocriptine treatment is a highly effective treatment if tumour complications develop. We are aware of eleven patients with complications caused by tumour enlargement in whom bromocriptine treatment has been used successfully [3, 7, 8, 16, 19, 23] against one failure [22].

In view of these reports we are at present not longer in favour of using routinely prophylactic bromocriptine treatment during pregnancy in patients with a macroprolactinoma. The development of headaches usually precedes the occurrences of visual field changes [17]. Also some groups observed sudden large increases in prolactin levels before the onset of symptoms of tumour enlargement [2, 23]. Our current policy of management of patients with macroprolactinomas is to instruct them to report headaches or any other neurological symptom immediately. From the beginning of pregnancy prolactin levels are monitored every two to four weeks. In addition visual field examinations are performed every four weeks. When sudden large increases in prolactin levels are observed or a headache or any other sign of tumour enlargement develops, bromocriptine treatment is started, unless the pregnancy is so advanced that induction of labour carries no risk for mother or fetus.

Before embarking on pregnancy suprasellar extension should be ruled out by high quality CT scanning. Treatment with bromocriptine often rapidly shrinks such tumours. We suggest therefore, that such patients are treated for a certain period with bromocriptine and encouraged to conceive only if suprasellar extension has resolved. As prolactinomas often rapidly increase to their pre-treatment size after discontinuing bromocriptine treatment, these patients probably would benefit from prophylactic treatment during pregnancy.

References

[1] Aubert et al.: The ontogenesis of human prolactin from fetal life to puberty. In: Prolactin and Reproduction (P. G. Crosignani, C. Robyn, eds.). London 1977.

[2] Batrinos et al.: Prolactin and placental hormone levels during pregnancy in prolactinomas. Int. J. Fertil. **26** (1981) 77.

[3] Bergh et al.: Clinical course and outcome of pregnancies in amenorrhoeic women with hyperprolactinaemia and pituitary tumours. Br. Med. J. **1** (1978) 875.

[4] Clements et. al.: Studies on Human sexual development IV. Fetal pituitary and serum, and amniotic fluid concentrations of prolactin. J. Clin. Endocrinol. Metab. **44** (1977) 408.

[5] Coelingh Bennink: The suppression of hyperprolactinaemia during pregnancy. Acta Endocrinol. Suppl. (Copenh.) **225** (1979) 181.

[6] Corenblum et al.: Possible anti-tumour effect of 2 bromo-ergocryptine (CB-154 SANDOZ) in 2 patients with large prolactin-secreting pituitary adenomas. Clin. Research. **33** (1975) 614A.

[7] Corenblum: Successful outcome of ergocryptine-induced pregnancies in twenty-one women with prolactin-secreting pituitary adenomas. Fertil. Steril. **32** (1979) 183.

[8] Burzaco et al.: Bromocriptine en la expansión de tumores hipofisarios durante el ambarazo. Clin. Invest. Ginec. Obstet. **2** (1978) 90.

[9] Davies et al.: DNA synthesis and the secretion of prolactin and growth hormone by the pituitary gland of the male rat: Effects of diethylstilboestrol and 2-bromo-a-ergocryptine methanesulphonate. J. Endocrinol. **61** (1974) 411.

[10] Gluckman et al.: Prolactin in umbilical cord blood and the respiratory distress syndrome. J. Pediatr. **93**, 4 (1978) 1011.

[11] Goluboff, Ezrin: Effects of pregnancy on the somatotroph and the prolactin cell of the human adenohypophysis. J. Clin. Endocrinol. **29** (1969) 1533.

[12] Hauth et al.: A role of fetal prolactin in lung maturation. Obstet. Gynecol. **51** (1978) 81.
[13] Ho Yuen et al.: Prolactin, estradiol, and thyroid hormones in umbilical cord blood of neonates with and without hyaline membrane disease: A study of 405 neonates from midpregnancy to term. Am. J. Obstet. Gynecol. **142** (1982) 698.
[14] Kullander: Effect of 2 br-alpha-ergocryptin (CB 154) on serum prolactin and the clinical picture in a case of progressive gigantomastia in pregnancy. Ann. Chir. Gynaecol. Fenn. **65** (1976) 227.
[15] Lloyd et al.: Effects of oestrogen and bromocryptine on in vivo secretion and mitosis in prolactin cells. Nature **255** (1975) 497.
[16] Maeda et al.: Effective bromocriptine treatment of a pituitary macroadenoma during pregnancy. Obstet. Gynaecol. **61** (1983) 117.
[17] Magyar and Marshall: Pituitary tumors and pregnancy. Am. J. Obstet. Gynecol. **132** (1978) 739.
[18] Martin-Perez et al.: Lack of dependency between androgen production and prolactin in man. Acta Endocrinol. Suppl. (Copenh) **225** (1978) 174.
[19] Pepperell: Ovulation induction. Fertil. Steril. **40** (1983) 6.
[20] del Pozo et al.: Induced human gestational hypoprolactinemia: Lack of action on fetal Adrenal Androgen Synthesis. J. Clin. Endocrinol. Metab. **51** (1980) 936.
[21] van Petten, Bridges: The effects of prolactin on pulmonary maturation in the fetal rabbit. Am. Obstet. Gynecol. **134** (1979) 711.
[22] Rjosk et al.: Prevention and therapy of visual complications during pregnancy in patients with prolactinomas. In: Pituitary adenomas (Biology, physiopathology and treatment). (Eds: Derome et al.) Paris 1979.
[23] van Roon et al.: Rapid regression of a suprasellar extending prolactinoma after bromocriptine treatment during pregnancy. Fertil. Steril. **26** (1981) 173.
[24] Rosenberg et al.: Decidual production of prolactin in late gestation: Further evidence for a decidual source of amniotic fluid prolactin. Am. J. Obstet. Gynecol. **138** (1980) 681.
[25] Turkalj et al.: Surveillance of bromocriptine in pregnancy. JAMA **247** (1982) 1589.
[26] Winters et al.: Fetal plasma prolactin levels. J. Clin. Endocrinol. Metab. **41** (1975) 626.

Natural regression after pregnancy of a CT visualized microprolactinoma

S. F. Garzarelli, R. Corsini, V. Vallerino

Introduction

The status of prolactin (PRL) regulation following regression of pituitary PRL-secreting adenomas during bromocriptine therapy is not fully elucidated. Individuals harbouring PRL-secreting adenomas have disordered hypothalamic control of PRL secretion before and after transsphenoidal adenectomy has restored the PRL concentrations to normal [1] [2]. Bromocriptine is a dopaminergic agonist which lowers the circulating PRL levels and in individuals with a prolactinoma the drug also possesses antitumour effects [3]. The use of this drug that restores or induces ovulation has enabled women with a prolactinoma to ovulate and conceive. Some publications suggest that pregnancy may be extremely hazardous [4] because during normal pregnancy, the volume of the pituitary gland increases by approximately 70% [5]. In the presence of a prolactin-secreting pituitary tumour or lactotrophe hyperplasia, pregnancy may be associated with a dramatic enlargement of the pituitary gland [6]. For this reason surgical treatment has usually been initiated after the identification of these tumour, particularly if pregnancy is desired because surgical cure rates are superior when the lesions are small [7]. Surgical removal whenever the diagnosis is made prevents the study of the natural history of this disease. Recently, other investigators advocate conservative management since these tumours have been reported to grow very slowly or not at all [8] [9].

One patient is presented who, by current criteria probably had a prolactin-producing pituitary tumour which underwent apparent spontaneous regression after pregnancy following bromocriptine therapy.

Case report

A 31 year old patient was initially seen in 1977 and presented with galactorrhoea and amenorrhoea following withdrawal in March, 1976, of combination oral contraceptives. The amenorrhoea started in June 1970. The basal PRL level in 1977 was 87 ng/ml; visual field examination by the Goldman technique was normal. Pituitary function studies with thyrotropin-releasing hormone (TRH), luteinizing hormone-releasing hormone (LH-RH) and metoclopramide (MCP) were undertaken and the results are shown in table 1.

Table 1 Pituitary function studies before pregnancy (1978)

	time (min) 0	30	60	90	120	
response to 200 μg of TRH and 100 μg of LHRH intravenously						
Prolactin (ng/ml)	80	75	95	80	85	*
TSH (μU/ml)	5	8	8	8	6	
LH (mIU/ml)	9	8	8	7	7	*
FSH (mIU/ml)	8	6	7	7	7	*
response to 10 mg of metoclopramide intramuscularly						
Prolactin (ng/ml)	85	90	98	96	89	*

zero time data in the above and other tables were the mean of two samples drawn 15 minutes apart.
* blunted responses.

An "upper limit of normal size" sella turcica on the routine lateral skull X-ray film without any other specific radiographic abnormality, was noted.

CT examination carried out with a 5005 perfected with a 2085 EMI CT System, using xenon multidetectors, 13 mm slice thickness and 160 × 160 matrix, showed an unclear image that however suggested the possible existence of a microprolactinoma (fig. 1).

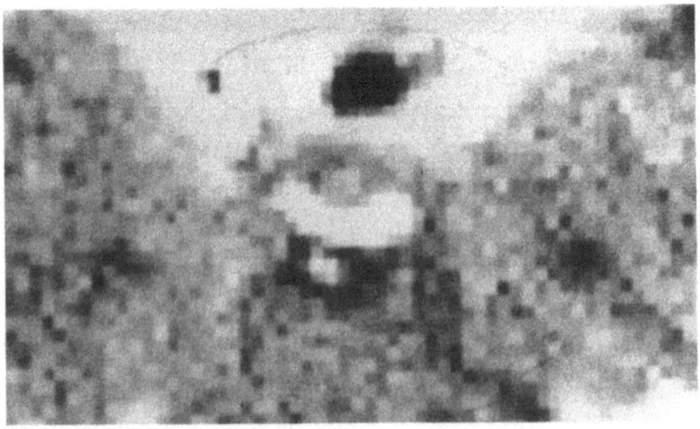

Fig. 1 CT picture of pituitary; the existence of the tumour is in doubt, an unclear image seemed to be present inside the sella.

At this point the patient was referred to a Neurosurgeon who advised surgery and strongly suggested against attempting to become pregnant. Since the patient feared surgery and also greatly desired a child she did not accept the surgeon's advice and came to us for an alternative. On this basis we decided to initiate medical treatment. Bromocriptine therapy (5 mg/day) was commenced with suppression of PRL levels and resumption of cyclic menstruation, followed by conception soon after. She stopped therapy immediately after a positive pregnancy test. She delivered normally and lactation was suppressed with bromocriptine. She continued therapy for 6 months after delivery. One month after withdrawal of the drug pituitary function was assessed by tests with TRH, LH-RH and MCP. These results are shown in table 2.

Table 2 Pituitary function studies 6 months after delivery immediately after suspension of bromocriptine therapy (1979)

	time (min)					
	0	30	60	90	120	
response to 200 μg of TRH and 100 μg of LHRH intravenously						
PRL (ng/ml)	42	45	51	47	43	*
LH (mIU/ml)	15	82	82	59	60	
FSH (mIU/ml)	13	30	29	26	23	
GH (ng/ml)	4	3	2	1	1	
TSH (μU/ml)	4	8	12	10	9	
response to 10 mg of metoclopramide intramuscularly						
PRL (ng/ml)	45	56	51	52	50	*

* blunted responses.

The CT scan revealed no growth of the tumour and the visual field examination was normal. Thereafter a slight increase in basal PRL occurred but cyclic ovulatory menstruation continued. The patient after this control did not return because she felt well. She came for a visit at the end of 1983, and was menstruating with galactorrhoea. We repeated pituitary function tests with TRH, LH-RH, MCP and Nomifensine. These results are shown in table 3.

Hormone assay and test protocols

The polypeptide hormones were assayed by double antibody radioimmunoassay (RIA) methods: commercially available kits were used. Normal responses are a 100% increment over baseline for LH and FSH to LH-RH, for PRL and TSH to TRH and for PRL to MCP. With regard to the growth hormone response to TRH an increase should not have been and indeed not seen. A normal response of PRL to nomifensine was a 30–39% reduction in basal PRL levels.

Table 3 Pituitary function studies 5 years after suspension of bromocriptine therapy (1984)

	time (min)						
	0	30	60	90	120	180	
response to 200 μg of TRH and 100 μg of LHRH intravenously							
PRL (ng/ml)	43	54	53	39	42		*
LH (mIU/ml)	15	130	125	140	120		
FSH (mIU/ml)	20	25	30	35	20		
response to 10 mg of metoclopramide intramuscularly							
PRL (ng/ml)	45	56	51	52	50		*
response to 200 mg of nomifensine orally							
PRL (ng/ml)	35	41	38	31	33	36	*

* blunted responses.

Discussion

This observation over a 5 year span demonstrates that the regression of hyperprolactinaemia after pregnancy in a woman with a suspected microprolactinoma treated with bromocriptine in order to conceive was associated with a defect in the regulation of PRL secretion. Hypothalamic dysfunction with hyperprolactinaemia rather than microadenoma might be implicated as the cause of the galactorrhoea-amenorhoea and spontaneous resolution of this dysfunction could create a similar clinical situation. However, the initial pituitary function tests demonstrated a blunted LH response to LH-RH with blunted PRL responses to TRH and MCP. In the second set of studies performed 6 months after delivery, when cyclic ovulation and the PRL levels were restored, the PRL responses to both TRH and MCP remained blunted in the presence of normal responses of gonadotropin.

In vitro, adenomatous lactotropes have a decreased number of dopaminergic receptors as compared to the number in non-adenomatous cells [10]; while in vivo there is evidence of enhanced dopaminergic activity at the level of the hypothalamus [11] if there is a prodactinome. After PRL levels were reduced but not restored to normal in our patient there remained a persistent defect in the PRL response to TRH and MCP. Despite these findings ovulation was normal with cyclic menstruation. After 5 years of normal cyclic menstruation, the defect in the PRL response to TRH, MCP and nomifensine persists. These hormonal findings together with a doubtful CT image and a long clinical history of amenorrhoea-galactorrhoea make a PRL producing tumour a more likely possibility.

The natural history of PRL-secreting pituitary adenomas and the effects of pregnancy on pituitary tumours are poorly understood. A more extensive knowledge would help to develop guidelines for the management of patients with pituitary tumours. The fall in the PRL concentration from 90 to 40 ng/ml most likely represents a spontaneous infarction and/or necrosis of a PRL secreting pituitary adenoma. Pituitary haemorrhage might produce the same clinical findings as those of necrosis. However, most cases of pituitary apoplexy usually involve extensive haemorrhage and produce altered consciousness and other central nervous system symptoms (i.e. acute headaches, ocular palsies, hyperpyrexia, visual loss) [12]. Although haemorrhage is a well documented complication of pituitary adenomas in general [13] this entity has not been reported in PRL-secreting microadenomas with secondary reduction in serum PRL concentration. In contrast to the possible catastrophic event of pituitary haemorrhage, a tumour may undergo spontaneous asymptomatic infarction, which has been reported in patients with acromegaly [14]. Our patient most likely represents a case of asymptomatic selective tumour infarction of the majority of galactotrophic cells since the PRL concentration was reduced, but we do not exclude the possibility of the positive effects of pregnancy together with bromocriptine on the hypothalamic regulation of PRL secretion.

We do not have an answer to this problem because up to now proof of the existence of a pituitary adenomas requires histological examination. Operative pretreatment (before pregnancy) has several limitations: need for highly specialized centers; unsatisfactory results on hyperprolactinaemia [15]; frequent postoperative global or partial hypopituitarism (possibility of hypothalamic damage, i.e. necrosis) with the resultant need for chronic endocrinologic treatment [15] and the possibility of tumour-related complications during pregnancy even with pretreatment [16].

In conclusion, despite the limitations, the data in this report may support an effort to avoid unnecessary operations before pregnancy in patients suffering from microprolactinoma, and we can add this case to the numberous cases present in the literature, of normal and sometimes therapeutic pregnancy seen in women suffering from hyperprolactinaemia.

Acknowledgements

The authors are grateful to Dr. M. Giusti for his help in preparing this work.

References

[1] Barbarino, A., L. De Marinis, G. Maira, et al.: Serum prolactin response to thyrotropin-releasing hormone and metoclopramide in patients with prolactin secreting tumors before and after transsphenoidal surgery. J. Clin. Endocrinol. Metab. **47** (1978) 1148.
[2] Camanni, F., E. Ghigo, E. Ciccarelli, et al.: Defective regulation of Prolactin secretion after successful removal of prolactinomas. J. Clin. Endocrinol. Metab. **57** (1983) 1270.
[3] McGregor, A. M., M. F. Scanlon, K. Hall, et al.: Reduction in size of a pituitary tumor by bromocriptine therapy. N. Engl. J. Med. **300** (1979) 291.
[4] Editorial: Pituitary tumours and pregnancy. Lancet **1** (1976) 404.

[5] Erdheim, J., E. Stumme: Über die Schwangerschaftsveränderung der Hypophyse. Beitr. Pathol. Anat. **46** (1909) 1.
[6] Rjosk, H. K., R. Fahlbusch, K. von Werder: Influence of pregnancies on prolactinomas. Acta Endocrinol. **100** (1982) 337.
[7] Domingue, J. N., I. L. Richmond, C. B. Wilson: Results of surgery in 114 patients with prolactin-secreting pituitary adenomas. AM. J. Obstet. Gynecol. **137** (1980) 102.
[8] Davajan, V., O. A. Kletzky, C. M. March, et al.: The significance of galactorrhea in patients with normal menses, oligomenorrhea, and secondary amenorrhea. AM. J. Obstet. Gynecol. **130** (1978) 894.
[9] Haesslein, A. C., E. J. Lamb: Pituitary tumors in patients with secondary amenorrhea. Am. J. Obstet. Gynacol. **125** (1976) 759.
[10] Bression, D., A. M. Brandi, M. P. Martres, et al.: Dopaminergic receptors in human prolactin-secreting adenomas: a quantitative study. J. Clin. Endocrinol. Metab. **51** (1981) 1037.
[11] Quigney, M. E., S. J. Judd, G. B. Gilliland, et al.: Functional studies of dopamine control of prolactin secretion in normal women and women with hyperprolactinemic pituitary microadenoma. J. Clin. Endocrinol. Metab. **50** (1980) 994.
[12] Locke, W., A. V. Scally: The Hypothalamus and Pituitary. In: Health and Disease. C. Thomas, Publisher, Springfield, Illinois 1972.
[13] Uihlein, A., W. M. Balfour, P. F. Donovan: Acute hemorrhage into pituitary adenomas. J. Neurosurg. **14** (1957) 140.
[14] Ewer, R. H., T. G. Kotheimer: Spontaneous burned-out acromegaly with preservation of normal growth hormone responses: diagnostic historical, theoretical, and treatment aspects. Johns Hopkins Med. J. **127** (1970) 199.
[15] Derome, P. J., F. Peillon, R. H. Bard, et al.: Adenomes a prolactine: resultats du traitement chirurgical. Nouv. Presse Med. **8** (1979) 577.
[16] Gemzell, C., C. F. Wang: Outcome of pregnancy in women with pituitary adenoma. Fertil. Steril. **31** (1979) 363.

Prolactin levels and ovarian function after surgical treatment of prolactinomas

G. Tscherne, W. Urdl, L. M. Auer, G. Clarici, G. Leb, A. Warnkross

Introduction

Amenorrhoea is caused by hyperprolactinaemia in up to 20% of cases [14, 15]. The determination of prolactin levels is therefore essential in the differential diagnosis in accordance with the known WHO-schedule for classification of amenorrhoea. Serious cases, that is to say, with prolactin levels above 100 ng/ml, are associated with a prolactinoma to a high degree, depending on the quality of diagnosis. There are quite different reports about the frequency [15].

For the Gynaecologist the successful treatment is related to ovarian function and interfertility. The possibility of establishing ovulatory cycles with subsequent pregnancy by normalizing the prolactin secretion was a remarkable advance in infertility therapy [14]. In cases with prolactinoma there are still controversial opinions about treatment, about the benefits of surgical or conservative therapy or combined regimens. In order to judge the effect of surgical treatment we studied prolactin levels and ovarian function after operation.

Patients and methods

Among 25 amenorrhoeic patients with prolactin levels above 100 ng/ml 19 pituitary adenomas were diagnosed. 15 women underwent surgical treatment in the form of transsphenoidal selective adenomectomy. 13 microadenomas and 2 macroadenomas were removed.

The indication for surgical treatment was desired pregnancy in 6 cases, insufficient conservative treatment in 2 cases of infertility and the adenoma itself in 7 cases.

Prolactin was measured by a commercial kit (Fa. Serono), the normal level being up to 25 ng/ml. Ovarian function was judged by determination of LH and FSH (Riagnost, Fa. Hoechst), registration of onset of menses and basal body temperature.

Results

In 3 cases only, prolactin decreased to normal levels, followed by spontaneous menses and ovulatory cycles, indicating normalised ovarian function (fig. 1). Preoperative prolactin levels were between 200 and 300 ng/ml. One woman with ovulatory oligomenorrhoea and a desire for pregnancy became pregnant after a short low dose bromocriptine therapy.

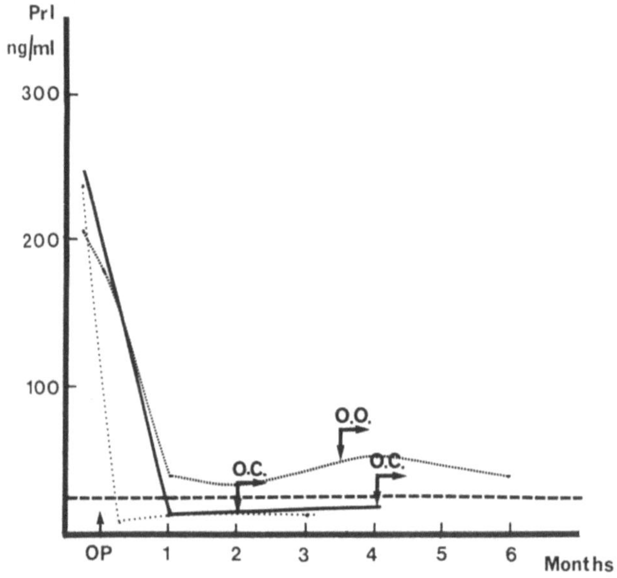

Fig. 1 Serum prolactin levels after surgery of prolactinoma. Onset of menses followed by ovulatory cycles (ovulatory oligomenorrhoea in one case).

Prolactin levels remained elevated after surgery in 12 cases, no menses occurred.

In 5 patients aged from 20 to 33 years (average 26 years) without a desire for pregnancy there was a significant decrease in prolactin, but not to normal levels (fig. 2). In all these cases prolactin was above 300 ng/ml before operation. Additional bromocriptine therapy (5 mg a day), initiated 2–6 months after operation led to normal ovulatory cycles in 3 cases, to menses in 2 cases, where no basal body temperature was measured or treatment was not carried out regularly.

Figure 3 shows the curves of 6 infertile patients, aged from 24 to 32 years (average 28 years). The prolactin decreased, but not to a normal level. By additional bromocriptine treatment (5–10 mg a day) menses and ovulatory cycles were established in 4 cases, in 2 patients menses occurred, and normal corpus-luteum-function was

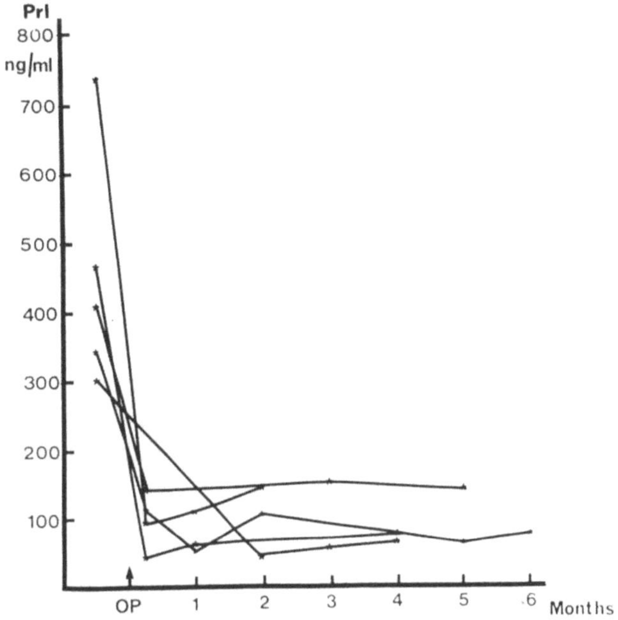

Fig. 2 Serum prolactin levels after surgery of prolactinoma. 5 patients without a desire for pregnancy.

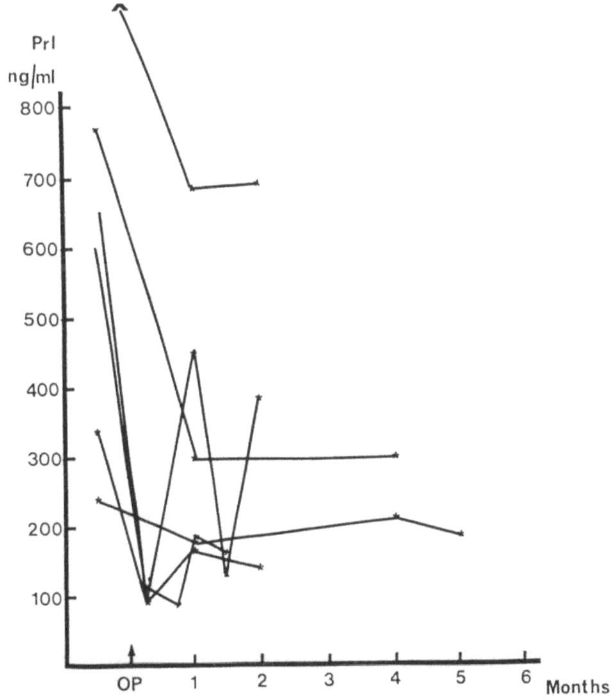

Fig. 3 Serum prolactin levels after surgery of prolactinoma. 6 patients with a desire for pregnancy.

induced by additional clomiphene therapy. All 6 women became pregnant. One further infertile patient with panhypopituitarism after operation of a macroprolactinoma has not yet become pregnant.

Thus of the 8 women with a desire for children 7 became pregnant and a total of 11 pregnancies resulted.

The onset of menses and ovulatory cycles signaling normalization of ovarian function occurred after varying intervals, depending on the duration of amenorrhoea, the age of the women and the form of additional treatment. Corresponding to this was normalization of FSH and LH before the onset of mensis.

With interruption of bromocriptine therapy, prolactin again rose and amenorrhoea reappeared (fig. 4). The increase in prolactin to similar levels as before withdrawal of bromocriptine was observed in all 5 patients with no desire for children during a period of up to 5 years.

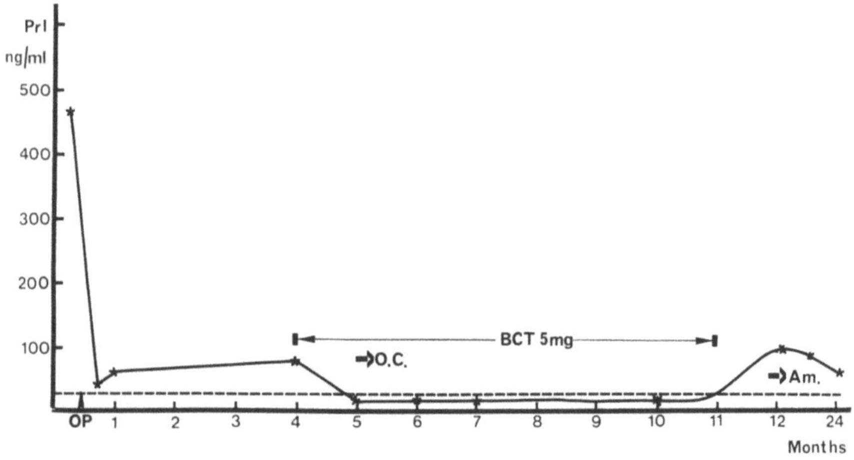

Fig. 4 P. H., 23 y. Serum prolactin levels after surgery of prolactinoma; normalization by additional bromocriptine treatment, reappearance of amenorrhoea after cessation of bromocriptine.

Discussion

Normalization of prolactin secretion and ovarian function after surgical treatment of prolactinomas has been reported in 40–70% of cases [4, 7, 10]. Results are obviously better in patients with small microadenomas than with larger adenomas and high levels of prolactin [12]. The relatively small percentage of normalization after adenomectomy in our own patients may be caused by the fact that there was severe hyperprolactinaemia in all cases (up to 1800 ng/ml). The remaining hyperprolactinaemia after surgery may be explained by hyperplasia of the lactotrophs in the pituitary tissue surrounding the adenoma or different disturbances in the portal vessel system of the hypophysis or in the hypothalamus [12].

The effectiveness of additional bromocriptine in the treatment of postoperative hyperprolactinaemia was confirmed by normalization of prolactin and ovarian function in all but one of our patients. Thus the prognosis for infertile patients is very favourable. The normalization of gonadotropin secretion and the onset of bleeding is to be expected after varying intervals depending on the seriousness of the amenorrhoea. Bromocriptine therapy may be necessary for months, the dose should be increased until normalization of prolactin levels is attained. In some cases additional clomiphen may be necessary to establish normal corpus-luteum function.

Permanent improvement of ovarian function depends on a continuation of bromocriptine therapy. Concerning the question of prolonged bromocriptine treatment versus observation alone it must be kept in mind that hyperprolactinaemic amenorrhoea may cause osteoporosis and breast cyst formation.

Thus, in the light of our present knowledge, the indication for surgical treatment of prolactinomas must be considered very carefully and individually in every case. Criteria for the decision as to treatment are the age of the patient, the clinical symptoms and, as the most important factor, whether there is a desire for children or not.

In infertile patients macroprolactinomas should be removed in every case, also large microadenomas with high levels of prolactin (above 300–400 ng/ml) to prevent possible complications in pregnancy [2, 5, 9]. Since bromocriptine treatment is possible during pregnancy also without evident risk, conservative treatment of prolactinomas has increased [3, 6, 11, 13, 16]. The precondition for the decision is an exact diagnosis including examination by a third generation CT scanner.

In cases without a desire for children microadenomas may be treated conservatively under CT scan control and regular prolactin determination. A negative aspect of long-term treatment of prolactinomas by bromocriptine is the possibility of fibrosis of the tumour [1, 8]. Further considerations are the difficulties of predicting the progress of the tumour, the question about "responders" and "non-responders" and also the opinion of the patient herself. The exploration of exact criteria is the task of continued investigations based on interdisciplinary cooperation.

References

[1] Auer, L. M., G. Clarici, G. Leb, et al.: Surgical results and long term follow-up in female and male prolactinomas. Proc. 1st Int. Symp. on Prolactinomas, Graz 1984.

[2] Bergh, T., S. J. Nillius, L. Wide: Clinical course and outcome of pregnancies in amenorrhoeic women with hyperprolactinaemia and pituitary tumors. Br. Med. J. **2** (1978) 875–880.

[3] Bergh, T., S. J. Nillius, P. Enoksson, et al.: Bromocriptine-induced pregnancies in women with large prolactinomas. Clin. Endocrinol. **17** (1982) 625–631.
[4] Chang, R. J., W. R. Keye Jr., J. R. Young, et al.: Detection, evaluation and treatment of pituitary microadenomas in patients with galactorrhea and amenorrhea. Am. J. Obstet. Gynecol. **128** (1977) 356–363.
[5] Hammond, C. B., A. F. Haney, M. R. Land, et al.: The outcome of pregnancy in patients with treated and untreated prolactin-secreting pituitary tumors. Am. J. Obstet. Gynecol. **147** (1983) 148–157.
[6] Jacobs, H. S., S. U. Thobani: Long term follow-up of medically treated hyperprolactinaemia (including prolactinoma) – evidence for cure. In: Advances in Diagnosis and Treatment of Infertility (V. Insler, G. Bettendorf, eds.), p. 263. Elsevier North Holland, New York 1981.
[7] Landolt, A. M.: Surgical treatment of pituitary prolactinomas: postoperative prolactin and fertility in seventy patients. Fertil. Steril. **35** (1981) 620–625.
[8] Landolt, A. M.: Structure and ultrastructure of prolactinomas. Proc. 1st Int. Symp. on Prolactinomas, Graz 1984.
[9] Magyar, D. M., J. R. Marshall: Pituitary tumors and pregnancy. Am. J. Obstet. Gynecol. **132** (1978) 739–751.
[10] Nelson, P. B., M. Goodman, J. C. Maroon, et al.: Factors in predicting outcome from operation in patients with prolactin-secreting pituitary adenomas. Neurosurgery **13** (1983) 634–641.
[11] Nillius, S. J.: Management of prolactinomas in pregnancy. Proc. 1st Int. Symp. on Prolactinomas, Graz 1984.
[12] Pelkonen, R., B. Grahne, E. Hirvonen, et al.: Pituitary function in prolactinoma. Effect of surgery and postoperative bromocriptine therapy. Clinical Endocrinology **14** (1981) 335–348.
[13] Pepperell, R. J.: Long-term follow-up of Hyperprolactinaemia in women. Proc. 1st Int. Symp. on Prolactinomas, Graz 1984.
[14] Rjosk, H. K.: Sterilität durch Hyperprolaktinämie: Klinik, endokrine Befunde, Therapie. Urban & Schwarzenberg, München–Wien–Baltimore 1983.
[15] Schneider, H. P. G., H. G. Bohnet: Die hyperprolaktinämische Ovarialinsuffizienz. Gynäkologe **14** (1981) 104–118.
[16] Turkalj et al.: Surveillance of bromocriptine in pregnancy. J A M A **247** (1982) 1589.

Pregnancies after treatment of prolactinomas: course and complications

W. Urdl, G. Tscherne, L. M. Auer, G. Clarici, G. Leb, H. Warnkross

Introduction

For women with amenorrhoea or anovulation as a result of hyperprolactinaemia, caused by a prolactinoma, a spontaneous pregnancy is a very rare phenomenon [8]. Most of these women nowadays can become pregnant due to various improvements in the treatment of prolactinomas. This has been made possible since we have been able to measure prolactin levels radioimmunologically [12, 24] and since the introduction of microsurgical techniques for the treatment of prolactin-producing pituitary adenomas [4, 6, 10], and because there are pharmocotherapeutic possibilities of influencing the tumour-caused or functional hyperprolactinaemia with dopaminergic drugs [7, 27]. In 1909 Erdheim and Stumme could already prove, that the normal pituitary gland enlarges about 1,7 times because of the raised oestrogen level during pregnancy [5]. Later on it could be demonstrated, that also the adenomatous tissue enlarges under the influence of a raised oestrogen level [19]. This can lead to clinical symptoms such as visual field defects and headaches caused by compression of the chiasma opticum or owing to the compression of the IIIth or VIth cerebral nerves. Dramatic events like an irreversible loss of sight, irreversible cerebral nerve-palsy caused by haemorrhage inside the adenoma or fatal intrecerebral bleedings are published as case-reports only [3, 15, 19, 20, 29]. In 1978 Magyar and Marshall reported on 91 pregnancies in 73 women with untreated prolactinomas: visual field defects occurred in 25%, severe headaches in 26% of the women and only 61% remained without complications. Whereas in 78 pregnancies of 73 women with treated prolactinomas only 4% developed headaches and 5% visual disturbances [16].

The aim of this study was to examine the frequency of complications in the pregnancies of these women, who became pregnant after surgery or medical treatment of their prolactinomas or after a combination of these therapeutic procedures and to determine factors influencing the frequency of complications. In addition there we examined, whether differences could be found referring to the course of the pregnancy and fetal outcome in comparison with pregnancies in normoprolactinaemic women.

Selection of patients and methods

Between 1978 and 1983 in the Department od Obstetrics and Gynaecology of the University of Graz a prolactinoma was shown to be present in 16 women, who were examined endocrinologically because of an amenorrhoea-galactorrhoea syndrom. This amounts to a prolactinoma-rate of 33.5% when compared with the total number of patients with hyperprolactinaemia (n = 45). In 11 of these 16 women pregnancy was desired. From 10 of these 11 women 14 pregnancies occurred (tab. 1). 2 women became pregnant after medical treatment with bromocriptine (Parlodel®) only, and 8 after a combination of transsphenoidal microsurgery and postoperative therapy with bromocriptine [1]. In 2 of these patients an additional dose of clomiphene-citrate was necessary to bring about ovulation and therefore pregnancy. One patient, who had suffered from panhypopituitarism after subfrontal operation of a macroprolactinoma in 1975 and transsphenoidal microsurgery of a recurrent prolactinoma in 1979, could not became pregnant despite normalization of her strongly increased postoperative prolactin-levels, with high doses of bromocriptine and the additional treatment with gonadotropins till now.

As soon as pregnancy was diagnosed bromocriptine therapy was withdrawn. Prolactin controls and visual field investigations were made at four week intervals in addition to the usual examinations during pregnancy. Serum levels of serum-prolactin were estimated using a commercially available radio-immunoassay test-kit (Serono).

In cases with complications such as headaches and/or visual field disturbances, or even in cases of a rapid increase in the prolactin levels, the above mentioned controls were carried out at least once a week.

Results

Out of 16 patients who were treated because of a prolactinoma, 11 desired pregnancy. In 10 of these 11 patients 14 pregnancies were possible (tab. 1).

The exploration of the sella turcica showed a *microadenoma* in 8 of the 10 women, of which 7 became pregnant after transsphenoidal microsurgery followed by bromocriptine treatment. This postoperative therapy was necessary in all cases because of continuously high prolactin-levels. One patient conceived after bromocriptine-therapy alone. The average prolactin level during pregnancy in this group with microprolactinomas was 462 ng/ml (28.3–750 ng/ml). So far 11 pregnancies have occurred in this group: 6 women have been delivered of 6 healthy and mature babies after pregnancies without any complications. A 34 year old woman, who conceived after bromocriptine therapy alone, bore a premature boy with 2030 gr and 44 cm by caesarian section. A 36 year old woman delivered a healthy and ma-

Table 1 Prolactinomas n = 16 (36 p. c.). Desire for pregnancy: 11 / Pregnancies: 14

Pat.	Age	Adenoma Micro	Macro	Op.	Op. + Bct.	Bct.	Add. Th.	Preg.	Complic.	Labour	Labour Op.
R. A.	36	+			+		Clomiphen	+		+	Forceps
W. M.	30	+			+		Clomiphen			++	
Sch. J.	24	+			+					+	
L. J.	24	+			+					+	
P. G.	30		+		2 × Op. +		Gonadotr.				
U. E.	26		+		+				Headaches	++	
F. M.	32	+			+			+		+	
B. A.	30	+			+			+			
P. B.	30	+			+			+			
W. M.	34	+				+				+	Caes. Section
G. R.	38		+			+			Headaches, Visual f. Defect	+	Caes. Section
		8	3		9	2		4		10	

Department of Obstetrics and Gynaecology of the University of Graz ture child with the aid of forceps; in both cases on account of obstetric indications (foetal distress). All the children in this group are healthy and without any anomalies. 3 women in this group are now in their late phase of pregnancy without problems.

A *macroadenoma* was revealed in two women, who desired pregnancy: One patient whose adenoma had been operated transsphenoidally became pregnant twice after postoperative treatment with bromocriptine and has delivered two healthy and mature babies.

Both pregnancies were complicated by severe headaches, resistant against treatment, from the middle trimester. The complaints occurred after an excessive rise in the prolactin levels, with a maximum of 4780 ng/ml. In both pregnancies the patient was free from headaches within 48 hours after treatment with bromocriptine and the prolactin level fell to a range of about 300 ng/ml within one week. In this case we administered a bromocriptine dose of between 5 and 10 mg per day.

The second patient, a 38 year old woman, became pregnant after conservative treatment with bromocriptine alone. The suggested transsphenoidal operation of a macroprolactinoma with a diameter of 12 mm had been refused. Also in this pregnancy severe headaches and, in addition, a bitemporal visual field defect on both sides developed in the second trimester. These symptoms also followed an increase in the prolactin level, with a maximal range of 1886 ng/ml. After bromocriptine (5–7.5 mg per day) she was free of complaints within 48 hours and her visual field defect disappeared within one week. The prolactin levels fell to a range of about 120 ng/ml, in the same period. This woman delivered a healthy and mature boy by caesarian secretion because of an obstetric indication (foetal distress).

The mean prolactin level during pregnancy in both cases with macroprolactinomas and complications was 1164.6 ng/ml (850–4780). In comparison with the group with microadenomas without complications and the meanvalue of 462.3 ng/ml (28.3–750) there was a significant difference ($p<0.05$).

The average birth weight of the 11 babies, so far born, lay at 2915 gr (2030–3800 gr). Three of these children had to be delivered operatively (27%), two by caesarian section (section-rate: 18%) and the third by forceps (forceps-rate: 9%). One boy showed a one-sided cryptorchism, but the other children were free of anomalies. Among the described 14 pregnancies there were no twins. The premature birth rate (babies with a birth weight below 2500 gr) lay at 9%. In the 14 pregnancies of these study we saw no abortions. In one case a danger of a premature birth was resolved promptly with tocolytic drugs. One ongoing pregnancy is complicated by EPH-gestosis (7.1%).

Discussion

Each pregnancy for women with prolactinomas must always be considered a risk. This is true for cases of either medically or surgically treated microadenomas, but especially for pregnancies combining surgically and/or medically treated macroadenomas. Therefore the course of pregnancy in these women ought to be supervised carefully in the above mentioned manner.

Out of 14 pregnancies after treatment of a prolactinoma in 3 pregnancies complications like headaches (14.2%) and visual field defects (7%) occurred. Such complications during pregnancy were seen in two women after treatment of a macroprolactinoma. The prolactin levels during these complicated pregnancies were significantly higher than in the comparable group with *micro*adenomas. Complications occurred at times after a steep increase in the prolactin level. These findings are in accordance with the results of other investigators [9, 16].

Therapy in pregnancy must start as soon as neurological or ophthalmological symptoms, or even headaches in connexion with an excessive rise in the prolactin level occur. Then the first step must be the application of dopaminergic drugs [22, 23, 28]. This is based on observations in animal tests, controlling the growth of a pituitary tumour with ergotalkaloids [18]. Some tumour remissions were reported in non-pregnant women with supra- and parasellar expanded prolactinomas [17]. In 1978 Bergh et al. reported on improvements in the visual field defects by means of bromocriptine therapy during pregnancy [2]. If severe symptoms occur, this therapy can be combined with dexamethasone [13, 23].

The suppression of the placental oestrogen production by influencing the foetal adrenocortical tissue seems to be the decisive glucocorticoid effect.

In contrasdt Ho Yuen reported in 1978 the case of a hyperprolactinaemic female who developed bitemporal visual field defects in the second half of pregnancy, though she had been treated with bromocriptine during the entire pregnancy [11]. This is supported by an observation of Rjosk et al., who observed further deterioration of vision under bromocriptine therapy [21]. In their patient rapid restitution of the visual fields occurred only after premature caesarian section. That induction of labor leading to rapid fall in circulating oestrogens may reverse visual field defects has also been shown by Thorner et al. [25]. As a last resort to preserve visual function emergency surgery may be necessary during pregnancy [14].

In 1410 pregnancies in women who conceived while taking bromocriptine the incidence of foetal abnormalities recorded was not different from that of the untreated population [26]. Nevertheless treatment with dopaminergic drugs is usually stopped when pregnancy is diagnosed.

References

[1] Auer, L. M., G. Clarici, G. Leb, et al.: Surgical results and long term follow-up in female and male prolactinomas. Proc. 1st Int. Symp. on Prolactinomas, Graz 1984.

[2] Bergh, T., S. J. Nillius, L. Wide: Clinical course and outcome of pregnancies in amenorrhoeic women with hyperprolactinaemia and pituitary tumors. Br. Med. J. **2** (1978) 875–880.

[3] Christensen, E., H. Larson: Fatal subarchnoid hemorrhages in pregnant women with intracerebral and intramedullary vascular malformations. Acta Psychiatr. Neurol. Scand. **29** (1954) 441–451.

[4] Derome, P. J., F. Peillon, R. H. Bard, et al.: Adenomas a prolactine: resultats du traitement chirurgical. Nouv. presse. Med. **8** (1979) 577–583.

[5] Erdheim, J., E. Stumme: Über die Schwangerschaftsveränderungen in der Hypophyse. Beitr. Pathol. Anat. **46** (1909) 1–132.

[6] Fahlbusch, R., H. K. Rjosk, K. von Werder: Operative treatment of prolactin producing adenomas. In: Treatment of pituitary adenomas (R. Fahlbusch, K. von Werder, eds.), pp. 225–237. Thieme Verlag, Stuttgart 1978.

[7] Frantz, A. G., D. L. Kleinberg, G. L. Noel: Studies on prolactin in man. Recent Prog. Horm. Res. **28** (1972) 527–590.

[8] Gemzell, C., C. F. Wang: Outcome of pregnancy in women with pituitary adenomas. Fertil. Steril. **31** (1979) 363–372.

[9] Griffith, R. W., I. Turkalj, P. Braun: Pituitary Tumors during pregnancy in mothers treated with bromocriptine. Br. J. Clin. Pharmacol. **7** (1979) 393–396.

[10] Hardy, J., H. Beauregard, F. Robert: Prolactin secreting pituitary adenomas: Transsphenoidal microsurgical treatment. In: Progress in prolactin, physiology and pathology (C. Robyn, M. Harter, eds.), pp. 361–370. Elsevier/North Holland Biomedical Press, Amsterdam 1978.

[11] Ho Yuen, B.: Bromocriptine, pituitary tumors and pregnancy. Lancet **2** (1978) 1314.

[12] Hwang, P., H. Guyda, H. G. Friesen: A radio immunoassay for human prolactin. Proc. Natl. Acad. Sci. USA **68** (1971) 1902–1906.

[13] Jewelewicz, R., E. A. Zimmermann, P. W. Carmel: Conservative management of a pituitary tumors during pregnancy following induction of ovulation with gonadotropins. Fertil. Steril. **28** (1977) 35–40.

[14] Kajtar, P., G. H. Tomkin: Emergency Hypophysectomy in pregnancy after induction of ovulation. Br. Med. J. **4** (1971) 88–90.

[15] Lamberts, S. W. J., J. G. M. Klijn, S. A. De Lange: The incidence of complications during pregnancy after treatment of hyperprolactinemia with bromocriptine in patients with radiologically evident pituitary tumors. Fertil. Steril. **31** (1979) 614–619.

[16] Magyar, D. M., J. R. Marshall: Pituitary tumors and pregnancy. Am. J. Obstet. Gynecol. **132** (1978) 739–751.

[17] McGregor, A. M., M. F. Scanlon, K. Hall, et al.: Reduction in size of pituitary tumor by bromocriptine therapy. N. Engl. J. Med. **300** (1979) 291–293.

[18] McLeod, R. M., J. E. Lehmeaer: Suppression of pituitary growth and function by ergot alkaloids. Cancer Res. **33** (1973) 849–855.

[19] Peillon, F., E. Vila Porcile, L. Olivier, et al.: L'action des oestrogenes sur les ademomes hypophysaires chez l'hommes. Documents histopathologiques en microscopie optique et electronique et rapport de l'experimentation. Ann. Endocrinol. (Paris) **31** (1970) 259–270.

[20] Rand, C. W.: Two cerebral complications of pregnancy: Brain tumor and spontaneous subarachnoid hemorrhage. Clin. Neurosurg. **3** (1957) 104–141.

[21] Rjosk, H. K., R. Fahlbusch, J. H. Greite, et al.: Prevention and therapy of visual complications during pregnancy in patients with prolactinoma. (Abstr.) In: Pituitary adenomas, biology, physiopathology and treatment (P. J. Derome, C. P. Jedynak, F. Peillon, eds.), p. 340. Asclepios France, Paris 1979.

[22] Rjosk, H. K., K. v. Werder: Schwangerschaft und Wochenbett nach behandelter Hyperprolactinaemie. Der Gynäkologe **15**/I (1982) 22–29.

[23] Schneider, H. P. G., H. G. Bohnet: Die hyperprolactinaemische Ovarialinsuffizienz. Der Gynäkologe **14**/II (1981) 104–118.

[24] Sinha, J. N., F. W. Selby, U. J. Levis, et al.: A homologous radio immun-assay for human prolactin. J. Clin. Endocrinol. Metab. **36** (1973) 509–516.

[25] Thorner, M. O., G. M. Besser, A. Jones, et al.: Bromocriptine treatment of female infertility: report of 13 pregnancies. Br. Med. J. **4** (1975) 694–697.

[26] Turkalj, I., P. Braun, P. Krupp: Surveillance of bromocriptine during pregnancy. Br. J. Clin. Pharmacol. **7** (1979) 393–396.

[27] Turkington, R. W.: Inhibition of prolactin secretion and successful therapy of the Forbes-Albright syndrome with L-dopa. J. Clin. Endocrinol. **34** (1972) 306–311.

[28] Urdl, W., G. Tscherne, A. W. Kowatsch, et al.: Die Behandlung prolaktinombedingter Komplikationen in der Schwangerschaft. Ein kasuistischer Beitrag. In: Fortschritte der Fertilitätsforschung, 12 (1983) S. 290.

[29] Winter, E. W.: Hypophysentumor und Schwangerschaft. Arch. Gynäkol. **147** (1931) 95–112.

Psychosomatic findings in patients with elevated prolactin

O. Jürgensen, B. Bardé

Introduction

Sobrinho [1] and Nunes [2] apparently were the first in the world who reported on psychosomatic factors in over a 100 women with elevated prolactin in 1978 and 1980. Our own investigations were initiated in 1979 completely independantly and without even knowing their work. Apparently we were the first to include males in our study. Originally we meant to find out whether amenorrhoea associated with elevated prolactin differs from merely functional amenorrhoea in psychosomatic aspects.

Material and method

Included in the study were 27 females aged 18 to 42 years and 11 males aged 17 to 69 years. Sixteen of the 27 females and all the males had prolactinomas. Prolactin was known to be elevated from 1 to 5 years duration, basic values ranging from 2000 mu/ml to more than 5000 mu/ml serum. All patients were submitted to a free psychoanalytical interwiev and to an object relation test (ORT-Philipson) [3]. Main subjects of investigation were: Conscious and unconscious imaginations of the disease, past and present object relations, defense-structures, ego-function and psychiatric diagnoses.

Results

Conscious imaginations of the disease

The conscious ideas and fears related to the disease did not differ in patients with or without pituitary adenoma. The individual meaning attached to the disorder was generally fatal, in contrast to its medically rather benign course.

Conclusions about the *unconscious meaning* (tab. 1) of the disease in males and females alike were drawn by the following items which must be omitted here: Biografic events and their assimilation by the subject, structures of defense, thoughts, fears and fantasies as revealed by the ORT.

Table 1 The unconscious meaning of hyperprolactinaemia in 38 patients

	women	men
Hostile maternal introjection	9	5
Representation of repressed murderous instincts	5	–
Representation of isolated instinctual omnipotence	2	2
Tumour as neg. Self-Representation ("malformed monster")	2	–
Identification with primary objects which died of brain-disease	3	1
Redemption of fatal disease by idealised objects (Chief of Dept., clinic)	2	–
Disease not connected with narcissistic defense	4	1
Disease experienced as a castrating stigma	–	2
Total	27	11

In 9 women and 5 men the disease equalled the unconscious meaning of a hostile sadistic maternal introjection. The majority of those patients was diagnosed as depressive. All members of this group had pituitary adenomas which in females and males alike seemed to represent a hostile maternal persecutor with no chance of escape.

Among the 5 males who thus felt persecuted there is one whose father was assasinated as a former nazi in a prisoners' camp. His mother separated from the patient when she got remarried. Another patient of this group was a former constructor of crematoria in concentration camps. A close relative of the patient incidentally got killed in such a stove constructed by the patient. Consciously this patient lived a pleasant life free of feelings of guilt. But his repressed fears became evident in the ORT were he depicted scenes of either suicide or homicide. Further unconscious phenomena attached to the disease are depicted in table 1 and will not be commented on here but are published elsewhere [4, 4a].

Object relations

Object relations referring to the relationships with parents and partners were unhappy and distorted in the majority of patients. More than half of the female patients had mothers who abused them and intruded into their adult lives and even into their marriages. Two females were abandoned by their mothers up to the age of 6.

As far as fathers were concerned, in 7 females and 2 males they were absent due to war, death or divorce. Eleven more fathers though, physically present, were devalued by alcohol-addiction, psychosis, mental breakdown or simply considered meaningless by their wives. In only 25% of all patients their relationships with parents appeared to be sufficiently affectionate.

The quality of their relations with their partners followed exactly the pattern of parent-relations though originally intended as a better substitute for a poor home.

In contrast, the relationship with children was different in our female patients. To them children conceived during bromocriptin-therapy represented symbols of survival or redemption, which was true especially for depressive patients to whom children were substitutes for disappointing parents or partners.

Ego-function

Ego-function was unimpaired in 19/38 patients. In 5 females and 2 males ego function was impaired by repressive retreats and addiction. In another 5 females and 3 males there was impairment with respect to emotional performance. Two females and 2 males showed ego-deficiencies concerning reality-testing and perception. They were diagnosed as borderline-personalities or schizophrenics.

Psychiatric diagnoses (table 2)

Accordingly, pregenital, disorders prevailed in our clientel with 15 female and 2 male cases of manifest depression. In 4 females and 7 males there were even more serious symptoms of regression like oral fixation, anorexia, borderline, false self and schizophrenia. Included is a man who later committed suicide with an aggressive plant poison. His symptoms had started at the age of 7 with obesity. At the age of 15 he had brain surgery for a pituitary adenoma, and at the age of 22 he had a

Table 2 Psychiatric diagnoses in 38 patients with hyperprolactinaemia

	women	men
Depression, partially combined with paranoid traits	15	2
Somatization instead of depression	1	–
Oral symbiotic fixation in extreme obesity	1	–
Other narcissistic disorders (borderline, schizoid traits etc.)	4	7 (!)
Obsessive-compulsive character	2	1
Chronic anorexia	1	–
Hystrical structure	3	1
Total	27	11

recurrence-operation. As a student of physics he lived completely isolated. He had neither friends nor a girl friend to communicate with. He detested his parents' concern for his health. His greatest fear was that the disease might turn him into a woman. And he considered himself a source of important secrets which he would never reveal to anybody. Unfortunately, the interview with him might have touched on those secrets which finally killed him. Obsessive-compulsive structures of character were observed in 2 women and 1 man. Altogether in only 3 females and one male the diagnosis of hysterical – i.e. fairly normal structure was made.

Onset of symptoms

The beginning of symptoms was traced back by our female patients over many years. With the exception of one case of renal failure the disease was never related to one single event, but appeared chronic in character, and in the majority of cases could be traced back to the age of menarche. In many cases the diagnosis was made in the course of an infertility work-up, usually combined with feelings of envy and inferiority towards fertile siblings. In many other cases amenorrhoea followed events of separation or loss.

In contrast, in our male patients the manifestation of the disease appeared late in life and was serious in character involving threatening loss of vision. Impotence and obesity were less marked longstanding symptoms which were frequently overlooked. Our male patients' lives and object-relations up to the point of diagnosis appeared even more distorted than the females'.

Summary and conclusions

For more detailed information we refer to our publications in 1982, 1983 and 1985 [4, 4a, 5].

1. Thirty-four out of 38 patients with hyperprolactinaemia showed severe psychopathology with a prevalence of depressive or prepsychotic disorders.
2. Conscious and unconscious fantasies attached to the disease were of a fatal outcome, in contrast to its medical benignity.
3. Object relations appeared to be unhappy and distorted in the majority of patients concerning relationships with parents and partners. The relationships with children in our female patients differ from this pattern insofar as children represent symbols of redemption and survival.
4. The beginning of the disease appeared to be chronic, corresponding to a continuous rather than a single traumatisation by life-events like separation and loss.
5. Lifelong deformation of intrapsychic structures might affect neurotransmitter-metabolism resulting in hyperprolactinaemia [6] in females and males alike thus representing an endocrine non sex-linked equivalent of depressive disease. [7].

References

[1] Sobrinho, L. G., J. F. Sousa, E. F. Henriques: Étude de la psychodynamique de patientes porteuses d'une galactorrhée non puerpérale avec ou sans tumeur hypofisaire. Rev. Fr. Endocrinol. Clin. Nutr. Metab. **19** (1978) 507.
[2] Nunes, M. C. P., L. G. Sopbrinho, C. Calhaz-Jorge, et al.: Psychosomatic factors in patients with hyperprolactinemia and or galactorrhea. Obstetr. and Gynecology **55** (1980) 591.
[3] Phillipson, H.: A short introduction to the object relation technique. Tavistok Center London (Windsor), NFER Publ. Comp., London 1973.
[4] Jürgensen, O., B. Bardé: Psychodynamic findings in women with elevated Prolactin. In: The Young Woman. Excerpta Medica, Int. Congr. Series 618 (Dennerstein, Senarclens, eds.), p. 138. Excerpta Medica, Amsterdam 1983.
[4a] Bardé, B.: Zur Psychodynamik der Hyperprolaktinämie. Inauguraldissertation, Frankfurt 1985 [Institut für Psychoanalyse].
[5] Jürgensen, O., B. Bardé: Zur Psychodynamik der Hyperprolaktinämie. Gynäkologe **15** (1982) 190–197.
[6] Reichlin, S.: Etiology of pituitary adenoma. In: The pituitary adenoma (Post, ed.), p. 29. Plenum medical book company, New York–London 1980.
[7] Czernik, A.: Zur Psychophysiologie und Neuroendokrinologie von Depressionen. Springer, Berlin–Heidelberg 1982.

List of contributors

Aleshire, S., Clinical Chemistry Section, Dept. of Pathology, Vanderbilt University Medical Center, Nashville, Tennessee 37232, USA
Auer, L. M., Universitätsklinik für Neurochirurgie, Landeskrankenhaus, A−8036 Graz
Becker, D. P., Division of Neurosurgery, Medical College of Virginia, Box 613, MCV Station, Richmond, Virginias 23298, USA
Bobest, M., Markusovszky Hospital, Neurosurgical Dept., Ham an K. u. 28, H−9700 Szombathely
Bozadjieva, E., Medical Academy, Institute of Endocrinology, Gerontology and Geriatrics, Boul. Ch. Michailov 6, 1303 Sofia, Bulgaria
Buchfelder, M., Neurochirurgische Universitätsklinik, Erlangen−Nürnberg, Schwabachanlage 6, D−8520 Erlangen
Cecotto, C., Ospedale Generale Regionale di Udine, Divisione Neurochirurgia, I−33100 Udine
Faglia, G., University of Milan, Chair of Endocrinology, School of Medicine, I−20100 Milano
Fahlbusch, R., Neurochirurgische Universitätsklinik Erlangen−Nürnberg, Schwabachanlage 6, D−8520 Erlangen
Ferrari, E., E., Dept. of Internal Medicine, University of Pavia, I−27100 Pavia
Flückiger, E., Sandoz AG, Pharma Dept., CH−4002 Basel
Galvan, G., Landeskrankenanstalten, Abt. für Nuklearmedizin und Endokrinologie, A−5020 Salzburg
Garzarelli, S., Ospedali Civili di Sampierdarena, Divisione Ostretico-Ginecologica, I−16126 Genova
Gen, M., Dept. of Neurosurgery, Hiroshima University School of Medicine, Kasumi 1−2−3 Minamiku, 1734 Hiroshima, Japan
Gottswinter, J., Medizinische Poliklinik der Universität Heidelberg, Abt. Innere Medizin VI, Luisenstr. 5, D−6900 Heidelberg
Heshmati, H. M., CHU Pitié-Salpêtrière, Dept. of Endocrinology, F−75013 Paris
Höfler, H., Pathologisches Institut der Universität Graz, Auenbruggerplatz 25, A−8036 Graz
Jacobs, H., Cobbold Laboratories, Thorn Institute of Clinical Sciences, The Middlesex Hospital Medicine School, GB−London W1N 8AA
Jautzke, G., Klinikum Steglitz der Freien Universität Berlin, Abt. Pathologie, Hindenburgdamm 30, D−1000 Berlin 45
Jürgensen, O., Städtelstr. 3, D−6000 Frankfurt/Main 70
Jungmann, E., Klinikum der Johann-Wolfgang-Goethe-Universität − Zentrum Innere Medizin, Abt. für Endokrinologie, Theodor-Stern-Kai 7, D−6000 Frankfurt/Main 70
Landolt, A. M., Neurochirurgische Universitätsklinik, Rämistr. 100, CH−8081 Zürich
Leb, G., Medizinische Universitätskllinik Graz, A−8036 Graz
Leicht, E., Medizinische Klinik und Poliklinik der Universität des Saarlandes, Innere Medizin II, D−6650 Homburg/Saar
L'Hermite, M., Hôpital Brugman, Place van Gehuchten 4, B−1020 Bruxelles
Luger, A., 2. Medizinische Universitätsklinik, Garnisongasse 13, A−1190 Wien

Lundberg, P. O., Dept. of Neurology, University Hospital, S–751 85 Uppsala
Maira, G., Institute of Neurosurgery, Catholic University, I–00168 Roma
Mashiter, K., Hammersmith Hospital, Endocrine Unit, GB–London W12 OHS
Montini, M., Division of Endocrinology, Unit Hospital, Largo Barozzi 1, I–24100 Bergamo
Muhr, C., Dept. of Neurology, University Hospital, S–751 85 Uppsala
Nakagawa, Y., Neuropathologisches Institut der Freien Universität Berlin, Hindenburgdamm 30, D–1000 Berlin 45
Nesselrooij, J. van, Institute CIVO – Toxicology and Nutrition TNO, Utrechtseweg 48, NL–3704 HE Zeist
Nillius, S. J., Dept. of Obstetrics and Gynecology, University Hospital, S–751 85 Uppsala
Ohta, M., Dept. of Neurosurgery, Hiroshima University, School of Medicine, Kasumi 1–2–3 Minamiku, 1734 Hiroshima, Japan
Parent, A. D., Dept. of Neurosurgery, University of Mississippi Medical Center, 2500 North State Street, Jackson, Mississippi 39216, USA
Pásztor, E., National Institute of Neurosurgery, Amerikai u. 57, H–1145 Budapest
Pepperell, R., Dept. of Obstetrics and Gynecology, University of Melbourne, Parkville, Victoria 3052, Australia
Pérez-Alvarez, M., Ciudad Sanitaria "La Paz", Neurochirurgia, Castellana 261, E–Madrid 34
Popović, V., 27 Mart 28, YU–11000 Beograd
Roosen, N., Neurochirurgische Universitätsklinik, Moorenstr. 5, D–4000 Düsseldorf 1
Scanarini, M., Divisione di Neurochirurgia, Ospedale Civile, I–35100 Padova
Schatz, H., Klinikum des Justus-Liebig-Universität, Zentrum für Innere Medizin, Rodthohl 6, D–6500 Gießen
Schneider, G., Radiologische Universitätsklinik Graz, A–8036 Graz
Schrell, U., Neurochirurgische Universitätsklinik Erlangen–Nürnberg, Schwabachanlage 6, D–8520 Erlangen
Stracke, Klinikum der Justus-Liebig-Universität, Zentrum für Innere Medizin, Klinikstr. 36, D–6500 Gießen
Symon, L., Gough Cooper Dept. of Neurolog. Surgery, The National Hospital, Queen Square, GB–London WC1E 3BG
Tscherne, G., Geburtshilfl.-gynäkologische Universitätsklinik Graz, A–8036 Graz
Urdl, W., Geburtshilfl.-gynäkologische Universitätsklinik Graz, A–8036 Graz
Watanabe, K., Southern Tohoku Research Institute for Neuroscience, 18–Inaebayashi Yatsuyamada, Fukuyama-cho, Koriyama, Fukushima, Japan
Werder, K. von, Universitätsklinikum links der Isar, Medizinische Klinik Innenstadt, Ziemsenstr. 1, D–8000 München 2
Wit, W. de, Orionlaan 42, NL–3721 HE Bilthoven

Authors' index

Subject index

Bei Fragen zur Produktsicherheit wenden Sie sich bitte an:
If you have any questions regarding product safety,
please contact:

Walter de Gruyter GmbH
Genthiner Straße 13
10785 Berlin
productsafety@degruyterbrill.com